# Contents

# Foreword

Kazutaka Kogi

We are facing rapid changes in work life as a consequence of the globalizing economy. Changes in employment and demographic structures, introduction of new technologies, and the current global financial crisis are having deep impacts on health and safety of workers worldwide. These changes are creating new challenges in occupational health practice for effectively managing work related health and safety risks and promoting health of workers in diverse working situations. Increasing attention is drawn to comprehensive risk management at the workplace and improved access to occupational health services as a result of these situations.

It is encouraging that various new attempts are being made to improve work methods and the working environment and secure active participation of employers and workers in workplace health activities. This effort is clearly reflected in the activities of our International Commission on Occupational Health (ICOH). Through its 35 scientific committees and its task and working groups, ICOH activities are focusing on proactive risk assessment procedures and the extension of occupational health services to underserved sectors. A particular emphasis is placed on the development of basic occupational health services and the application of participatory approaches, particularly for improving small-scale workplaces. ICOH makes joint efforts with other international organizations in line with the International Labor Organization (ILO) global strategies and the World Health Organization (WHO) global plan of action for healthy workplaces for all workers. It is also encouraging that cooperation with national and regional associations is advancing in these aspects.

The new developments reported in this book represent an important step forward in our collaborative efforts. These developments confirm the need for the combined efforts of employers, workers, and society toward workplace health promotion. The positive experiences in needs assessment and in the planning and implementation of sustainable improvement processes reported from many countries are particularly important. We can learn useful lessons that can facilitate action-oriented healthy workplace programs despite the many constraints in increasingly diverse work life settings.

International cooperation is emerging to meet the goals of using good practices in reducing safety and health risks at work, and designing and using multidisciplinary healthy workplace programs and related training and information materials. ICOH likewise places high priority on developing action-oriented toolkits. Further, we must intensify efforts to make fuller use of known health promotion best practices in order to provide specific guidance and support for workplace settings. Thus, by utilizing these best practices that have been appropriately adjusted to specific settings, we can ensure that workplace health promotion and health protection become an integral and successful part of management practices and thereby extend their impact to a wide range of sectors.

It is gratifying that experiences from different regions are compiled together in this book. This gives us useful insights into locally workable interventions toward a healthy and safe environment as well as toward worklife changes. I am sure that workplace health successes, including those reported in this publication, provide us with practical hints for actions at the regional, national, and local levels. ICOH places high priority on ethical standards and social justice in our daily practice, and the lessons learned through these health promotion practices and shared in this publication will help us incorporate reliable changes into the workplace culture and practices. There is an acute need for concerted action to improve workers' health in many difficult conditions, and I hope this book will be recognized as a valuable contribution to occupational health and well-being of workers in different regions.

Kazutaka Kogi
President
International Commission on Occupational Health (ICOH)

# Foreword

## Joana Godinho

This book provides a global account of the status of health promotion in the workplace, showing that employees and organizations are moving toward healthier practices, albeit slowly. This business move is expected to contribute not only to a healthier workforce but also to increased productivity and reduced healthcare costs.

The World Health Organization (WHO) has been a global leader in advancing much of the current thinking about the importance of healthy lifestyles and environments to keep chronic diseases at bay, especially cardiovascular diseases and cancer, some of the main global killers. To gain and maintain such a lifestyle, people need to live and work in health promoting communities and workplaces, which give them opportunities and incentives for healthy practices, such as eating a balanced diet with plenty of fruits and vegetables, getting sufficient sleep, engaging in physical activity daily, and managing stress without having to resort to excessive alcohol intake, smoking, or abusing drugs. These healthy practices contribute to decrease their risk of disease, disability, and premature death—and help the private and public sectors to keep organizational and healthcare costs under control.

No country in the world can be competitive in the world economy with unhealthy workers. On the other hand, the workplace setting can play a major role in encouraging people to adopt healthier lifestyles. Health and safety legislation confined to the prevention of physical accidents provided the historical drivers for health promotion in the workplace. Countries with health insurance linked to employment, such as the United States, may have had more of an incentive to engage in health promotion in the workplace, as referred to in Chapter 20. For health promotion in the workplace to gain further ground, it is necessary to identify additional incentives for workers and organizations to engage in healthy practices as a sound business move. There is still a great deal to be done, not the least in continuing to investigate the impact of health promotion in the workplace on organizational costs and returns.

This publication highlights how 21 countries are addressing these challenges by focusing on the following areas regarding health promotion in the workplace: the prevailing health issues and risk practices; national healthcare systems; historical and cultural influences on both physical and mental health; key drivers for establishing global workplace health promotion programs; examples of best practices; key outcomes and success indicators; and available evidence.

Joana Godinho
Senior Health Specialist, Human Development
The World Bank
Washington, DC

# Preface

The field of workplace health promotion (WHP) has enjoyed significant growth on a global scale over the last decade. Responding to the chronic disease trends as well as the healthcare cost and productivity challenges, governments, health insurances, and social partners (employer and employee representative groups) are increasingly turning to health promotion strategies. While stakeholders often still need to be convinced of the business value of workplace health promotion, this growth and early development stage is an extremely exciting prospect for health promotion professionals worldwide. Envision yourself in a start-up company that has a highly innovative and promising product with global relevance and that you truly love. On top of this positive atmosphere, the field seems to attract deeply motivated and caring individuals in whichever country you go. All of this bodes well for health promotion, but can we convince the venture capitalists—to stay with the start-up analogy—and make it mainstream?

Although workplace health promotion is a young field, dedicated professionals have implemented many excellent programs over the years in various countries. This publication attempts to document many of these. As such a global account of WHP has not yet been recorded, this book fills a real need. As globalization accelerates and the workforce becomes more mobile, there is a thirst for knowledge with regard to health trends and behaviors in other countries, as well as cultural aspects of WHP. Multinational employers are faced with the challenge of developing global health and well-being strategies and supporting local sites in the implementation of programs. This presents a daunting task given the multiple levels and facets of cultures and countries.

This book contains WHP profiles of 21 countries from 6 continents: Asia, Africa, North America, South America, Europe, and Australia. These include high-, middle-, and low-income countries. We have succeeded in featuring all major countries, minus a few exceptions. Each chapter covers the following categories:

- general facts on the country
- prevailing health issues and risk behaviors
- healthcare systems
- influence of culture and mentality
- key drivers for establishing workplace health promotion programs
- program examples and good practices
- outcomes and success indicators

- existing research findings
- conclusion

These chapters have been written by distinguished professionals who are regarded as health promotion pioneers in their given country. All of the contributing authors are members or friends of the International Institute for Health Promotion (IIHP), which is based at American University in Washington, DC. The book idea was originally discussed within the IIHP and immediately found tremendous resonance and support. We, as founders of the IIHP, are proud of the IIHP's connection to this book and are truly grateful to all contributing authors for their dedication.

Being the first edition, the publication process was an adventure for us and strewn with many unforeseen challenges, especially due to the global nature of the project. We are truly excited to finally make the book a reality after many years of reflection and discussion and we welcome your feedback and suggestions for improvement.

—Wolf Kirsten and Robert C. Karch

# Acknowledgments

The publication of this book represents a global collaboration. Thirty-five authors from 21 countries contributed, with many more individuals helping in the background. We are deeply grateful to all of the contributing authors, many of whom we have known for numerous years through the International Institute for Health Promotion (IIHP). All of the authors submitted high-quality manuscripts—some on a very short timeline—and were most responsive to editorial changes. Given the fact that for most, English is not their native language, we were impressed with the quality of their writing. Hats off to you! In addition, we would like to congratulate the authors for being gracious representatives of their home countries.

We would also like to thank Joana Godinho from the World Bank and Kazutaka Kogi from the International Commission of Occupational Health (ICOH) for crafting powerful forewords on short notice. Both are consummate professionals who fully understand the undeniable link between healthy citizens and productive societies.

To the International Health Consulting team—Robin McClave, Pia Schneider, and Tanya Kalas—we give special thanks for your encouragement and input. You were immensely helpful and kept us on track along the way. In addition, the country-specific data information provided by Melissa Johnson and the development of instructional content for each chapter assisted by Mary Ellen Rose added two unique and valuable dimensions to this text for which we are very appreciative.

Karen Karch did an amazing job editing all the chapters. Her tireless effort, and, in particular, her editorial sensitivity in working with cultural nuances from authors and transcripts from so many non-English speaking countries, are extremely laudable, deeply appreciated, and central to our ability to get the full manuscript out of the door to our publisher. Also, a big thank you to the staff at Jones & Bartlett Learning, especially Mike Brown, Catie Heverling, Teresa Reilly, Sophie Fleck, and Kate Stein for guiding us along the way and creating the final product.

# Introduction: Setting the Context for Workplace Health Promotion

Wolf Kirsten

## Global Health Trends

Employers and employees throughout the world are facing immense challenges with an ongoing economic crisis, an increasingly fast-paced business environment, growing demands for productivity, and a global rise in chronic diseases. This book will highlight health trends and challenges at the workplace. The workplace has recently received considerable attention with regard to health promotion, mainly due to two reasons:

1. The significant impact of unhealthy employees on the business. Numerous studies have documented the negative economic consequences of poor employee health, health risks, and dissatisfaction in form of absenteeism, presenteeism, accidents, and healthcare costs (Mills, Kessler, Cooper, & Sullivan, 2007).
2. The recognition of the workplace as a useful setting to advance public health. The World Health Organization (WHO) has advanced the settings approach and recently outlined a comprehensive framework on how to promote health at the workplace (World Health Organization [WHO], 2010a).

A longer standing tradition exists with regard to how work can affect the health of workers, that is, the impact of the physical or psychosocial working environment. From a global perspective, next to the World Health Organization and the International Labor Organization (ILO), the International Commission on Occupational Health (ICOH) has been the most prominent organization advocating policies and programs on how to minimize the health impact of work (International Commission on Occupational Health [ICOH], 2009). Job-related accidents and illnesses claim more than two million lives annually (International Labor Organization [ILO], 2005). This number is rising in developing countries due to rapid industrialization. In addition, 268 million nonfatal workplace accidents occur each year in which the victims miss at least 3 days of work as a result, as well as 160 million new cases of work-related illness (ILO, 2005). The working world is changing rapidly, for example, the International Data Corporation (IDC) projects that by 2013 a third of the world's workforce will be mobile workers (International Data Corporation [IDC], 2009). This will require new methods and strategies in the field of workplace health promotion, such as how to reach mobile workers or how to address the new health challenges.

The alarming increase of chronic disease has left its mark on the workplace. According to the WHO (2008), noncommunicable diseases cause 38 million deaths annually (70% of all global deaths when adding injuries). Eighty percent of these deaths occur in low- and middle-income countries. The forecast is even worse: death rates from noncommunicable diseases are likely to increase by 17% globally over the next 10 years, with the greatest increase projected in the African region (27%) followed by the eastern Mediterranean region (25%) (WHO, 2008). The WHO identifies four major noncommunicable diseases (cardiovascular diseases, diabetes, cancers, and chronic respiratory diseases) and four related risk factors to address (tobacco use, unhealthy diets, physical inactivity, and the harmful use of alcohol). The Oxford Health Alliance's global campaign 3Four50 (www.3four50.com) focuses on three key risk factors (tobacco use, poor diet, and lack of physical activity) and four chronic diseases (heart disease, type 2 diabetes, lung disease, and many cancers) which are responsible for more than 50% of deaths in the world. The obesity epidemic is probably one of the most highlighted public health challenges. Each year, 2.6 million people are dying as a result of being overweight or obese (WHO, 2010b). Once associated with high-income countries, obesity is now also prevalent in low- and middle-income countries. In light of the aging trend in many countries, the chronic disease profile will become even more pronounced and create a growing challenge for international organizations, national governments, and employers alike. A British insurance provider, Bupa, issued a report on the future workforce of the United Kingdom (Bupa, 2009) that painted a bleak picture. Employees will be:

- older,
- with more long-term conditions or "lifestyle" conditions,
- caring for others,
- obese with diabetes and/or heart problems,
- in the kind of jobs more likely to have an impact on psychological health, and
- working in knowledge-intensive or service industries.

The economic impact of noncommunicable disease is staggering. According to the joint report by the World Health Organization and the World Economic Forum "Preventing Noncommunicable Diseases in the Workplace through Diet and Physical Activity," the financial impact of lifestyle-related diseases to countries in 2015 amounts to the following (WHO/World Economic Forum [WEF], 2008):

| | |
|---|---|
| China: | $558 billion |
| India: | $237 billion |
| Russia: | $303 billion |
| United Kingdom: | $33 billion |
| Brazil: | $9.3 billion |
| Pakistan | $6.7 billion |

# Trends in Workplace Health Promotion

While U.S. employers have addressed individual employee health for a long time, it has been somewhat of a taboo in Europe, where health is regarded as a personal issue and not a concern of the employer. This is partially cultural but mainly due to the differing healthcare systems. In the United States, the employer feels the direct cost impact of poor employee health while in most European countries (and many other countries worldwide) the state carries the burden in some form or the other. This has led to a higher prevalence of health promotion programs in the United States (Buck Consultants, 2009) (see Figure I-1).

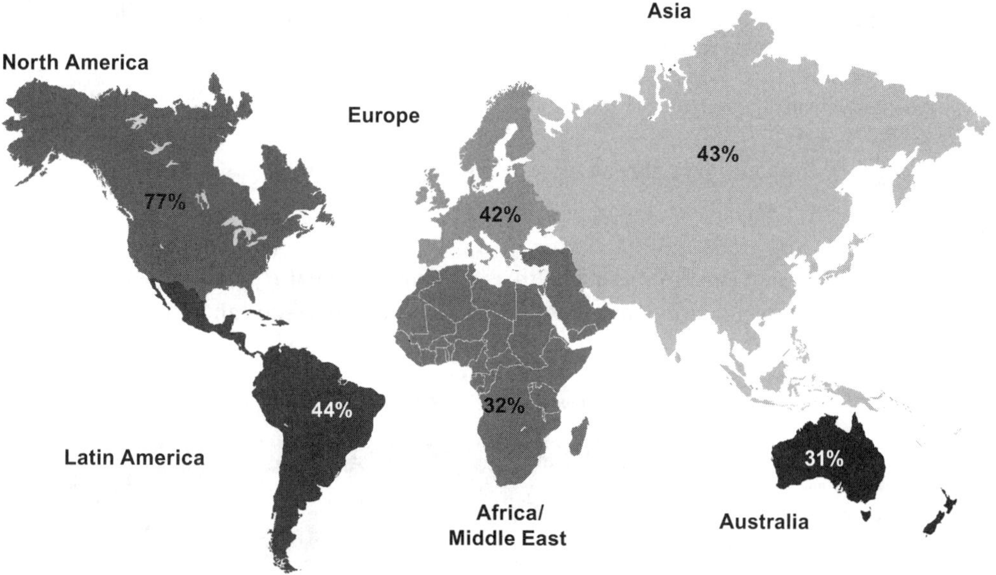


Figure I-1 Global prevalence of health promotion programs.

Source: Buck Consultants, 2009

In the United States, employers continue to struggle with healthcare costs in light of the daunting demographic and disease trends. In the rest of the world, employers mainly feel the impact of poor health through absenteeism and presenteeism. The Global Survey of Health Promotion and Workplace Wellness Strategies (Buck Consultants, 2009) asked 1,103 organizations about the main objectives for implementing health promotion programs (see Figure I-2).

| | Africa | Asia | Australia | Canada | Europe | Latin America | United States |
|---|---|---|---|---|---|---|---|
| Improve productivity/presenteeism | 1 | 2 | 1 | 1 | 1 | 1 | 2 |
| Reduce employee absences | 2 | 3 | 2 | 2 | 3 | 3 | 3 |
| Improve workforce morale/engagement | 4 | 1 | 3 | 4 | 2 | 4 | 4 |
| Maintain work ability | 3 | 6 | 6 | 7 | 4 | 2 | 8 |
| Further organizational values/mission | 5 | 4 | 8 | 6 | 6 | 6 | 5 |
| Attract and retain employees | 6 | 7 | 4 | 5 | 5 | 7 | 7 |
| Improve workplace safety | 7 | 5 | 5 | 8 | 7 | 5 | 6 |
| Reduce healthcare/insurance costs | 9 | 9 | 11 | 3 | 11 | 11 | 1 |
| Promote corporate image or brand | 8 | 8 | 6 | 9 | 8 | 9 | 9 |
| Fulfill social/community responsibility | 10 | 10 | 8 | 10 | 9 | 8 | 10 |
| Comply with legislation | 11 | 11 | 10 | 11 | 10 | 10 | 11 |
| Supplement government-provided health care | 12 | 12 | 12 | 12 | 12 | 12 | 12 |

Figure I-2 Top employer objectives driving wellness initiatives.

Source: Buck Consultants, 2009

According to the survey, the main health issues driving health promotion programs were stress, physical activity, nutrition and healthy eating, work/life issues and chronic disease (see Figure I-3).

| | Africa | Asia | Australia | Canada | Europe | Latin America | United States |
|---|---|---|---|---|---|---|---|
| **Stress** | 1 | 1 | 1 | 1 | 1 | 3 | 5 |
| **Physical activity/exercise** | 4 | 2 | 2 | 4 | 2 | 1 | 1 |
| **Nutrition/healthy eating** | 10 | 3 | 4 | 5 | 6 | 2 | 2 |
| **Work/life issues** | 3 | 6 | 3 | 2 | 3 | 11 | 9 |
| **Chronic disease (e.g., cardiac, diabetes)** | 8 | 7 | 5 | 8 | 10 | 6 | 3 |
| **High blood pressure** | 9 | 5 | 7 | 10 | 11 | 4 | 4 |
| **High cholesterol** | 13 | 4 | 8 | 9 | 13 | 5 | 7 |
| **Workplace safety** | 6 | 8 | 6 | 6 | 5 | 8 | 11 |
| **Depression** | 5 | 11 | 10 | 3 | 7 | 13 | 10 |
| **Tobacco use/smoking** | 12 | 14 | 12 | 11 | 4 | 10 | 8 |
| **Psychosocial work environment** | 10 | 10 | 13 | 7 | 8 | 9 | 15 |
| **Obesity** | 15 | 12 | 9 | 15 | 14 | 7 | 6 |
| **Personal safety** | 6 | 9 | 14 | 12 | 9 | 15 | 13 |
| **Sleep/rest/recovery** | 17 | 13 | 11 | 13 | 12 | 12 | 14 |
| **Maternity/newborn health** | 18 | 17 | 16 | 16 | 15 | 14 | 12 |
| **Substance abuse** | 14 | 18 | 15 | 14 | 16 | 18 | 16 |
| **Infectious diseases/AIDS/HIV** | 2 | 16 | 17 | 18 | 18 | 17 | 17 |
| **Public sanitation** | 16 | 15 | 18 | 17 | 17 | 16 | 18 |

Figure I-3 Health issues driving wellness strategies.

Source: Buck Consultants, 2009

The global survey showed that a large portion of employers, from 33% to 47% depending on the objective, do not know the impact of their health promotion initiatives on the organization's strategic objectives (see Figure I-4). Only 22% of surveyed organizations report measuring financial outcomes of their health promotion programs.

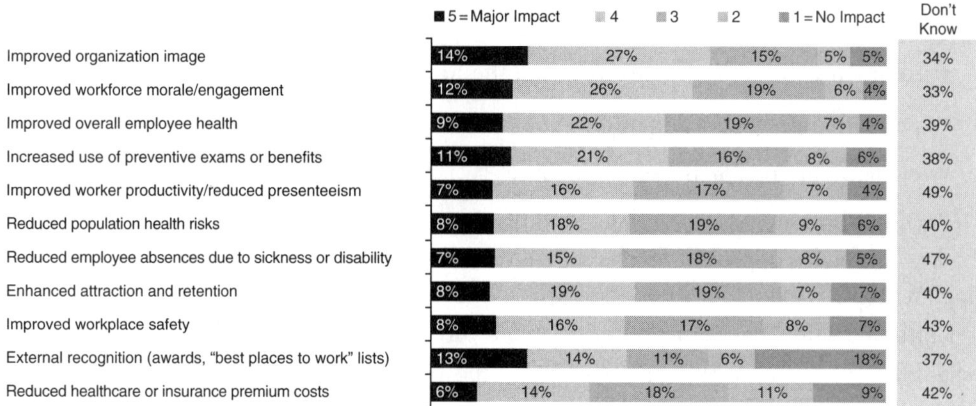


Figure I-4 Impact of wellness initiatives on organizations.

Source: Buck Consultants, 2009

These findings underline the need for enhanced evaluation and better instruments that can be used across countries and healthcare systems. The survey supports similar findings of other smaller surveys (Watson Wyatt Worldwide, 2006) that show that employers worldwide are increasingly recognizing the value of health promotion. However, on a global scale, only a minority of companies are adopting a health promotion approach. There are still countless companies, especially in developing countries and small employers, that have not yet implemented basic occupational health and safety services (Jamison et al., 2006). This scenario does not bode well for developing and emerging countries, which are facing a chronic disease crisis. The country profiles in this book highlight these challenges and examine how major emerging economies, such as China and India, are trying to address the trend.

## What Is "Workplace Health Promotion"?

It is important to clarify what workplace health promotion is, because the term is highlighted in the title of this publication and features prominently throughout the book. Many terms, such as worksite wellness, health and well-being, health and productivity management, health enhancement, disease prevention, etc., are used internationally and often confusion arises around these. Two of the most recognized definitions have been published by the International Association for Worksite Health Promotion (IAWHP) and the European Network for Workplace Health Promotion (ENWHP). The IAWHP defines workplace health promotion as "a corporateset of strategic and tactical actions that seek to optimize worker health and business performance through the collective efforts of employees, families, employers, communities, and society-at-large" (International Association for Worksite Health Promotion [IAWHP], 2009). The ENWHP takes a slightly different approach with the definition in the Luxemburg Declaration.

> Workplace Health Promotion (WHP) is the combined efforts of employers, employees, and society to improve the health and wellbeing of people at work. This can be achieved through a combination of:
>
> - improving the work organization and the working environment
> - promoting active participation
> - encouraging personal development (ENWHP, 1997, 1)

The World Health Organization does not have a definition for workplace health promotion and takes a broader approach by defining a healthy workplace as one that considers the following (WHO, 2010a):

- health and safety concerns in the physical work environment
- health, safety, and wellbeing concerns in the psychosocial work environment, including organization of work and workplace culture
- health promotion opportunities in the workplace
- ways of participating in the community to improve the health of workers, their families, and other members of the community

Furthermore, the WHO presents a model and framework for a healthy workplace, which includes avenues of influence, process, and core principles (see Figure I-5).

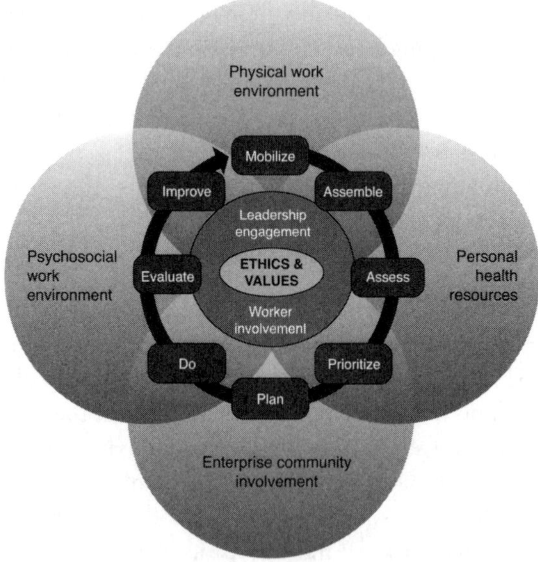


Figure I-5 Healthy workplace model.
Source: World Health Organization, 2010a

Based on these definitions, it is essential to understand that workplace health promotion is not merely targeting and improving health risks and behaviors of the employees, but also addressing the working environment as well as integrating with occupational health programs and medical services. The inclusive and multidisciplinary nature of workplace health promotion creates its challenges, as this requires breaking down existing barriers between disciplines. A common corporate challenge is the lack of communication between occupational health services (OHS), health, safety and environment (HSE), and human resources (HR). Too often, health promotion services are caught between these departments and do not receive adequate support. Overall, disciplines are gradually changing their conventional approaches and recognizing the need for a more proactive approach to workplace health. This includes the medical community, which has traditionally been resistant to external influence. For example, the Indian Association for Occupational Health (www.iaohindia.com) and the American College for Occupational and Environmental Medicine (www.acoem.org) have recently taken on workplace health promotion in their portfolio of activities.

## Good Practices in Workplace Health Promotion

There are numerous initiatives to summarize and highlight successful programs and practices for other workplaces to replicate. A number of these will be featured in the following chapters. Comparing with other companies, or benchmarking, has become the norm; often benchmarking is approached from a competitive perspective, but it is also valuable in order to learn from others. The ENWHP recently gathered good practice models through their Move Europe initiative (www.enwhp.org). The selection process was based on the ENWHP quality criteria, which were developed in 1999 (ENWHP, 1999). The criteria were divided into six sectors:

1. Workplace health promotion and corporate policy
2. Human resources and work organization
3. Planning of workplace health promotion
4. Social responsibility
5. Implementation of workplace health promotion
6. Results of workplace health promotion

The Wellness Councils of America (WELCOA) outlined the features of a "well workplace" (WELCOA, 2010):

- capturing CEO support
- creating cohesive wellness teams
- collecting data to drive health efforts
- carefully crafting an operating plan
- choosing appropriate interventions

- creating a supportive environment
- carefully evaluating outcomes

Additional significant good practice criteria and models have been developed in Canada (Canadian Healthy Workplace Criteria), Singapore (Singapore Health Award), and Brazil (Prêmio Nacional de Qualidade de Vida). Most recently, URAC, the United States–based accreditation and certification agency formerly known as the Utilization, Review, Accredition Commissions, and the Global Knowledge Exchange Network on Healthcare (GKEN), have initiated the first global health promotion awards program, which includes a workplace award. The inaugural winning programs are described at www.aihpa.org. All of these programs agree that the commitment and support of leadership is one of the most important predictors of success.

## The Future of Workplace Health Promotion

As evidenced by the Global Survey of Health Promotion and Workplace Wellness Strategies (Buck Consultants, 2009), the field of workplace health promotion is growing year by year and further growth is expected. Even the severe economic recession could not halt this growth, seeing as most companies surveyed did not cut their programs and some actually increased their investments (Buck Consultants, 2009). Given the current disease and demographic trends, the challenges will no doubt be greater for individuals, employers, and countries. The workplace setting provides a unique opportunity to tackle noncommunicable diseases and improve global health, for it is in the workforce where the largest majority of adults can be found in any given country—even within countries with unemployment rates as high as 20–30%. Although this has been recognized by numerous organizations—governmental, nongovernmental and private—healthcare systems do not seem to support a more proactive approach. In addition, financial constraints and short-term thinking in the corporate world create barriers for the implementation of health promotion strategies. The consequence for our field is a need for enhanced documentation and outcome data that is relevant to the given system and environment. These data should include presenteeism as a measure, especially as the self-report instruments have matured and are now being used internationally, such as the Work Limitations Questionnaire (WLQ), the Stanford Presenteeism Scale (SPS), and the Health and Work Performance Questionnaire (HPQ). One of the most impressive studies was commissioned by Dow Chemical in 2005 (Collins et al., 2005). A survey of 12,397 employees found that for all chronic conditions studied, the cost associated with presenteeism greatly exceeded the combined costs of absenteeism and medical treatment combined—at least three times as much in all cases except diabetes (see Figure I-6).

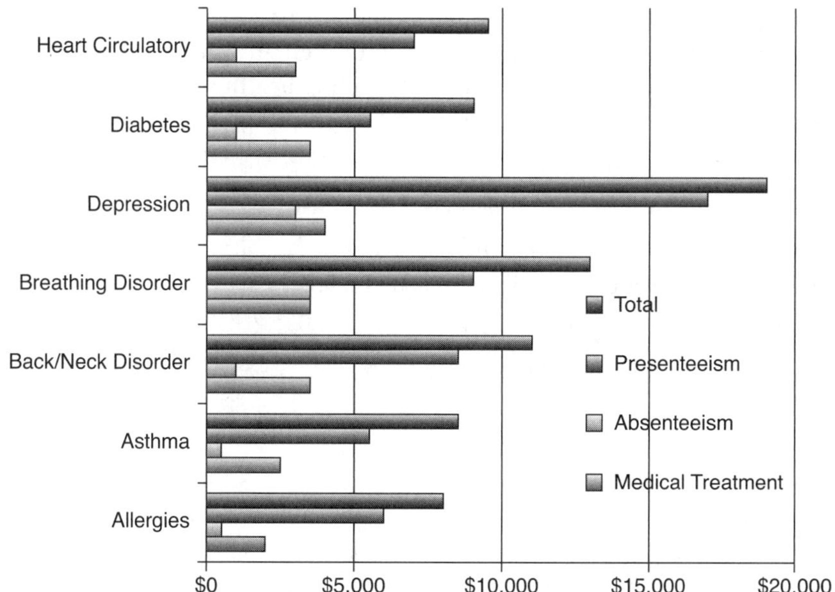


Figure I-6 The economic impact of presenteeism, absenteeism, and medical costs due to chronic health conditions.

Source: Adapted from Collins et al. (2005)

Another documented need is improved integration of health-related programs, such as health promotion, occupational health, disease management, workers' compensation, disability case management, and human resources. In addition, corporate social responsibility (CSR) strategies should also be linked to employee health programs as synergies exist. The overall integration is a common challenge, especially in large multinational companies, with regard to communication structures and data collection. A seamless tracking and improvement process from healthy to at-risk to sick or disabled employees will be beneficial in order to achieve positive outcomes. It is particularly important to address the health of all employees, not only the sick and disabled ones. Interventions need to be more tailored to the individual and consider personality types and preferences. Substantial progress has been made in this regard with the lightning-fast developments in technology. The emergence of virtual worlds will likely enhance the tailoring of health messages in the near future.

Culturally adapted messages and programs are still lacking. Not much has been done on a global scale aside from translations, spelling adjustments (e.g., labor vs. labour), and measurement conversions (e.g., pounds vs. kilograms). Cultural adaptation and sensitivity programs have not kept track with the growth in global health promotion strategies. In order to achieve marked and sustainable behavior change, more diligence and investment is required on the part of employers and program providers.

Finally, workplace health promotion will assume a greater role in improving employees' overall well-being at the workplace. Employers are often struggling with sagging employee morale and dissatisfaction, making a holistic approach to health and well-being necessary.

In summary, future needs for the field of workplace health promotion are the following:

1. Evaluation and measurement
2. Integration of health-related programs
3. Focus on all employees—sick and healthy
4. Tailoring of interventions utilizing new technologies
5. Cultural adaptation and sensitivity
6. Holistic approach to health and well-being

## References

Buck Consultants. (2009). *Report of working well: A global survey of health promotion and workplace wellness strategies.* San Francisco, California: Author.

Bupa, The Oxford Alliance, RAND Europe, & The Work Foundation. (2009). *Healthy work—Challenges and opportunities to 2030.* London: Bupa.

Collins, J., Baase, C., Sharda, C., Ozminkowski, R. J., Nicholson, S., Billotti, G. M., et al. (2005). Assessment of chronic health conditions on work performance, absence and total economic impact for employers. *Journal of Occupational and Environmental Medicine, 47,* 547–557.

European Network for Workplace Health Promotion. (1999). *Quality criteria of workplace health promotion.* Retrieved February 21, 2010, from http://www.enwhp.org/enwhp-initiatives/1st-initiative-quality-criteria.html

European Network for Workplace Health Promotion. (1997). *Luxembourg Declaration on Workplace Health Promotion.* Luxemburg: ENWHP.

International Association for Worksite Health Promotion. (2009, March 26). *Atlanta announcement on worksite health promotion.* Retrieved October 19, 2009, from http://www.acsm-iawhp.org/files/AtlantaAnnouncement.pdf

International Commission on Occupational Health. (2009). About ICOH. Retrieved December 10, 2009, from http://www.icohweb.org/site_new/ico_about.asp

International Data Corporation. (2009). *Worldwide mobile worker population 2009–2013 forecast.* Framingham, MA: IDC.

International Labor Organization. (2005). *World Day for Safety and Health at Work 2005: A background paper.* Geneva: ILO.

Jamison, D. T., Alleyne, G., Breman, J. G., Claeson, M., Evans, D., Jha, P., et al. (Eds.). (2006). *Disease Control Priorities in Developing Countries* (pp. 413–432). Washington, DC: Oxford University Press/World Bank.

Mills, P. R., Kessler, R. C., Cooper, J., & Sullivan, S. (2007). Impact of a health promotion program on employee health risks and work productivity. *American Journal of Health Promotion, 22,* 45–53.

Watson Wyatt Worldwide. (2006). *Research report: Adopting a global health care benefits strategy: 2006 survey of multinationals on health care.* Retrieved October 20, 2009, from http://www.watsonwyatt.com/research/resrender.asp?id=W-916&page=1

Wellness Council of America. (2010). *WELCOA's seven benchmarks.* Retrieved February 21, 2010, from http://welcoa.org/wellworkplace/index.php?category=16

World Health Organization. (2008). *2008–2013 action plan for the global strategy for the prevention and control of noncommunicable diseases.* Retrieved February 21, 2010, from http://whqlibdoc.who.int/publications/2009/9789241597418_eng.pdf

World Health Organization. (2010a). *WHO healthy workplace framework and model.* Retrieved February 21, 2010, from http://www.who.int/occupational_health/healthy_workplace_framework.pdf

World Health Organization. (2010b). *WHO obesity fact file.* Retrieved February 20, 2010, from http://www.who.int/features/factfiles/obesity/en/index.html

World Health Organization/World Economic Forum. (2008). *Preventing noncommunicable diseases in the workplace through diet and physical activity: WHO/World Economic Forum report of a joint event.* Retrieved February 20, 2010, from https://members.weforum.org/pdf/Wellness/WHOWEF_report.pdf

## Additional References

American College for Occupational and Environmental Medicine. http://www.acoem.org

The European Network of Workplace Health Promotion's initiative, Move Europe. http://www.enwhp.org

Indian Association for Occupational Health. http://www.iaohindia.com

The Oxford Health Alliance's global campaign, 3Four50. http://www.3four50.com

# About the Editors

## Wolf Kirsten, MSc

Wolf Kirsten is the founder and president of International Health Consulting based in Berlin, Germany (www.wolfkirsten.com). His company mission is to help international corporations, organizations, and governments improve the quality of life of their respective populations through innovative, culturally appropriate, and cost-effective health promotion programs.

Mr. Kirsten has published and edited extensively on the global aspects of health promotion in various international publications. He has assisted numerous international corporations with the implementation and coordination of their health promotion programs. His consulting portfolio extends from China to North America and Europe to the Middle East, advising companies such as Nokia, Johnson & Johnson, Cisco, and Saudi Aramco. He also advised the Ministry of Health of the Kingdom of Bahrain and crafted a national health promotion strategy. Mr. Kirsten teaches post-graduate courses in health promotion at the Freie Universität in Berlin and the Hochschule Magdeburg and is a sought-after speaker and trainer.

He is the cofounder and board member of the International Institute for Health Promotion (IIHP), which he managed for eight years in Washington, DC, and he is on the board of the International Association of Worksite Health Promotion (IAWHP).

Mr. Kirsten received his master of science in health promotion management and graduated *magna cum laude* from American University in Washington, DC. He is a German native and lived abroad for many years, including in the United States, England, and China.

## Robert C. Karch, EdD

Dr. Karch is a professor in the School of Education, Teaching, and Health at American University in Washington, DC. He brings more than 30 years of academic leadership experience, extensive project management expertise, and a wealth of real-world business acumen to any project he undertakes (www.robertkarch.com). His well-established and award-winning record for innovative academic program development in the areas of health promotion management and chronic disease interventions are perhaps unparalleled in higher education.

To date, more than 400 students have received their master of science (MS) degree in health promotion management from the innovative interdisciplinary graduate program that Dr. Karch created and established at American University in 1980. Moreover, his professional work has greatly contributed, both nationally and internationally, to the advancement of knowledge with respect to not only the social, environmental, cultural, and organizational aspects of health promotion, but also the role and importance of self empowerment of employees within workplace settings.

Aside from directing the MS program, he also teaches the capstone courses for the MS, Strategic Planning for Health Promotion and Critical Issues in Health Promotion, as well as a course in global health and global health policy. Dr. Karch is also the founder and executive director of the National Center for Health and Fitness (established in 1980) and the International Institute for Health Promotion (established in 1996) at American University.

Over the past 25 years, Dr. Karch has been the principal investigator on more than a dozen projects with a combined value in excess of $28 million. All of those projects directly focused on changing and then sustaining health related behaviors in human subjects. In many of those studies, Dr. Karch and his research colleagues applied advanced financial models to statistically significant outcomes so as to document the financial return on such program investments.

Over the past 25 years, Dr. Karch has lectured, given keynote addresses, scholarly papers, conducted intense training courses and consultative services for corporations, governmental agencies, and private sector groups in dozens of countries throughout the world on the topic of health promotion.

# Contributing Authors

**Kerstin Baumgarten, PhD**
Hochschule Magdeburg-Stendal (University of Applied Sciences)
Department of Social and Health Sciences
Stendal, Germany

**Finn Berggren**
President, Gerlev Physical Education and Sports Academy
Cofounder and Steering Board Member, HEPA Europe—European Network for Health Enhancing Physical Activity
Denmark

**Bob Boyd, OAM**
President, National Wellness Institute of Australia, Inc.
Director, Wellness Communication Solutions
Brisbane, Queensland, Australia

**Wei-Qing Chen, MD, PhD**
Department of Biostatistics and Epidemiology
School of Public Health
Sun Yat-sen University
Guangzhou, China

**Katy Cherry, BSc**
Freelance Health Writer and Health Promotion Specialist
London, United Kingdom

**Volney Vasquez Henríquez, MSc**
Founder and President, Promondo Company
Santiago, Chile

**Antero Heloma, MD, PhD**
National Institute for Health and Welfare (THL)
Helsinki, Finland

**Vladimir Hobza, PhD**
Faculty of Physical Culture
Palacky University of Olomouc
Olomouc, Czech Republic

**Peter Thomas Honeyman, MB, BS, FACOEM**
Independent Consultant Occupational Physician
Israel

**Gerhard Huber, PhD**
Institut für Sport und Sportwissenschaft der Universität Heidelberg
Universität Heidelberg
Heidelberg, Germany

**Tanya Kalas**
Health Promotion Specialist
International Health Consulting
Berlin, Germany

**Robert C. Karch, EdD**
Professor, School of Education, Teaching, and Health
Executive Director, National Center for Health and Fitness
International Institute for Health Promotion
American University
Washington, DC, United States

**G. L. Khanna, PhD**
Dean, Faculty of Applied Sciences
Manav Rachna International University
Faridabad, India

**Wolf Kirsten, MSc**
Founder and President
International Health Consulting
Berlin, Germany

**Linda Kovler, RN, BA, BSN, MOccH**
Global Health and Well-Being, Intel Electronics
Israel

**Dieter Lagerstrøm, PhD**
Associate Professor, Department of Public Health, Sport, and Nutrition
University of Agder
Kristiansand, Norway

**Rod Lees, B Soc Wk, Dip Ed Psych, Cert Teach**
Wellness Consultant and Personal Trainer
Events Coordinator, National Wellness Institute of Australia, Inc.
Brisbane, Queensland, Australia

**Cinthia Ortiz Leiteiro, RN, MBA**
Promondo Company
Santiago, Chile

**Low Soo Leng, MSc**
Health Promotion Board
Singapore

**Jian Li, MD, PhD**
Department of Safety Engineering and Ergonomics
University of Wuppertal
Wuppertal, Germany

**Annie Ling, PhD**
Health Promotion Board
Singapore

**Chew Ling, MBBS, MMed (Public Health), FAMS**
Health Promotion Board
Singapore

**Ricardo De Marchi, MD**
CEO of CPH Health
São Paulo, Brazil

**Vishal Marwah, MS, MBBS**
Global Cardiovascular Programs, Department of Cardiology
Mount Sinai School of Medicine
New York, New York, United States

**Giuseppe Masanotti, MD**
Professor, Faculty of Medicine
Public Health Department of Medical and Surgical Specialties
University of Perugi
Perugia, Italy

**Peter R. Mills, MB BS, MSc, MD, MCRP**
Specialist in Respiratory Medicine
The Whittington Hospital
Director, Glasslyn Health Solutions
London, United Kingdom

**Alan Pui Wee Ming, MPH**
Health Promotion Board
Singapore

**Takashi Muto, MD, PhD**
Professor, Department of Public Health
Dokkyo Medical University School of Medicine
Tochigi, Japan

**Lars Österblom, MSc**
Senior Organizational Development Consultant
Lars Österblom Consulting
Stockholm, Sweden

**Emmanuel Olufemi Owolabi, PhD**
Department of Physical Health Education
University of Botswana
Gaborone, Botswana

**Neo Seow Ping, BSc**
Health Promotion Board
Singapore

**Rimma A. Potemkina, MD, PhD**
State Research Center for Preventive Medicine
Ministry of Health and Social Development of the Russian Federation
Moscow, Russia

**Jalees K. Razavi, MBBS, DPHC, DIH, FRCPC, FACOEM, FACPM**
Director, Occupational Health, Imperial Oil Limited
Calgary, Alberta, Canada

**Thomas Skovgaard, PhD**
Associate Professor, Institute of Sports Science and Clinical Biomechanics
University of Southern Denmark
Odense, Denmark

**Radim Šlachta, PhD**
Faculty of Physical Culture
Palacky University, Olomouc
Czech Republic

**Gert L. Strydom, PhD**
Professor, School for Biokinetics, Recreation, and Sport Science
North West University (Potchefstroom Campus)
South Africa

**Cilas Wilders, PhD, BJur**
Instituut vir Biokinetika/Institute for Biokinetics
Fakulteit Gesondheidswetenskappe/Faculty of Health Sciences
NW Universiteit/University—Potchefstroom
South Africa

**Jan Winroth**
Senior Lecturer, University West
Trollhättan, Sweden

**Lek Yin Yin, B Soc Sc (Hons)**
Health Promotion Board
Singapore

# The International Institute for Health Promotion

The founding and development of the International Institute for Health Promotion (IIHP) in 1996 was a logical strategic international extension of the prior 16 years of academic and research activities conducted by the National Center for Health and Fitness (NCHF), founded at American University in 1980 by Dr. Robert C. Karch, coauthor of this text. The central purpose of NCHF was to provide leadership for the United States in the areas of health risk identification and lifestyle improving activities and to stay abreast of the growing and changing needs of the health and fitness industry and, in particular, health promotion professionals. To that end, in 1980, as a central activity of the NCHF, Dr. Karch also established an interdisciplinary Master of Science Program in Health and Fitness Management (now an MS in Health Promotion Management) at American University.

The onset of globalization and in particular the internationalization of the workforces of the world coupled with the increasing requests for information from the international community with respect to health promotion activities served as the impetus for the establishment of the IIHP at American University. Thus, starting in the 1988, the founder of the NCHF embarked on a systematic process of evaluating the merits of officially establishing a global network of institutions and individuals to respond to the ever increasing needs of the global community with respect to quality health promotion programs and the educational preparation of professionals entering this rapidly emerging discipline. The culmination of this process was the founding meeting for IIHP, developed by Dr. Karch and Wolf Kirsten, held at American University in June of 1996. Today the IIHP is comprised of some 200 institutions, organizations, and individuals that represent more than 50 countries.

To further implement the strategic objectives of the IIHP, the organization is actively establishing IIHP regional centers throughout the world so as to bring the collective resources of the membership of the IIHP closer to select regions as well as to each other.

## Mission Statement

The mission of the IIHP is to strategically maximize the intellectual resources of select academic institutions, private and public sector organizations, companies, and professionals in order to continually enhance and advance the education preparation and training of health promotion professionals.

The IIHP will accomplish this through the facilitation and development of collaborative educational strategies, focused research, and public and private sector initiatives and partnerships.

## Strategic Objectives

The membership of the IIHP is dedicated to fulfilling the organization's mission through the successful development and implementation of the following five strategic objectives.

1. To develop and recommend core curricula content for preparation of current and future health promotion professionals
2. To develop, recommend, and offer continuing educational programs for health promotion professionals
3. To develop a research program along with appropriate methodologies to advance the evidence base of quality health promotion programs
4. To develop and coordinate international exchange opportunities for students, faculty, and professionals within the field of health promotion
5. To encourage and assist public and private sector organizations in the development, implementation, management, and evaluation of health promotion policies and programs

Chapter 1

# Australia

Bob Boyd and Rod Lees

After reading this chapter you should be able to:

- Identify core strategies that are the focus of Australia's workplace health promotion efforts
- Describe Australia's historical evolution of workplace health promotion
- Explain the different approaches employed by corporate health promotion efforts throughout Australia
- Review the central disease-states and health issues driving Australia's health promotion needs
- Name the components of, and the associated funding sources for, Australia's healthcare system
- Discuss the impact of culture on Australia's health status and health promotion efforts

| Table 1-1 Select Key Demographic and Economic Indicators | |
|---|---|
| Nationality | Noun: Australian(s)<br>Adjective: Australian |
| Ethnic groups | White 92%, Asian 7%, Aboriginal and other 1% |
| Religion | Catholic 25.8%, Anglican 18.7%, Uniting Church 5.7%, Reformed 3%, Eastern Orthodox 2.7%, other Christian 7.9%, Buddhist 2.1%, Muslim 1.7%, other 2.4%, unspecified 11.3%, none 18.7% (2006 Census) |
| Language | English 78.5%, Chinese 2.5%, Italian 1.6%, Greek 1.3%, Arabic 1.2%, Vietnamese 1%, other 8.2%, unspecified 5.7% (2006 Census) |
| Literacy | Definition: age 15 and over can read and write<br>Total population: 99%<br>Male: 99%<br>Female: 99% (2003 est.) |
| Education expenditure | 4.5% of GDP (2005)<br>Country comparison to the world: 86 |

*continued*

| Table 1-1 **Select Key Demographic and Economic Indicators,** *continued* | |
|---|---|
| Government type | Federal parliamentary democracy |
| Environment | Soil erosion from overgrazing, industrial development, urbanization, and poor farming practices; soil salinity rising due to the use of poor quality water; desertification; clearing for agricultural purposes threatens the natural habitat of many unique animal and plant species; the Great Barrier Reef off the northeast coast, the largest coral reef in the world, is threatened by increased shipping and its popularity as a tourist site; limited natural fresh water resources |
| Country mass | Total: 7,741,220 sq km<br>Country comparison to the world: 6<br>Land: 7,682,300 sq km<br>Water: 58,920 sq km<br>*Note:* includes Lord Howe Island and Macquarie Island |
| Population | 21,515,754 (July 2010 est.)<br>Country comparison to the world: 54 |
| Age structure | 0–14 years: 18.4% (male 2,033,106/female 1,929,863)<br>15–64 years: 67.8% (male 7,397,562/female 7,197,829)<br>65 years and over: 13.5% (male 1,306,329/female 1,607,146)<br>(2010 est.) |
| Median age | Total: 37.5 years<br>Male: 36.8 years<br>Female: 38.3 years (2010 est.) |
| Population growth rate | 1.171% (2010 est.)<br>Country comparison to world: 108 |
| Birth rate | 12.39 births/1,000 population (2010 est.)<br>Country comparison to world: 162 |
| Death rate | 6.81 deaths/1,000 population (July 2010 est.)<br>Country comparison to world: 146 |
| Net migration rate | 6.13 migrant(s)/1,000 population (2010 est.)<br>Country comparison to the world: 11 |
| Urbanization | Urban population: 89% of total population (2008)<br>Rate of urbanization: 1.2% annual rate of change<br>(2005–2010 est.) |
| Gender ratio | At birth: 1.06 male(s)/female<br>Under 15 years: 1.05 male(s)/female<br>15–64 years: 1.03 male(s)/female<br>65 years and over: 0.84 male(s)/female<br>Total population: 1 male(s)/female (2010 est.) |

*continued*

| Table 1-1 **Select Key Demographic and Economic Indicators,** *continued* | |
|---|---|
| Infant mortality rate | Total: 4.67 deaths/1,000 live births<br>Country comparison to the world: 195<br>Male: 5.08 deaths/1,000 live births<br>Female: 4.33 deaths/1,000 live births (2010 est.) |
| Life expectancy | Total population: 81.72 years<br>Country comparison to the world: 8<br>Male: 79.33 years<br>Female: 84.25 years (2010 est.) |
| Total fertility rate | 1.78 children born/woman (2010 est.)<br>Country comparison to the world: 156 |
| GDP—purchasing power | $824.3 billion (2010 est.) |
| Parity | Country comparison to the world: 19 |
| GDP—per capita | $38,800 (2009 est.)<br>Country comparison to the world: 23 |
| GDP—composition by sector | Agriculture: 4.1% |
| Agriculture—products | Wheat, barley, sugarcane, fruits, cattle, sheep, poultry |
| Industries | Mining, industrial and transportation equipment, food processing, chemicals, steel |
| Labor force participation | 11.45 million (2009 est.)<br>Country comparison to the world: 44 |
| Unemployment rate | 5.7% (2009 est.)<br>Country comparison to the world: 51 |
| Industrial production | -4.1% (2009 est.)<br>Growth rate |
| Distribution of family income (GINI index) | 30.5 (2006) |
| Investment (gross fixed) | 28.5% of GDP (2009 est.)<br>Country comparison to the world: 32 |
| Public debt | 17.6% of GDP (2009 est.)<br>Country comparison to the world: 108 |
| Market value of publicly traded shares | $NA (December 31, 2009) |
| Current account balance | $-29.89 billion (2009 est.)<br>Country comparison to the world: 182 |
| Debt (external) | $920 billion (December 31, 2009 est.)<br>Country comparison to world: 11 |

*continued*

| Table 1-1 **Select Key Demographic and Economic Indicators,** *continued* | |
|---|---|
| Debt as a % of GDP | ——— |
| Exports | $160.5 billion (2009 est.)<br>Country comparison to the world: 23 |
| Exports—commodities | Coal, iron ore, gold, meat, wool, alumina, wheat, machinery, and transport equipment |
| Export—partners | Japan 22.2%, China 14.6%, South Korea 8.2%, India 6.1%, United States 5.5%, NZ 4.3%, United Kingdom 4.2% (2008) |
| Imports | $160.9 billion (2009 est.)<br>Country comparison to the world: 21 |
| Import—commodities | Machinery and transport equipment, computers and office machines, telecommunication equipment and parts; crude oil and petroleum products |
| Import—partners | China 17.94%, United States 11.26%, Japan 8.36%, Singapore 5.54%, Thailand 5.8%, Germany 5.3%, United Kingdom 4.3% (2009) |
| Stock of direct foreign investment at | |
| Home | $295.9 billion (December 31, 2009 est.)<br>Country comparison to the world: 15 |
| Abroad | $226.7 billion (December 31, 2009 est.)<br>Country comparison to the world: 15 |

Source: CIA. (2010). *The world factbook.* Retrieved August 31, 2010, from www.cia.gov

# Introduction

Australia is, by international standards, a very healthy country. The World Health Organization (WHO) stated that "Australia consistently ranks in the best performing group of countries for healthy life expectancy" (Department of Health and Aging, n.d.)

However, Australia still has major health issues. The increasing prevalence of problems such as obesity and diabetes and the inability of past methods to deal with these and other major health issues has some in the health field predicting that life expectancy rates will level out and may even start to diminish. In addition, life expectancy of the indigenous population is 17 years less than the nonindigenous population. Inequality in life expectancy also exists between rich and poor as well as between rural and city dwellers. A healthcare system that is under increasing strain is placing more and more pressure on both the private sector and government at all levels to take steps to improve the health of all Australians.

Historically, health promotion strategies have largely followed the medical model of prevention; that is, primarily risk reduction through behavior change targeted at a specific health problem. However, the limited success of this approach to deal with many major lifestyle-related health problems in the long term is now fueling the push for a different approach. Could this be the trigger for greater acceptance of the wellness movement, which emphasizes life enrichment of the whole person rather than purely risk reduction?

Wellness as a term, way of life, and health paradigm has been very slow to be embraced by individuals, organizations, the healthcare system and both levels of government since its first flicker of life in Australia more than 30 years ago. In fact, the current health crises and the media attention they are receiving may also prove to be what is needed for many more decision makers to realize the importance of the workplace as a health promotion setting. Perhaps this may also reignite the workplace health promotion flame which sparked in the late 1970s, caught fire in the mid-1980s (mainly government agency promoted), but failed to burn any brighter until relatively recently with the emergence of a growing number of private providers offering health services to the workplace.

"It is estimated that currently over 1,500 corporate and government employers provide health assessments and intervention programs for over 400,000 employees" (National Preventative Health Taskforce, 2009, p. 52). This data appears to be an increase of that reported in the 1991 survey (return percentages reported only) commissioned by the National Coordinating (formerly Steering) Committee for Health Promotion in the Workplace (1993). Yet this current figure represents only about 3.6% of Australian workers (National Preventative Health Taskforce, 2009). More fuel is necessary to start the "bush fire" in order for workplace health promotion to deliver the outcomes it is capable of achieving in reducing the growing cost of ill health in Australia.

## Prevailing Health Issues and Risk Behaviors

The National Preventative Health Taskforce was established in April 2008 by the Australian central government. The theme was, "Australia: the Healthiest Country by 2020." The initial discussion paper outlined a number of prevailing health issues and risk behaviors that need to be addressed. The central issues nominated are obesity, tobacco, and alcohol. The reason for this is that, "put together, smoking, obesity, harmful use of alcohol, physical inactivity, poor diet and the associated risk factors of high blood pressure and high blood cholesterol cause approximately 32% of Australia's illness" (National Preventative Health Taskforce, 2008, p. 7).

### Smoking

Out of a total population of around 20 million, there are at least 2.9 million adult Australians who smoke on a daily basis. While this constitutes a 30% decline since 1976, approximately half of these smokers who continue to smoke for a prolonged period will die early.

Smoking-related illness costs up to 5.7 billion AUD (Australian dollars) per year in lost productivity. In addition, the smoking rate for young people is still cause for concern. Of similar concern is the over 50% smoking rate of indigenous Australians (National Preventative Health Taskforce, 2008, p. 8).

### Obesity

The number of Australians who are overweight or obese has been increasing dramatically since 1980, and it is predicted that if the trend continues, nearly 75% of Australians will be overweight or obese by 2025. The current estimated figure of overweight and obesity stands at over 60% (National Preventative Health Taskforce, 2008, p. 7). Of particular concern is the percentage of children who are either overweight or obese. The 2007 National Children's Nutrition and Physical Activity Survey reports this percentage as 25% (National Preventative Health Taskforce, 2008, p. 7). This is a huge increase from the 1960s figure of 5%. Thus, it is reasonable to predict that life expectancy figures for Australia will fall in the future.

### Alcohol

While the majority of the Australian population drink alcohol at levels below long-term risk or harm, a major problem exists with young adults and Australia's Aboriginal population. The annual costs of harmful consumption of alcohol are huge. They consist of costs associated with crime, health, loss of productivity, and road trauma. Collectively, this adds up to a total of over 10 billion AUD.

The taskforce's emphasis on smoking, obesity, and alcohol is not at the exclusion of ongoing concerns related to other major health issues, such as the aging of the Australian population, cancer (skin, breast, and prostate), diabetes, road-related accidents and fatalities, and mental health issues. For example, the key findings from the National Survey on Mental Health and Wellbeing found that 1 in 5 Australians aged 16–85 years had a mental health disorder in 2007 (Australian Bureau of Statistics, 2007).

## Healthcare System

The Australian healthcare system is based on a combination of a universal public health system called Medicare and a private health insurance sector. Medicare provides health care that is designed to be largely affordable and accessible to all Australians and can be provided free of charge at the point of care. Doctors in private practice are free to determine the number of rebatable services they provide and the fees they charge to patients. Individuals, who are charged by the doctor for a consultation, claim the standard fee back through Medicare. The Medicare benefits paid are based on a percentage of the Medicare schedule fee.

Medicare also provides free in-hospital services in public hospitals for patients who choose to be treated as public patients. Under Medicare, public patients in public hospitals are not charged for medical services or hospital accommodation costs. This, however, has caused a supply and demand problem, leading to extensive waiting periods in some cases.

The Pharmaceutical Benefits Scheme is the other component of the public healthcare system. This scheme subsidizes a high proportion of prescription medication bought from pharmacies.

The overall public healthcare program is financed through the general taxation system, which includes the Medicare levy, based on an individual's taxable income. This is set at 1.5% above a threshold income level and 2.5% for those people without private health insurance (Department of Health and Ageing, n.d.).

The Private Health Insurance Administration Council (PHIAC) is an independent statutory authority that regulates the private health insurance industry. The overall policy is controlled by the Australian government. Private health insurance covers individuals and families for hospital treatment in the private hospital sector, as well as for a range of ancillary treatments such as dentistry, optometry, physiotherapy, etc. The PHIAC *Annual Report 2007–08* indicated that "44.7% of Australians were covered with private health insurance" (Private Health Insurance Administration Council, 2008, p. 3). The level of coverage for individuals and families depends on the specific policy and the premium paid.

Private health insurance continues to be offered on a community-rated basis wherein discrimination between policy holders on the basis of age, health, gender, race, etc, is prohibited by legislation. In support of this principle, insurers must participate in risk equalization arrangements that share the cost burden of higher-risk policy holders across all insurers. Some categories of Australians, such as members of the armed forces and veterans, are covered by additional special arrangements, while remaining eligible for mainstream Medicare coverage.

Compulsory workers' compensation insurance also covers work-related injuries and illnesses. The annual premium for this insurance is paid by an employer and is calculated by the past number and cost of claims. A small number of (mostly) large organizations are self-insurers. In addition, injuries from motor vehicle accidents may be covered by compulsory third-party motor vehicle insurance. This insurance premium is paid by vehicle owners as a component of vehicle registration.

## Influence of Culture and Mentality

Knowledge and understanding of the culture and mentality of the Australian population is critical when interpreting its health data as well as when investigating the history and the current status of workplace health promotion.

It is said that Australians have very strong attitudes and beliefs that have been developed by the difficulty in subduing the land. Australian settlers experienced great hardship and had to support each other in order to survive. The battle against the elements by Australia's working class led to the nickname "Aussie battlers." *Mateship* has been a central tenet of survival in the harsh environment. It can be defined as the code of conduct that stresses equality and friendship. Mateship has been extremely significant in relation to the armed forces and may also explain why sport plays such a central role in the Australian culture. One result of the prevalence of a mateship culture in Australian society is that Australians are expected to behave with humility and not think of themselves as better than their peers. A consequence of this is that even living a healthy lifestyle could be seen as putting oneself above the rest of the group.

Supporting the underdog and the belief in a "fair go" are key parts of Australian culture and Australian society. This can be seen in the existence of strong public health and education systems and the existence of equal opportunity legislation. It is an idea that involves everyone having an equal chance to achieve their goals and reach their potential.

There are, however, problems associated with this culture and mentality. Peer pressure can be extremely influential. The culture of binge drinking associated with the youth culture and sport (particularly codes of football) is a major problem and a regular topic of concern for health organizations. Peer pressure plays a big role in this, as it also does in the uptake of smoking by youth. Peer pressure and the existing Australian culture may also influence the relatively slow uptake and low level of involvement of employees in many workplace health promotion programs.

Australian society is one of great contrasts when it comes to attitudes of health. On one hand, Australians worship sporting success and a healthy, fit body, and on the other hand, a large stomach (beer gut) is seen as a status symbol by some members of society.

## Drivers of Workplace Health Promotion

Unlike the situation that exists in other parts of the world, especially the United States, Australian employers do not have any responsibility regarding the payment for their employees' health insurance. The majority of employers do, however, have responsibility for the payment of a worker's compensation scheme premium. This premium covers the cost of workplace accidents and injury (physical and psychological) as well as any injury sustained while the worker is travelling to and from work. Some employers have chosen for their organizations to be self-insured. However, they are still legally committed to the same level of care of their employees as those employers who are covered by the worker's compensation scheme. Occupational health and safety is therefore a strong workplace health driver in Australia. This is enshrined in both national and state government legislation. The Australian Safety and Compensation Council (ASCC) is Australia's national body that leads and coordinates national efforts to prevent workplace death, injury, and disease in Australia (Australian Government, n.d.).

The traditional driver for workplace health promotion programs has been through health and safety legislation. It has, however, been largely confined to the prevention of physical accidents at work, the emphasis being on safety, not health per se. Employers are legally required to provide for the safety of their employees but not legally required to provide specifically for their health, with the exception that unsafe practices and work environments can affect one's health (in other words, risk management, not health promotion).

Until recently, the issue of psychological injury has been largely ignored. The driver from the psychological injury perspective has been the cost associated with worker's compensation claims. While these claims are fewer in number than the physical injury claims, in general, they are twice the cost. This has led to the introduction of a number of programs offering support to organizations and to individuals within an organization who are suffering from psychological injury with the view of developing preventative strategies.

# Programs and Good Practices

A brief trip through history is necessary to understand the current position of workplace health promotion in Australia.

## Pioneers

Dr. Brian Furnass, a physician who worked in the 1970s as the director of the university health services at the Australian National University, became very interested in the concept of wellness and visited the United States in 1975 to research the wellness movement. Dr. Furnass and his coauthors of the book, *The Magic Bullet: The Social Implications and Limitations of Modern Medicine,* had a clear vision that the practice of medicine relied too much on the magic bullet (taking a tablet) and too little on assisting people with the more difficult task of living well.

A small number of private companies offering executive medical and health checks existed in the major cities from the late 1970s. For example, the Heart Beat Centre, based in Brisbane, was offering these services and more as health management programs to industry. Companies involved in that program were given Australian business awards for innovative workplace initiatives early in the 1980s (personal papers).

In 1982, the Australian College of Occupational Medicine (ACOM) released its first position paper on health promotion in industry. In association with trade unions and the Confederation of Australian Industry, ACOM released its second "Health Promotion in Industry" report in 1990 (The Australian College of Occupational Medicine, 1990). It provided direction to industry on cost-effective use of resources directed to worker health and safety.

In the mid-1980s, medical insurance companies were establishing fitness centers for policy holders and selling health programs to businesses as part of company insurance packages. During this time, the Commonwealth Department of Sport, Recreation, and Tourism published a booklet linking fitness and productivity. Funding was made available by this department in 1984–1985 for employee fitness and recreation initiatives. This department also promoted the national "Health and Fitness at Work—It Works" program. Contained in the program booklets was a list providing details of more than 20 workplace health promotion programs around Australia (Department of Sport, Recreation, and Tourism, n.d.).

In the late 1980s, the newly established National Steering (later Coordinating) Committee on Health Promotion in the Workplace published a newsletter to encourage more health promotion programs at work and to provide better access to resources for those in the workplace wanting to develop programs. This Committee also promoted a national program called "Health at Work." The program information kit listed the details of a number of current programs around the country (National Coordinating Committee for Health Promotion in the Workplace, n.d.).

In the 1990s, governments at all levels in Australia continued to publish documentation on an ad hoc basis about the benefits of maintaining a healthy workforce. This coincided with the gradual development of commercial organizations offering to companies a range of health services, primarily health assessments for employees.

## Twenty-First Century

From the beginning of the 21st century, there has been an increase in awareness and knowledge of the need for faster return to work after injury. That, coupled with the increased awareness of the true cost of workplace issues such as stress, absenteeism, presenteeism and the concern for work–life balance, highlighted the need for the development and implementation of more appropriate responses.

The National Preventative Health Taskforce notes that "given the huge preventable losses of workplace productivity due to obesity, tobacco, and alcohol, the private and public sectors have key roles as employers and the promotion of much healthier workplaces" (National Preventative Health Taskforce, 2008, p. viii). The report goes on to suggest that a new program offered by the Victorian government offers an excellent example to model.

### The WorkHealth Program

This Victorian WorkHealth program is a government-funded program that gives employers the opportunity to offer their employees workplace-based health checks. The funding is based on the size of the firm. For businesses with an annual payroll of less than 10 million AUD, employers are fully reimbursed by the state government. If the business has an annual payroll greater than 10 million AUD, employers are required to make a contribution of 30.00 AUD per worker towards the cost of the health checks (WorkHealth, n.d. b).

### Australian Unity

One example of a WorkHealth program is that offered by Australian Unity, a national health, financial services, and retirement living organization with more than 1,200 employees across 17 main sites. Its program covers a range of activities including an online health assessment tool with health information and newsletters, a health expo offering health assessments, health information seminars, and healthy cooking demonstrations. In addition, there is a range of employee-led programs. These programs cover funded community work, social events, an employee assistance program, ergonomic assessments, massage, and physical activity events (WorkHealth, n.d. a).

## Queensland Department of Education, Training, and the Arts Workforce Health Management Program

One of the best programs associated with the reduction of psychological injuries within an organization is the Workforce Health Management program offered to the staff of the technical training institutes within the Department of Education, Training, and the Arts in Queensland. The program was designed to develop a range of prevention, response, and recovery activities as a means of reducing the number and cost of psychological injuries. The program relied on the development of local committees and offered a wellness program, additional capability development for rehabilitation coordinators, mental health first aid training, early intervention, and intensive case management. None of the staff referred to the program in 2005–2006 progressed to a psychological-based worker's compensation injury. Return on investment (ROI) based on the number and potential cost of affected staff without program intervention was calculated to be 5:1.

## Greenslopes Private Hospital Staff Wellness Program

Greenslopes Private Hospital in Brisbane was accredited as a WHO Health Promoting Hospital in 2005. The Greenslopes Private Hospital staff wellness program commenced in 2001. Revenue from the state-of-the-art on-site gymnasium, established in 2003, supplemented by grants from hospital executives, is the main funding for the program. Permanent staff are able to salary sacrifice their gym membership, meaning that their gym membership can be deducted from their salary. The program was integrated with human resources, occupational health and safety, staff development, the social club, and library into the new Worklife@GPH initiative in 2005. The program has won the following awards: ACCI/BCI National Work and Family Award 2005 (<500 employees) and National Human Resources Award for Best Health and Wellbeing Strategy (winner—2006 and 2007, finalist—2008 and 2009). Wellness services available to staff through the program include Club Wellness (gymnasium), Wellness Assist (free confidential counseling), Financial Wellness (free financial planning), Greenslopes Nutrition at Work, Wellness2Go (wellness ideas for department meetings), Night Owl (specifically for night-shift workers), health promotion events, health risk management, vaccinations, corporate sporting events, massage therapy, weight management, work–life balance, team building, car servicing, and access to a justice of the peace. A wellness advisory group and a team of wellness ambassadors ensure the program is needs based, participatory, and empowering. The program is regularly evaluated at both the organizational and individual levels to ensure it meets the needs of employees and maximizes ROI (K. Walton, personal communication, September 21, 2009).

## Blue Care Lifestyle Program

Blue Care is an organization that provides care, support, and education to all members of the community, including frail aged, people with disability, and people requiring nursing or allied health support following release from hospital. The Central Queensland Fraser Coast district of Blue Care has entered into a partnership with Central Queensland University to provide a staff wellness program (Caring for the Carers) for more than 11,000 of their staff employed over an area roughly one third the size of the state. The program promotes "a lifestyle wellness journey much richer than the standard diet and exercise regimes" ("Caring for the Blue Care carers," 2009). The 12-month program, commenced in August 2009, is being developed and coordinated by a Central Queensland University masters student. The student is supported by trained volunteer ambassadors in the 29 Blue Care hubs across the region. Utilizing an online wellness inventory and relevant online questionnaires, an employee's health and wellness status and level of motivation to change are assessed. The inventory then guides the employee to "create a tailored personal wellness plan and provides resources to help reach wellness goals" (Blue Care, 2008, p.8). A major resource is remote access to accredited wellness coaches.

## Queensland University of Technology Wellness Matters Program

The Queensland University of Technology Wellness Matters program had its beginnings in the mid-1990s. With the assistance of the head of the School of Human Movement Studies, the Health Promotion subcommittee of the University Health and Safety committee, after years of applying, gained funding for the appointment of a full-time health promotion coordinator. The program is based within the university human resources department and the manager reports to the deputy HR director of health and safety.

Program services delivered to Queensland University of Technology's more than 6,000 full-time-equivalent employees situated on 3 campuses include seminars and workshops, health and wellness appraisals, an extensive and varied range of physical activity sessions, Just Walk It program, Walk Australia program, Make My Day program, personal wellness coaching, personal training, special interest groups such as Queensland University of Technology bicycle user group, weekly health challenges and tips, and community healthy activity involvement.

The program is offered as an individual staff member or as a faculty/division program such as the faculty of Built Environment and Engineering BEEWell program. An advisory board and a large number of volunteer wellness ambassadors assist in delivery, evaluation, and reshaping program offerings to meet employees' and the university's health and wellness requirements. Faculty/division often provide additional program funding to the centrally provided budget (for the last 8 years), otherwise activities run on a cost-recovery basis (Queensland University of Technology, 2009).

## Other Programs

There are numerous other small, medium, and large company programs that could have been reported here, but many are not reported or recorded anywhere. Many companies contract external organizations to provide a full range of services. The number of these organizations has risen dramatically since 2002. Once again, there is no compilation of these organizations. There is a need for an inventory of current Australian programs and organizations. It is hoped that in the near future this will happen in Australia, or that more Australian companies will input their program data into existing surveys of workplace health promotion programs, such as the annual Buck Consultants' Global Health Promotion and Workplace Wellness Survey (Buck Consultants, 2009).

# Outcomes and Indicators

The National Preventative Health Taskforce discussion paper (2008) provides a number of examples where health promotion programs in Australia have been successful. One example is the reduction in smoking (75% of men in the 1950s to less than 20% in 2009). This has dramatically reduced the deaths of men from lung cancer and heart disease. Road trauma deaths on Australian roads have dropped 80% since 1970. Australia's commitment to improving immunization levels has resulted in eliminating a number of serious health problems. Immunization is one aspect of the healthcare system that has been readily integrated into workplace health. A growing number of workplaces, including some that do not have a structured health promotion program, provide flu shots for employees every winter. Reductions in sick leave, attributed to this practice, are quoted to be as high as 36%.

This raises another pressing issue. Publication of workplace health promotion program outcome claims are a matter of concern. Generally, there is a distinct lack of scientifically based evaluation of workplace programs in Australia. This is due to a number of factors. First, there is a relative immaturity in the area (in research and development, not time). Second, there is the fact that historically, nearly all university health promotion degree courses were initially structured to provide students with the skills to evaluate the more common traditional community health programs. Third, workplace health promotion is not a well established or recognized profession in Australia, and many organizations, while well intentioned, employ other professionals (health or business) to manage/coordinate their programs. This may be due to a lack of knowledge on the organization's part or a lack of suitably qualified professionals in the job marketplace at the time. Consequently, more sophisticated workplace relevant evaluation tools such as cost benefit ratio, ROI, and net present value are not a component of many currently existing programs.

Unfortunately, the lack of application of higher order, specific workplace health promotion program evaluation measures often leads to the reporting of questionable and unsubstantiated claims regarding the outcomes of programs. One immediate positive effect of such reporting of these successes could be to encourage other companies considering implementing a workplace program to do so. However, if similar results, often expected in the same short time period, are not forthcoming, the organization may cancel the program. This has been known to create an attitude by management of "been there, done that, and it didn't work" if a program is mooted in the future.

The dearth of reported, evidence-based results from Australian workplace health promotion programs was especially evident when the National Preventative Task Force primarily referenced overseas research (United Kingdom and United States) to support its position that workplaces could be settings for action in making Australia the healthiest country by 2020. That position was, "A large number of studies now point to the economic return on investment that can accrue through investments in employee health programs" (National Preventative Health Taskforce, 2009, p. 51).

The other major issue regarding workplace health promotion programs is that many are self-funded. Governments at all levels over the years have run hot and cold on the issue, and so consistent government funding has not been available. On the other hand, private enterprise understandably requires assurances regarding its ROI before committing to funding a program. Hence, in the absence of government support and funding, ROI was and still is a key factor in the sustainability of health promotion programs in the workplace in Australia.

Yet the ROI of many programs was not and still is not evaluated. For many organizations, an investment in a health promotion program is an add-on and readily sacrificed during difficult economic circumstances, especially if there is no evidence to show ROI. It is often seen as nice to have, but not an essential part of organizational business. In fact, sometimes a program is initiated just so someone can "tick a box." Thus, while many health and wellness program providers quote various dollar values regarding ROI, there is speculation about the accuracy of much of this information relevant to Australian workplaces.

There are some who still argue that prevention programs do not work, and that it is impossible to bring about behavior changes in a whole population. While some of this criticism comes from those with a vested interest (tobacco companies, etc.), others are concerned about controlling people's behavior through legislation and the often long delay in achieving results. Many practitioners in the field would agree that it will take up to 5 years for sufficient cultural change to occur in a workplace to allow the full benefits of a program to be evident and truly evaluated. For some organizations, this is far too long (most programs are initially funded from 6 weeks to 1 year) and funding is then placed elsewhere.

## Existing Research

Subsequent to the demise of the National Coordinating (formerly Steering) Committee for Health Promotion in the Workplace and its associated state bodies in the mid-1990s, there has been no government-funded workplace health promotion body in Australia. The Health & Productivity Institute of Australia (HAPIA), a peak nongovernment body for corporate wellness providers has been established only recently. The publication of a national workplace health promotion newsletter (commenced in 1989) also ceased with the demise of the National Coordinating Committee. Consequently, in the past, the small number of science-based workplace health promotion research projects that were carried out were primarily reported in more relevant and more prestigious overseas publications. Therefore, little workplace health promotion information was readily available in the public domain. Consequently, many Australian companies never heard of workplace health promotion, let alone became aware of the benefits a successful and sustainable program could provide.

For more than 2 decades, there have been reports published biennially on the status of health in Australia, the most recent being in 2008 (Australian Institute of Health and Welfare, 2008). However, advances in information searching technology have been influential in increasing the awareness of Australians about workplace health promotion around the globe. Reports including *Preventing Noncommunicable Diseases in the Workplace Through Diet and Physical Activity: WHO/World Economic Forum Report of a Joint Event* (WHO, 2008); *Working Towards Wellness: The Business Rationale* (World Economic Forum, 2008b); *Working Towards Wellness: Practical Steps for CEOs* (World Economic Forum, 2008a); and *Building the Case for Wellness* (PricewaterhouseCoopers, 2008) are now more readily accessible and are being studied by more individuals who are in positions to further the Australian workplace health promotion field. Whereas 30 years ago it was rare to do so, now many Australian companies access workplace health promotion material from overseas organizations such as WELCOA; Partnership for Prevention; The National Business Group on Health; The Institute for Health and Productivity Management; European Network for Workplace Health Promotion; The Health Communication Unit at the Centre for Health Promotion, University of Toronto; and University of Michigan Health Management Research Center, to name a few.

The downside of this is similar to the premise one size does not fit all. What works in other countries, especially the United States, does not necessarily work in Australia due to cultural, social, business, and financial dissimilarities. This highlights the necessity for Australia to further develop its own specific workplace health promotion research, culture, community, scientific base, organization(s), and publishing outlet(s).

There has been a recent increase in Australian-based workplace health promotion research reports. These include *The Case for Work/Life Balance: Closing the Gap Between Policy and Practice* (Hudson, 2005), *The Health of Australia's Workforce* (Medibank Private, 2005), *Sick at Work* (Medibank Private, 2007), *Economic Modelling of the Cost of Presenteeism in Australia* (Econtech, 2007), *The Cost of Workplace Stress in Australia* (Medibank Private, 2008), *Workplace 2012: What Does It Mean for Employers?* (Mercer, 2008), and *The Future@Work Health Report* (Wesley Corporate Health, 2006). This latter report outlines the key findings of Wesley Corporate Health's health data on 8,600 employees as well as Australian and overseas workplace health studies. It presents the health and business case for a healthy workplace environment and reveals workplace strategies to address the major health risks affecting today's workforce.

## Conclusion

There is still a great deal to be done if Australia is going to win the battle against the major health risks its society faces. Like most other western nations, it is losing the battle against the lifestyle-generated diseases. A problem with risk reduction programs is that many Australians have an attitude of, "It could never happen to me." They have become immune to information about the dangers of particular lifestyle choices and generally believe that it must only apply to someone else. A new approach is needed.

The National Preventative Health Taskforce (2009) road map for action provides some cautious hope. Among its recommendations are a number relating to workplaces (pp. 52–53):

- The National Partnership on Preventative Health has allocated 290 million AUD to fund states and territories to facilitate delivery of healthy living programs in workplaces.
- The Australian government will develop a national healthy workplace charter with peak employer groups.
- The proposed establishment of a national leadership program—a network of senior employer and employee champions of work health initiatives.
- A process to identify models of good practice in public sector organizations for replication—public sector organizations to set an example. Investigation into incentive processes for workplaces to implement programs. These proposed incentives would come from changes to tax laws and tax concessions (fringe benefit tax and GST free), and/or legislation for a program levy requiring employers to commit a percentage of payroll to implementing workplace health promotion programs.

A further suggestion was for the "development of a national trial of integrated workplace health programs based on the U.S. National Institute for Occupational Safety and Health (NIOSH) WorkLife Initiative involving partnerships between state and territory occupational health service, volunteer enterprises, and nominated research centres" (National Preventative Health Taskforce, 2009, p. 52). However, the question has to be asked—Why use an international model when enough evidence-based programs exist in Australia to develop the best aspects of all into a unique Australian program template? It is recognized that U.S. and Australian drivers of workplace health promotion are dissimilar.

A positive of the proposed national trial is that it should provide the vehicle for initiating much-needed Australian workplace health promotion scientific research. However, the recommended action is traditional and historical in its occupational health and safety approach. If indeed Australia is seeking a fresh approach, one such approach would be *not* to work through the occupational health and safety domain. Why not capitalize on the emerging awareness of the wellness paradigm?

Dr. Don Ardell, a prolific writer in the health and wellness field in the United States, consistently argues that the traditional medical approach to worksite health promotion programs has failed to deliver the change in lifestyles required for a healthy society. He claims that "worksite risk reduction or prevention programs are a good thing for employees from a medical standpoint, but they do not offer favorable opportunities for staff and others to learn life enrichment skills" (Ardell, 2009). The National Wellness Institute of Australia supports the view that a balanced focus on nine components of wellness (i.e., physical, social, emotional, work, spiritual values, intellectual, cultural, environmental, and financial) is important for workplace health promotion programs to be successful and sustainable (National Wellness Institute of Australia, n.d.).

Parallel to the call by the National Preventative Health Taskforce to all Australians to take action to make Australia the healthiest country (National Preventative Health Taskforce, 2009), workplace health professionals have the opportunity to heed this call to advance their field. Now is the most opportune time since the loss of momentum in the mid-1990s to do so. The newly formed Health and Productivity Institute of Australia, which aims to be the "peak body of Corporate Wellness Providers in Australia" (Health and Productivity Institute of Australia, n.d.), can have a pivotal role to play in this process. Increased interaction by stakeholders with overseas workplace health and wellness professionals through conferences, webinars, research groups, and discussion boards and forums via web-based modalities such as IDWellness, will further enhance the development of the emerging profession (IDWellness, n.d.).

# Summary

Despite being a healthy country by international standards, Australia still has major health issues. While in the past there have been notable successes through traditional health promotion programs, a different approach needs to be considered. Could that be wellness?

Except for a 10-year period in the 1980s, Australian workplaces have not been utilized as a major setting to implement health promotion. The historical drivers for health promotion in the workplace have come through health and safety legislation, largely confined to the prevention of physical accidents. Until recently, the issue of psychological injury has been largely ignored in the workplace programs.

The Australian healthcare system (private and public, e.g., Medicare) removes the necessity for employers to budget for employee medical costs. There is, however, a new awareness by employers of the true cost of worker's compensation claims from workplace issues such as stress, presenteeism, and poor work–life balance. This has triggered renewed interest in workplace health promotion programs.

Concurrently, there is a government push to address the increasing cost of worsening health issues. The National Preventative Health Taskforce has established a central focus on reducing obesity, smoking, and the harmful use of alcohol. Strategies recommended in the taskforce's road map to make Australia the healthiest country by 2020 include many relevant to workplace health promotion. The future of workplace health promotion in Australia depends on the profession promoting itself as a respected vehicle to help achieve the government's vision.

Fostering the quantity and science of Australian workplace health promotion research is one way to achieve this goal. The development of a powerful professional body representing the majority of individuals and organizations involved in Australian workplace health promotion is another.

## Review Questions

1. What are the central issues of the National Preventative Health Taskforce?
2. What are the components of the Australian healthcare system and how are they funded? Regulated? Managed?
3. How does the Australian culture of mateship affect population health and health promotion efforts?
4. What is the traditional focus of Australia's workplace health promotion programs?
5. Name five major historical publications that contributed to the current position of Australia's workplace health promotion status.
6. What is the significance of outcome indicators for Australia's workplace health promotion programs?
7. What view is supported by the National Wellness Institute of Australia in regard to workplace health promotion programs?
8. Identify three statistical facts that describe the health and wellness of Australia's population.
9. Describe the difference between Australia's universal public health system and its private health system.
10. Explain the components of an effective Australian workplace health promotion initiative.

## References

Ardell, D. (2009, May 15). *Ardell wellness report.* Retrieved September 20, 2009, from http://www.seekwellness.com

Australian Bureau of Statistics. (2007). *National survey of mental health and wellbeing: Summary of results* (No. 4326.0). Canberra, Australia: Author.

Australian College of Occupational Medicine. (1990). *Health promotion in industry.* Victoria, Australia: ACOM.

Australian Government. (n.d.). *The Australian Safety and Compensation Council.* Retrieved September 18, 2009, from http://www.workplace.gov.au/workplace/Individual/Employee/OHS/SafeWorkAustralia.htm

Australian Institute of Health and Welfare. (2008). *Australia's health 2008.* (Cat. no. AUS 99.) Canberra, Australia: AIWH.

Blue Care. (2008). Program helps keep life balanced. *Blue Print, 14*, 8–9.

Buck Consultants. (2009). *Global wellness.* Retrieved September 18, 2009, from https://www.bucksurveys.com/bucksurveys/dividNavSurveysdiv/Global Wellness/tabid/72/Default.aspx

Caring for the Blue Care carers. (2009, September 10). *Rockhampton Morning Bulletin,* p. 34.

Department of Health and Aging. (n.d.). *Australia's health system.* Retrieved September 20, 2009, from http://www.doctorconnect.gov.au/internet/otd/publishing.nsf/Content/work-Australias-health-system-2

Department of Sport, Recreation, and Tourism. (n.d.). *Health & fitness at work—It works! information folder*. Canberra, Australia: Author.

Econtech. (2007). *Economic modelling of the cost of presenteeism in Australia.* Sydney, Australia: Medibank Private.

Health and Productivity Institute of Australia. (n.d.). *About us.* Retrieved September 20, 2009, from http://www.hapia.com.au/about/html

Hudson. (2005). *The case for work/life balance: Closing the gap between policy and practice.* Canberra, Australia: Author.

IDWellness. (n.d.). *Home.* Retrieved September 2, 2009, from http://idwellness.org

Medibank Private. (2005). *The health of Australia's workforce*. Sydney, Australia: Medibank Private.

Medibank Private. (2007). *Sick at work.* Sydney, Australia: Medibank Private.

Medibank Private. (2008). *The cost of workplace stress in Australia.* Sydney, Australia: Medibank Private.

Mercer. (2008). *Workplace 2012: What does it mean for employers?* Adelaide, Australia: Mercer.

National Coordinating Committee for Health Promotion in the Workplace. (n.d.). *Health at work: Information kit.* Canberra, Australia: National Heart Foundation of Australia.

National Coordinating Committee for Health Promotion in the Workplace. (1993). Workplace health promotion in selected industries. *Health at Work Newsletter, 16,* 2–16.

National Preventative Health Taskforce. (2008). *Australia: The healthiest country by 2020—A discussion paper prepared by the National Preventive Health Taskforce.* Canberra, Australia: Australian Government Publishing Service.

National Preventative Health Taskforce. (2009). *Australia: The healthiest country by 2020—National preventative health strategy—The roadmap for action.* Canberra, Australia: Australian Government Publishing Service.

National Wellness Institute of Australia. (n.d.). *What is wellness?* Retrieved September 18, 2009, from http://www.wellnessaustralia.org

PricewaterhouseCoopers. (2008). *Building the case for wellness.* London, England: PricewaterhouseCoopers, LLC.

Private Health Insurance Administration Council (PHIAC). (2008). *Annual report 2007–08.* Canberra, Australia: Australian Government Publishing Service. Queensland University of Technology. (2009). *Wellness matters.* Retrieved September 19, 2009, from http://www.wellness.qut.edu.au

Wesley Corporate Health. (2006). *The Future@Work health report.* Brisbane, Australia: Author.

WorkHealth. (n.d. a). *Australian unity.* Retrieved September 19, 2009, from http://www.workhealth.vic.gov.au/wps/wcm/connect/WorkHealth/Home/How/Information+and+resources/Case+studies/Case+study/Australian+Unity

WorkHealth. (n.d. b). *What is WorkHealth?* Retrieved September 19, 2009, from http://www.workhealth.vic.gov.au/wps/wcm/connect/WorkHealth/Home/Why/What%20is%20WorkHealth/

World Economic Forum. (2008a). *Working towards wellness: The business rationale.* Cologny/Geneva, Switzerland: Author.

World Economic Forum. (2008b). *Working towards wellness: Practical steps for CEOs.* Cologny/Geneva, Switzerland: Author.

WHO (World Health Organization) and World Economic Forum. (2008). *Preventing noncommunicable diseases in the workplace through diet and physical activity: WHO/World Economic Forum Report of a Joint Event.* Geneva, Switzerland: Author.

Chapter 2

# Botswana

Emmanuel Olufemi Owolabi

After reading this chapter you should be able to:

- Identify core strategies that are the focus of Botswana's workplace health promotion efforts
- Describe Botswana's historical evolution of workplace health promotion
- Explain the different approaches employed by corporate health promotion efforts throughout Botswana
- Review the central disease states and health issues driving Botswana's health promotion needs
- Name the components of, and the associated funding sources for, Botswana's healthcare system
- Discuss the impact of culture on Botswana's health status and health promotion efforts

Table 2-1 **Select Key Demographic and Economic Indicators**

| | |
|---|---|
| Nationality | Noun: Motswana (singular), Batswana (plural)<br>Adjective: Motswana (singular), Batswana (plural) |
| Ethnic groups | Tswana (or Setswana) 79%, Kalanga 11%, Basarwa 3%, other, including Kgalagadi and white 7% |
| Religion | Christian 71.6%, Badimo 6%, other 1.4%, unspecified 0.4%, none 20.6% (2001 census) |
| Language | Setswana 78.2%, Kalanga 7.9%, Sekgalagadi 2.8%, English 2.1% (official), other 8.6%, unspecified 0.4% (2001 census) |
| Literacy | Definition: age 15 and over can read and write<br>Total population: 81.2%<br>Male: 80.4%<br>Female: 81.8% (2003 est.) |
| Education expenditure | 8.7% of GDP (2007)<br>Country comparison to the world: 10 |

*continued*

| Table 2-1 Select Key Demographic and Economic Indicators, *continued* | |
|---|---|
| Government type | Parliamentary republic |
| Environment | Overgrazing; desertification; limited fresh water resources |
| Country mass | Total: 581,730 sq km<br>Country comparison to the world: 47<br>Land: 566,730 sq km<br>Water: 15,000 sq km |
| Population | 1,990,876<br>Country comparison to the world: 147 |
| Age structure | 0–14 years: 34.8% (male 352,399/female 340,058)<br>15–64 years: 61.4% (male 613,714/female 608,003)<br>65 years and over: 3.9% (male 31,155/female 45,547) (2010 est.) |
| Median age | Total: 22 years<br>Male: 21.8 years<br>Female: 22.1 years (2010 est.) |
| Population growth rate | 1.937% (2010 est.)<br>Country comparison to the world: 83 |
| Birth rate | 22.89 births/1,000 population (2010 est.)<br>Country comparison to the world: 83 |
| Death rate | 8.52 deaths/1,000 population (July 2010 est.)<br>Country comparison to the world: 92 |
| Net migration rate | 5 migrant(s)/1,000 population<br>Country comparison to the world: 21<br>*Note:* there is an increasing flow of Zimbabweans into South Africa and Botswana in search of better economic opportunities (2010 est.) |
| Urbanization | Urban population: 60% of total population (2008)<br>rate of urbanization: 2.5% annual rate of change (2005–2010 est.) |
| Gender ratio | At birth: 1.03 male(s)/female<br>Under 15 years: 1.04 male(s)/female<br>15–64 years: 1.01 male(s)/female<br>65 years and over: 0.68 male(s)/female<br>Total population: 1 male(s)/female (2010 est.) |
| Infant mortality rate | Total: 12.59 deaths/1,000 live births<br>Country comparison to the world: 141<br>Male: 13.43 deaths/1,000 live births<br>Female: 11.73 deaths/1,000 live births (2010 est.) |

*continued*

**Table 2-1 Select Key Demographic and Economic Indicators,** *continued*

| | |
|---|---|
| Life expectancy | Total population: 61.85 years<br>Country comparison to the world: 178<br>Male: 61.72 years<br>Female: 61.99 years (2010 est.) |
| Total fertility rate | 2.54 children born/woman (2010 est.)<br>Country comparison to the world: 90 |
| GDP—purchasing power | $24.14 billion (2009 est.) |
| Parity | Country comparison to the world: 111 |
| GDP—per capita | $12,800 (2009 est.)<br>Country comparison to the world: 86 |
| GDP—composition by sector | Agriculture: 2.3%<br>Industry: 45.8% (including 36% mining)<br>Services: 51.9% (2008 est.) |
| Agriculture—products | Livestock, sorghum, maize, millet, beans, sunflowers, groundnuts |
| Industries | Diamonds, copper, nickel, salt, soda ash, potash, livestock processing, textiles |
| Labor force participation | 685,300 formal sector employees (2007)<br>Country comparison to the world: 151 |
| Unemployment rate | 7.5% (2007 est.)<br>Country comparison to the world: 69 |
| Industrial production growth rate | -19.9% (2009 est.)<br>Country comparison to the world: 161 |
| Distribution of family income (GINI index) | 63 (1993)<br>Country comparison to the world: 4 |
| Investment (gross fixed) | 26.7% of GDP (2009 est.)<br>Country comparison to the world: 39 |
| Public debt | 17.9% of GDP (2009 est.)<br>Country comparison to the world: 107 |
| Market value of publicly traded shares | $4.283 billion (December 31, 2009)<br>Country comparison to the world: 87 |
| Current account balance | $-758 million (2009 est.)<br>Country comparison to the world: 124 |
| Debt (external) | $1.651 billion (December 31, 2009 est.)<br>Country comparison to the world: 134 |
| Debt as a % of GDP | ——— |

*continued*

Table 2-1 **Select Key Demographic and Economic Indicators,** *continued*

| | |
|---|---|
| Exports | $3.382 billion (2009 est.)<br>Country comparison to the world: 120 |
| Exports—commodities | Diamonds, copper, nickel, soda ash, meat, textiles |
| Export—partners | NA |
| Imports | $4.24 billion (2009 est.)<br>Country comparison to the world: 126 |
| Import—commodities | Foodstuffs, machinery, electrical goods, transport equipment, textiles, fuel and petroleum products, wood and paper products, metal and metal products |
| Import—partners | NA |
| Stock of direct foreign investment at | |
| Home | NA |
| Abroad | NA |

Source: CIA. (2010). *The world factbook*. Retrieved August 31, 2010, from www.cia.gov

# Introduction

Botswana, a former British protectorate, became independent in 1966 and has since been a bastion and role model of democracy in Africa. Since independence, there has been uninterrupted civilian government, which prides itself on the rule of law and respect for human dignity. The main occupations are mining and agrarian farming. However, tourism is fast becoming a major income earner, with Botswana boasting of thousands of kilometers of nature reserves and wildlife areas.

While Botswana arguably has one of the highest rates of HIV and AIDS in the world (CIA, 2009), it has embarked on one of Africa's, if not the world's, most progressive, comprehensive, and ambitious programs in dealing with the pandemic. The healthcare system and the democratic system of governance have been described as an African success story and an enviable model by international organizations and acknowledged world leaders. The government of Botswana has made significant progress in its fight against HIV/AIDS. For example, Botswana was the first country in Africa to provide universal access to antiretroviral treatment and to implement routine HIV counseling and testing in all its health services. Not only are people living with HIV/AIDS being targeted and encouraged to use these services, but pregnant mothers are routinely tested and those infected are taken through prevention of mother-to-child transmission therapy. For the last 15 years, HIV/AIDS has been the major issue, both politically and healthwise, in Botswana, and this is reflected in its central place in Botswana health care and workplace health promotion (WHP) issues.

Botswana is a landlocked country sharing international borders with Namibia, South Africa, and Zimbabwe. The climate is semiarid, and over 85% of the land lies within the Kalahari Desert. The population was 1.327 million in 1991 and 1.681 million in 2001, with females accounting for 52% of the population. The projected population for 2010 was 1.8 million (Botswana Central Statistics Office, 2009a).

## Prevailing Health Issues and Risk Behaviors

Botswana is currently experiencing one of the most severe HIV/AIDS epidemics in the world. The country's adult HIV prevalence of 24.1% (UNAIDS, 2006) is arguably one of the highest in the world. According to the Second Generation Sentinel Surveillance 2007 results, HIV prevalence among pregnant women 15–49 was 33.4% (Botswana NACA, 2008). However, the 2008 Botswana AIDS impact survey III (BAIS) data indicated a national prevalence rate of 17.6% with females recording substantially higher rates than males as in the previous years. Also, the prevalence rates are higher among urban dwellers than among village dwellers. The incidence rate of new HIV and AIDS infections for the country is 2.9% (Botswana Central Statistics Office, 2009b). According to this recently released HIV and AIDS update, the HIV prevalence by age group ranged from 2.2% in the 1.5–4.0 years group to 40.6% in the 40–44 years age group. It was also observed that the prevalence increased with age and peaked between the 30 and 45 years (see Table 2-2).

Table 2-2 **Comparing BAIS* II of 2004 and BAIS III of 2008 Results**

| | HIV prevalence (percent of total population by age) | |
|---|---|---|
| **Age (yrs)** | **2004** | **2008** |
| 1.5–4.0 | 6.3 | 2.2 |
| 5.0–9.0 | 6.0 | 4.7 |
| 10.0–14.0 | 3.9 | 3.5 |
| 15.0–19.0 | 6.5 | 3.7 |
| 20.0–24.0 | 19.0 | 12.3 |
| 25.0–29.0 | 33.0 | 25.9 |
| 30.0–34.0 | 40.2 | 39.7 |
| 35.0–39.0 | 35.9 | 40.5 |

*continued*

Table 2-2 **Comparing BAIS* II of 2004 and BAIS III of 2008 Results,** *continued*

| | | |
|---|---|---|
| 40.0–44.0 | 30.3 | 40.6 |
| 45.0–49.0 | 29.4 | 29.8 |
| 50.0–54.0 | 20.9 | 24.8 |
| 55.0–59.0 | 14.0 | 22.8 |
| 60.0–64.0 | 12.0 | 15.4 |
| 65.0+ | 6.8 | 10.4 |
| Total | 17.1 | 17.6 |

* BAIS: Botswana AIDS Impact Survey, a 3-year surveillance and evaluation (Botswana Central Statistics Office, 2009b).

Molomo (2008) aptly presented AIDS as a development issue because it reverses all the gains and projections of national development. The impact of HIV and AIDS on individual and national development in Botswana has been immense. One of the major effects of HIV and AIDS is on the population size. The projected population for 2021 is expected to be nearly 18% lower than it would be in the absence of the pandemic, and the number of deaths is expected to double (Government of Botswana Country Report, 2007). Accompanying the increased number of deaths would be an estimated fourfold increase in the number of orphans.

The average life expectancy is declining instead of rising as projected. Although the average life expectancy of Batswana was expected to reach 67 years in 2000–2005, it was reprojected to fall to 41 years in this period (SADC, 1998). Indeed, average life expectancy fell from 66.8 years in 1996 to 47.4 years in 1999 (UNDP, 1999). Yet, in the last 15 years, Botswana has been one of the top countries in Africa with the highest and fastest growing economy and human development index (UNDP, 1999). According to Botswana NACA (2008), HIV and AIDS contributed 49% of the fall in national growth, with reduced productivity growth contributing 31% and reduced supply of labor, 20%.

Unfortunately, the people of Botswana do not seem to be reciprocating government efforts in combating the HIV and AIDS pandemic. Although government efforts and the provision of antiretroviral treatment have reduced the number of AIDS deaths by half (Botswana NACA, 2008), the current adult prevalence of 25.7% and the number of new infections still occurring every year pose serious challenges for the future. It would appear that young citizens, in particular, are finding it difficult to adapt their lifestyle, especially related to alcohol use and sexual relationships. However, the current estimate is a far cry from the prevalence of 36% in 2000. According to the *Daily News*, the official government daily newspaper, this put Botswana on top of the world's HIV/AIDS chart ("Residents welcome home based care programme,"

2000). The *Mmegi*, a Botswana daily newspaper, in its editorial opinion on World AIDS Day in 2009, lamented that challenges lie ahead in the country's seemingly endless battle against the pandemic ("Our anti-HIV/AIDS," 2009). It listed continuing alcohol abuse and high-risk sexual behavior as major challenges that need to be tackled from the bottom.

## The Motswana, Physical Inactivity, and Productivity

The average Motswana is largely sedentary as an adult; most view physical activities as a child's preoccupation. Many observations and reports have been made on the low work output and productivity of Batswana workers (Lloyd 1999; Ministry of Health, 1996; Owolabi & Shaibu, 1999). The popular saying that "in Botswana, there is no hurry," aptly attests to this fact. It may indeed be a reflection or manifestation of the low physical fitness level of the average Motswana. Studies conducted on Batswana youths reported lower levels of physical fitness when compared with their counterparts in other countries (Corlett, 1984a, 1984b; Owolabi, unpublished data). This tendency not to want to exert oneself at work or to tire easily, although frequently attributed to a negative mindset toward work and poor motivation from within and without, may be caused by low physical fitness level more than other factors. In a recent study widely reported in national newspapers (Kesaobaka, 2009), it was found that Batswana citizens recorded worry and high levels of overweight and obesity. A study of public department employees who are at risk of metabolic syndrome also showed concerning results (see Table 2-3).

**Table 2-3 Risk of Metabolic Syndrome Among Sampled Government Employees in Botswana**

| Variable | Benchmark | Male | Female | Total |
|---|---|---|---|---|
| SBP (systolic blood pressure)(mmHg) | > 140 | 25.1 (21.7)* | 9.5 (18.4) | 17.3 (20.05) |
| DBP (diastolic blood pressure) (mmHg) | > 90 | 25.0 (32.9) | 14.3 (37.1) | 19.7 (35.0) |
| Underweight | BMI = 18.00 | 0 (6.3) | 0 (3.5) | 0.0 (4.9) |
| Overweight | BMI = 25–29.4 | 31.2 (40.0) | 33.4 (32.3) | 32.3 (36.2) |
| Obese | BMI > 30 | 16.6 (9.1) | 33.3 (34.9) | 24.9 (22.0) |
| Waist circumference | M = 1.00 m; F = 0.87 m | 20.1 (14.9) | 38.1 (59.5) | 29.2 (37.3) |
| % Body fat | M = 20; F = 25 | 12.0 (14.7) | 15.2 (18.8) | 13.6 (16.8) |

* % of government employees (% of volunteer public samples 6 months earlier.

In a 3-year study by Owolabi and Keetile (2007), it was concluded that there was a high prevalence of overweight, obesity, and blood pressure among urban Batswana men and women. The females tend to be more obese, while the men tend to have higher systolic blood pressure. Waist circumference is highly related to BMI and blood pressure in both males and females ($p < 0.001$). Using the criteria of at least three cardiovascular disease risks, Owolabi and Keetile concluded that there is a low prevalence of metabolic syndrome.

In addition to lack of regular physical exercise and sports, the low physical fitness of the average Motswana might have been compounded by the popularity of excessive alcohol consumption as a recreational activity. In two studies (Kgosiemang, 2004; Ramatlala, 2002) carried out among university students, over 80% of sampled students across all age groups and gender viewed drinking alcohol and sexual activity as recreational. There is an urgent need for advocacy, legislation, encouragement, and enlightenment campaigns to promote physical activity for all.

## Healthcare System

The Batswana government is the main provider of health services and facilities through the Ministry of Health, with missionaries, the mining industry, and private/commercial health institutions complementing government health care. Health care is delivered through a decentralized system. The healthcare system in Botswana is based on three tiers: primary, secondary, and tertiary. The primary and secondary levels are located across all villages, towns, and rural communities; whereas the tertiary level is comprised of referral centers located in the cities of Gaborone (the national capital) and Francistown. Botswana has an extensive network of health facilities comprising hospitals, clinics, health posts (local, village-based health centers), and mobile health stops, all spread around 24 health districts (Botswana Central Statistics Office, 2007). Nationally, 84% of the population is within a 5 kilometer radius from the nearest health facility, while another 11% is within a 5–11 kilometer radius. In the urban centers, however, 96% of the residents are within a 5 kilometer radius from the nearest health facility.

Botswana's government provides necessary services for communities. Both preventive and curative care is provided for every form of health problem—communicable and noncommunicable, prevalent and the rare—and for the risk factors of many diseases. In 2006, 7.2% of GDP was spent on health services (World Health Organization, 2006).

Considering that the majority of the adult population is employed, the government of Botswana is motivating public and private organizations to set up health and wellness units within their structures and to lead by example. The health and wellness units are staffed by qualified health professionals. Furthermore, most of these organizations organize regular workshops and symposia for the various cadres of employees, focusing particularly on how to reduce the rate of new HIV infections and motivating safe and healthy behavior. Health professional associations have also been making a special contribution in this regard. Religious organizations and places of worship, such as churches and mosques, are also involved in the efforts of health promotion, particularly on matters relating to HIV and AIDS.

The government backs up its health efforts with legislation and policies, devoting a lot of its efforts and expenses on health promotion. This emphasis on health promotion percolates to every government department, as well as parastatals and private organizations. Most employers or corporate bodies tend to have a health and wellness, occupational health, or staff welfare department or unit, in addition to fully staffed and equipped medical facilities for first aid and emergencies. Furthermore, government and other employers contribute about 50% to the healthcare costs of individual employees and their families through a health insurance scheme. For some employing organizations, the contributions may be as high as 80%.

In the last 15 years, health promotion efforts have been put into education, community development, policy, and legislation. These efforts aim to prevent and control communicable and noncommunicable diseases. For example, to supplement internationally sourced funds in battling the HIV and AIDS pandemic, the Botswana government increased national funds from 165.0 million U.S. dollars in 2005 to 203.8 million in 2007 (UNAIDS, 2008).

## Influence of Culture and Mentality

Democracy, respect for individual differences and limitations, and freedom of individuals are visible traits among the people of Botswana. It can even be argued that these commendable traits are sometimes taken to extremes, such as when parents frequently find it hard to scold or punish their erring children, particularly when they are over 12 years old. This lack of discipline coupled with misplaced respect can be argued to be the root cause of some juvenile, youth, and adult delinquencies in Botswana (Nolan, 2009; Orufheng, 2009). These delinquencies include excessive alcohol misuse and abuse and social problems.

Although there is government legislation controlling who can buy alcohol and where it can be drunk, it is rare that efforts are made to enforce the regulation. Even in the university setting, every attempt by the university administration to explore the restriction of alcohol purchasing or drinking hours was met with vehement opposition, not only from the students but also from the staff. Furthermore, President Ian Khama attempted to pass legislation through an act of Parliament restricting the hours of drinking alcohol and the operations of alcohol sale centers. There was widespread opposition from every sector of the society including from the Parliament itself. Yet, alcohol abuse has been implicated in several studies for the majority of delinquent behaviors among the people of Botswana ("Our anti-HIV/AIDS," 2009; Owolabi & Kalui, 1997; Owolabi & Mogotsi, 1999).

There still is a paucity of knowledge among the populace, particularly among students, about the factors related to safe and acceptable consumption of alcohol. The cultural factors that seem to be hampering the battle against the HIV/AIDS scourge in particular include:

- Low rates of marriage and unstable, multiple, concurrent sexual partners.
- Teenage pregnancy and motherhood.
- Single parenthood, consensual cohabitation, and lack of interest in marriage.

Khunwane (2009) reported that National Coordinator Molomo of the Botswana National AIDS Coordinating Agency lamented the high prevalence of HIV and AIDS among the citizens of Botswana despite the huge financial and human resources investments in the last 10 years, attributing the situation to the penchant for multiple concurrent partnerships. Indeed, both males and females across age groups pride themselves in the extensiveness of their sexual networks. Even married men and women seem to pride themselves on these health-hindering attitudes. Unfortunately, there is no deliberate social structure in place to formally and informally discourage these dangerous, disruptive, and destructive values. There are religious organizations such as churches that preach and counsel their members on the risks of sexual recklessness, the need to be faithful in marriage, and the avoidance of premarital sex. However, not all churches believe in these strict injunctions about sexual relationships before and during marriage.

A few years back, attention was shifted from the predominant slogan of "condomize" to an emphasis on abstinence. However, the Botswana NACA's 2008 progress report cited low acceptability of abstinence as a major obstacle to achieving prevention targets. The arguments against abstinence range from the unfairness of depriving sexually active adults to the difficulty in preventing youth from freely choosing their sexual lifestyle.

## Drivers of Workplace Health Promotion

Before the HIV/AIDS crisis induced governmental efforts and encouraged private companies to protect their workers' health, many companies operating in Botswana, particularly those with parent companies in South Africa, already had informal work health promotion programs in place.

Indeed, almost every private and government corporation has a functioning health and wellness unit. These units—which come under other various names, such as welfare, occupational health, etc.—organize health and wellness seminars, workshops, and HIV/AIDS prevention discussions and activities at least once a year. They offer many services for their staff, including periodic counseling and health screening (e.g, testing for HIV), and free condoms. They all provide emergency medical care for their staff and cover part of their other medical expenses. Unfortunately, the focus of these health and wellness units seems to be mainly on HIV/AIDS prevention and care of the infected. One would, however, love to see these units expanded to take care of the myriad emerging health and wellness issues, such as metabolic syndrome, obesity, high blood pressure, diabetes, and cardiovascular health problems. Although a few of the workplace wellness units have incorporated exercise and physical activity into the workers' break and lunch periods, a large majority have limited their interventions and activities to counseling and care of the workers when they fall sick during work hours. Going by empirical evidence from published studies (Fine, Ward, Burr, Tudor-Smith, & Kingdom, 2004; Linnan et al., 2008), it could be submitted that the most common obstacle to health promotion in the workplace is the employers' perception of the lack of benefits from health promotion.

In summary, through its open and collaborative efforts to combat the most current health problems, the government of Botswana is the main driving force behind workplace health promotion in Botswana. Public and private employers are encouraged to ensure a healthy working environment for their employees. Government departments and ministries lead the way by catering to their workers' health.

## Programs

Although all government departments and private employers with more than 20 employees have a health and wellness unit, workplace health promotion programs are not formal or concrete. These units are staffed by special officers, but it is doubtful if such employees are adequately trained and qualified for implementing the workplace health promotion program. The driving force seems to be the urgency to deal with the rampaging HIV/AIDS scourge physically and economically pauperizing the population. Thus, a major focus is to assist the people living with HIV/AIDS to live a comfortable and integrated social life. This is done through periodic counseling and psychological support. Employees are also encouraged to seek free HIV/AIDS screening to determine their HIV/AIDS status whenever there is any inexplicable health problem or cause for concern. The health and wellness units in the various departments, both governmental and private, also supply free condoms. Their health/medical units give antiretroviral therapy or refer workers to antiretroviral therapy designated sites for free, regular dosage of drugs. Yet, the worksite has the potential to become a key channel for the delivery of interventions to reduce chronic and lifestyle-related diseases, particularly among the adult population. The worksite environment further encourages sustained peer support.

### University of Botswana

During the 2008/09 session, the total student population at the University of Botswana was 15,000, while the staff population was 2,700. The staff population comprises 31.3% academic, 51.7% support staff, and 17% industrial workers. The university houses a health and wellness coordination center headed by a qualified officer. The University Health and Wellness Office caters to both staff and students as per its mission, but most of the university's health and wellness centers cater only to students. The university has various health and wellness delivery units (i.e., providing centers). These include:

- University Health Services, staffed by trained and qualified doctors, pharmacists, and nurses. Their core functions are the provision of general health care, including reproductive, counseling, health education, and consultation. They also produce a few leaflets and pamphlets to educate students on contemporary health issues. Only in exceptional circumstances does University Health Services provide health care to staff. They keep data on students' health issues (from HIV/AIDS to pregnancy and other specific, common health issues); these data are used to counsel students and monitor emerging and acute health issues. Annual evaluation of performance is done in terms of students' attendance and the relative prevalence of a particular health problem.

- University Counseling Services. This service is provided by the Department of Career and Counseling. Full-time, professional counselors assist students and staff with their psychological problems. The center also trains students on peer counseling. The center's approaches include face-to-face meetings, seminars, workshops, the production and distribution of leaflets and pamphlets on contemporary issues, and online communications.
- Health education. Health education is provided by the health and wellness center through periodic workshops, seminars, the production of educational pamphlets, and peer education and other awareness activities. Issues currently covered include healthy nutrition habits, responsible alcohol use, balancing work and family life, responsible sexual activities and the advantages of abstinence, health relationships, and nurturing and caring for one's social, emotional, and spiritual health. The main focus is behavioral change among students. The evaluation of achievement on these services is left to reports by staff members and subjective measures of the effects of health educational efforts on students.
- Sports and recreation. These services are provided by the Department of Culture, Sports and Recreation, which has a full complement of qualified and full-time professionals. The university has extensive sports facilities including an Olympic-size swimming pool, 400-meter running track, indoor sports hall, and various other standard facilities for indoor and outdoor ball and team games. The department also sends out regular educational leaflets on the need for physical activities and recreation among students. In addition, there are occasional seminars and workshops to encourage student participation in sports and recreation. Less than 30% of the students make significant use of these facilities, and this number comprises mainly the university athletes. In theory, the facilities are available for both staff and students, but staff members rarely use these facilities, except for the occasional use of the swimming pool and tennis courts.

The HIV/AIDS Center was set up to battle the scourge of HIV/AIDS on Botswana citizens. As a workplace health promotion unit, its major focus is to address the prevalence of HIV/AIDS among students and reduce the emergence of new cases. Its mission also includes educating noninfected students about HIV/AIDS and accepting, not stigmatizing, affected students. Very recently, an HIV/AIDS research center was established as part of the university's health and wellness efforts.

The staff are largely left to fend for their own health needs. There is, therefore, no formal workplace health promotion (WHP) program or policy in place for the over 2,700 staff members. The university staff sports association is a voluntary organization of staff members who pay annual dues to sustain the association. This association meets only periodically to participate in competitions with staff of higher institutions from Botswana and abroad. Staff members also have some freedom to use university facilities outside of student use hours.

As a whole, the University's Center for Health and Wellness Coordination is striving to meet its objectives by coordinating the efforts of the various centers addressing health promotion, particularly among students. The center is trying to break down the barrier between positive attitude and safe practice. It is confident that over 90% of continuing students have all the knowledge they need for responsible and healthy living. The absence of specific, objective instruments to annually evaluate performance and achievements in the various health promotion services in the university is a major obstacle for the center.

## The Botswana Police Force

The Botswana Police Force (BPF) has been very alert in identifying and appropriately responding to emerging staff health issues. Although the core duty of the BPF is crime prevention and reduction, the officers are aware that only police officers who are sound and sane in all aspects of health can carry out these duties effectively and efficiently. They are also aware that police officers and their families are exposed to various physical, social, emotional, and mental hazards in the performance of their lawful duties. Hence, the commitment of the BPF is to continually identify the workplace threats to the health of officers and their families and make efforts to prevent, neutralize, and/or control them. The BPF uses the integrated wellness approach through its Occupational Health, Safety, Chaplaincy, and Social Welfare (OHSCSW) unit.

The various sections within the OHSCSW unit are formally involved with WHP issues. Each section is headed by a health and wellness coordinator, who is a senior police officer. Every unit's health and wellness coordinator reports directly to the health and wellness coordinator at the Botswana Police Service headquarters in the capital city.

There are several divisions of the BPF spread across the country. The divisions are subdivided into smaller command groups called districts. The districts are further divided into stations or units. This hierarchy ensures effectiveness of police functions across the country. OHSCSW officers located in the headquarters and divisions take control of WHP issues in their divisions. In the districts, specially trained focal persons are appointed to monitor and implement WHP issues. At the station level, there are WHP assistants rather than OHSCSW officers. These assistants are inadequately trained but able to report on WHP issues to the focal persons and district officers, and where the issue is urgent enough, directly to the divisional officers or the coordinator at headquarters. The heads of the various sections also meet regularly to discuss health surveillance reports on the police force. The police health surveillance is crucial in monitoring the workplace health environment and quickly addressing any emerging health issue in the BPF. The focal persons in the districts send quarterly reports on their activities and observations to the divisional OHSCSW officers.

Each section of the WHP unit has a core of appropriate and trained staff at the OHSCSW and district levels including social workers, counselors, and psychologists. However, there is shortage of staff in the academic-intensive areas such as the forensic laboratory. Efforts are being made to identify and recommend appropriate staff for training among the police cadre.

Prior to 2000, the police devoted most of their WHP to the HIV/AIDS pandemic, which had a devastating impact on the force. Indeed, the first Botswana Police Service HIV/AIDS policy was published in March 2000 in response to a 1993 presidential directive (Botswana Police Service, 2000). The police service's HIV/AIDS mission statement states that "the Botswana Police Service will ensure that all its employees and their families are well informed and encouraged to take practical steps to avoid new infections and to provide adequate care and support services to the infected and affected" (Botswana Police Service, 2000). Although HIV/AIDS was the main focus, officers and their families raised other workplace health issues as well. Thus there was a need to expand the mission and policy from a focus on HIV/AIDS to a broader and more inclusive focus. In the year 2000, there was an unusually high prevalence of suicide cases among the staff of the BPF, and this necessitated the formation of a national committee to investigate various suicide responses, including a needs assessment survey and appropriate interventions. The committee's recommendations gave birth to the establishment of a chaplaincy and social welfare section within the OHSCSW unit in 2006. The formation of the chaplaincy and social welfare section was an appropriate response because many of the suicide cases had spiritual origins and implications. Although the police force has its cadre of trained pastors and reverends, they occasionally invite popular religious leaders to preach and spiritually counsel their staff in groups and individually, depending on the need.

In 2005, in response to identified needs, an occupational health and safety policy was launched. The major focuses of the policy included employee development on health and safety matters; provision of personal protective equipment; identification and assessment of potential hazards; installation of rapid incident response strategies; documentation and proper record keeping of occupational health and safety-related information; provision of first aid; management of communicable diseases, etc. The policy articulates the allocation of roles and responsibilities of different levels for workers' health and safety matters, from the commissioner of police to the last employee.

The occupational health and safety policy is reviewed every 2 years in order to assure its continuing relevance and suitability. Generally, the operational procedures to achieve the objectives of the department include health promotion awareness; health screening and counseling, both on an individual and group basis; occasional seminars and workshops; provision of health-promoting materials such as condoms and occupational safety materials; and an annual weeklong health and wellness program during which professionals are invited to lead the different aspects.

Police duties are physically demanding, with lots of emergencies in addition to daily duties; hence police officers are expected to be in top physical fitness condition at all times. There are several sports clubs in the BPS as with many other public and private employers. These clubs are open to those who are interested and have the requisite skills to perform at the elite level demanded by each sport. However, there is no policy on workplace health promotion of physical activities and continuing physical fitness for police personnel. In the central Police College, regular physical activities and sports are part of the curriculum and are mandatory for all officers in training. There is no corresponding policy to ensure the continued participation in physical activities and sports after graduating from the Police College. The absence of a formal policy on regular participation in physical activity and physical fitness implies that the decision for personnel to participate is left to the heads of each police station/unit and is not mandatory. A formal WHP policy currently being formulated by the OHSCSW and the BPF will be presented as recommendations to the Botswana Police Service.

As with many WHP efforts in developing countries, there is no formal instrument or objective measurement criteria to evaluate the effectiveness and achievement of the WHP unit of the BPS at the end of each year. However, the unit relies on various reports from the divisions and districts to evaluate its successes and challenges and plan for the upcoming year. In most cases, these data are highly subjective and cannot be directly used to gauge the success of the WHP unit with any specificity.

### Debswana Diamond Company

Some private companies, in addition to having robust and effective WHP programs targeted at preventing, controlling, and mitigating the impact of HIV/AIDS on the workforce, provide free antiretroviral therapy to their employees. One of these companies is the Debswana Diamond Company. The Debswana Workplace AIDS and Awareness Program was introduced in 1991 (Botswana NACA, 2008). This company was the first mining company in Southern Africa to provide antiretroviral therapy to its employees. The Debswana Diamond Company also has clearly defined workplace policies, an AIDS management system, and HIV/AIDS awareness and education and training programs, among other programs.

## Outcomes and Indicators

Measures or specified outcomes to evaluate health promotion efforts and their effectiveness on workers' physical and mental health, regular attendance at work, and productivity are lacking. This may not be unexpected in the Botswana worksite environment as there is no trained leadership in occupational and worksite health and there are no occupational standards for workplace health promotion.

## Existing Research

The severity of HIV/AIDS has been felt in the workplace as high rates of absenteeism, hospitalization, presenteeism, and even death. Hence, most of the efforts and studies on health promotion have been focused on HIV/AIDS.

For example, the Botswana government undertakes periodic HIV/AIDS surveillance in order to establish trends in HIV prevalence and new cases and also to gather information for developing policy and programs to stem the HIV and AIDS pandemic. It also conducts annual HIV/AIDs surveillance among pregnant women aged 15–49 years. The data includes both prevalence rate and behavioral patterns, in order to understand the underlying and immediate causes of the epidemic. The government also implemented periodic nationally representative behavioral surveys known as Botswana AIDS impact surveys (BAIS); the first was in 2001, the second in 2004, and the latest in 2008. The BAIS was initiated to regularly update information on prevalence, incidence, and behavioral patterns towards HIV/AIDS among the population (Montlane, 2009). This chapter's section, "Prevailing Health Issues and Risk Behaviors," presents details on the BAIS and other HIV/AIDS surveillance studies. The indifference of the average Botswana citizen to regular physical activity and sports is demonstrated by the results of the studies also referred to in this earlier section.

## Workplace Health Promotion—A Survey Report

Owolabi conducted a study in 2005 (unpublished data) aimed at evaluating the relationship between employees' and employers' perceptions of the benefits of workers' participation in regular physical exercises and the provision of corporate fitness programs. Fifty companies employing from 20 to over 100 employees, across different types of industries, were used in the study. One hundred and sixty employees were sampled across all strata of management.

The major findings were that despite the fact that 95% of the subjects perceived a corporate fitness program to be very important in improving the health and productivity of employees, only 10% participated in regular physical exercises of any form. Although 60% of the sampled companies had private fitness and sports facilities, none had a corporate health promotion policy or program. Furthermore, although all the companies had welfare managers, none of them had occupational health or corporate fitness personnel. It was found that the indifference of most companies to employees' fitness programs was due to the lack of commitment of the chief executive officers to workplace health promotion. The companies' workplace health programs were mainly in the form of facilities and recreation rooms, which workers patronized in the evening and Saturday after work hours. None of the 50 companies sampled had health and wellness activities within work hours. The motivation for WHP depended on the managing director of the company and his/her interest in health and wellness and perception of its value to workers.

# Conclusion

Public health promotion is being largely propelled by the zeal and efforts of the government of Botswana. However, a large chunk of these efforts is directed to preventing and mitigating the impact of HIV and AIDS on the people of Botswana and on individual and national development. Despite the billions of dollars and international collaborations toward fighting and preventing new HIV/AIDS infections over the last 15 years, the current prevalence and incidence rates are not commensurate or encouraging. It is hoped that the people of Botswana will soon begin to reciprocate government efforts in the seemingly endless battle against HIV/AIDS.

Workplace health promotion, though appreciated and perceived as very important in maintaining and improving the health, wellness, and productivity of workers, is not formally in place. Government also seems to be the main driver of WHP. The government's efforts in stimulating and encouraging WHP via the multifaceted approach to eradicating the HIV/AIDS scourge from Botswana are highly commendable. However, in most companies, there are no formal health policies, no formal and measurable WHP programs, and no means to measure the outcomes and impact periodically. Most of the companies have designated welfare or health and wellness managers, but none have qualified occupational health or corporate health and wellness personnel.

The indifference of most companies to WHP is due to the lack of commitment of the chief executive officers. Most efforts are reactive rather than proactive. It would be beneficial if employers in both public and private companies in Botswana initiated bold WHP programs based on urgent contemporary issues rather than waiting for high incidence in the workplace, and then chasing curative solutions. The University of Botswana and other higher institutions should implement policies that promote participation in sports.

## Summary

Botswana is located in southern Africa, and it became independent from British protectorate in 1966. Botswana is arguably the role model of democracy in Africa. It has one of the highest rates of HIV/AIDS prevalence in the world, but the government has shown great determination in dealing with the scourge.

Botswana affords universal access to antiretroviral treatment and counseling. It also offers its citizens free HIV status testing and free condoms in all public places. Infected pregnant women are taken through prevention of mother-to-child transmission therapy. HIV/AIDS has been the main issue in Botswana discourse and its health focus since 1995. Because one cannot divorce the workplace health from community health, a large chunk of workplace health promotion (WHP) attention and activities are focused on preventing, counseling, and dealing with the HIV/AIDS issue.

The prevailing health issues and health risk behaviors include HIV/AIDS and its causes. Despite millions of dollars and the government's concentrated efforts in the last 10 years to reduce prevalence and new infections, at best the HIV/AIDS situation appears stabilized. The current prevalence rates range from 2.2% in the age group of 1.5–4.0 years to 40.6% in the age group from 40–44 years. There are several recorded negative impacts of high HIV/AIDS prevalence on the population and economy of Botswana.

Uninhibited alcohol use and uncontrolled and undisciplined sexual relationships have been found to fuel the HIV/AIDS prevalence. Physical inactivity and accompanying low productivity are other concerns for WHP.

Government is the main provider of health services and facilities, although missionaries, mines, and private commercial health institutions also provide services. Through government's motivation and its enthusiastic attack on the HIV/AIDS scourge, most public and private organizations set up health and wellness units/departments within their structures.

Government backs up its health efforts with necessary legislation and policies. A lot of effort is devoted to health promotion, which has been incorporated in education, community development, policy, and legislation. Culture and mentality play a big role in WHP issues in Botswana. These include low rates of marriage and unstable and multiconcurrent sexual partners, fairly high prevalence of teenage pregnancies and motherhood, single parenthood, and cohabitation.

Workplace health promotion in most employing organizations is not formal or clearly defined. The absence of specific, objective measuring instruments to annually evaluate performance and achievements is a major setback for the effectiveness and progress in WHP in Botswana. Furthermore, physical activity, which is a major platform in WHP to relieve workers' stress and enhance productivity, is glaringly absent in the WHP policy of most employing organizations in Botswana, including the Botswana Police Force.

## Review Questions

1. Explain the impact of HIV/AIDS on the development of Botswana.
2. Describe the three tiers of the healthcare system in Botswana and what each provides.
3. What is the role of workplace health promotion programs in Botswana?
4. Choose one of the case studies of Botswana workplace health promotion and describe its impact on employee health.
5. How are research indicators affecting health promotion research in Botswana?
6. Consider the current status of workplace health promotion in Botswana and list three challenges to successful implementation of future workplace health promotion initiatives.

# References


Botswana Central Statistics Office. (2007). *Access to health services in Botswana.* Gaborone, Botswana: Republic of Botswana.

Botswana Central Statistics Office (CSO). (2009a). *Population by sex and census districts (1991 and 2001).* Gaborone, Botswana: Republic of Botswana.

Botswana Central Statistics Office (CSO). (2009b). *Preliminary Botswana HIV/AIDS impact survey III results.* Gaborone, Botswana: Republic of Botswana.

Botswana Federation of Trade Unions (BFTU). (2007, March) *Policy on health & occupational safe environment in Botswana.*

Botswana NACA. (2008). *HIV/AIDS in Botswana: Estimated trends and implications based on surveillance and modeling.* Gaborone, Botswana: Republic of Botswana.

Botswana Police Service. (2000). *HIV/AIDS: Workplace policy.* Gaborone, Botswana: Botswana Police Service.

Central Intelligence Agency (CIA). (2009). *The world factbook 2009.* Washington, DC: Central Intelligence Agency. Retrieved May 30, 2009, from https://www.cia.gov/library/publications/the-world-factbook/index.html

Corlett, J. (1984a). Health-related fitness of young Batswana adults [Botswana notes and records]. *The Journal of Botswana Society, 16*, 59–61.

Corlett, J. (1984b). A power function analysis of physical performance by Botswana children. *Journal of Sports Science, 2*(2), 131–137.

Fine, A., Ward, M., Burr, M., Tudor-Smith, C., & Kingdom, A. (2004). Health promotion in small workplaces: A feasibility study. *Health Education Journal, 63,* 334–346.

Government of Botswana Country Report. (2007). United Nations General Assembly Special Session on HIV/AIDS.

Kesaobaka, J. (2009, December 9). Batswana are overweight. *Botswana Daily News,* p.1.

Khunwane, T. (2009, November 27). New HIV infections worry government. *Botswana Daily News,* p. 20.

Kgosiemang, P. G. (2004). *How students in tertiary institutions spend their leisure time.* Gaborone, Botswana: University of Botswana.

Linnan, L., Bowling, M., Childress, J., Lindsay, G., Blakey, C., Pronk, S., … Royall, P. (2008). Results of the 2004 National Worksite Health Promotion Survey. *American Journal of Public Health, 98*, 1503–1509.

Lloyd, R. (1999). Productivity week. *Productivity and Quality Forum, 4*(3), 1.

Ministry of Health. (1996). *Community home based care for people with AIDS in Botswana: Operational guidelines (NACP 30).* Gaborone, Botswana: Ministry of Health.

Molomo, B. C. (2008). Foreword. *National AIDS Coordinating Agency—2008 progress report of the national response to the UNGASS.* Gaborone, Botswana: Republic of Botswana.

Montlane, L. (2009, November 5). BAIS results satisfactory. *Botswana Daily News,* p. 3.

Nolan, S. (2009, December 11). Violence against women is criminal. *Botswana Guardian,* p. 9.

Orufheng, D. (2009, December 11). Alcoholism: A national epidemic. *Botswana Guardian,* p. 10.

Our anti-HIV/AIDS strategy cannot be compromised on ideological reasons [Editorial comment]. (2009, December 1). *Mmegi, Botswana Daily Newspaper,* p. 8.

Owolabi, E. O., & Kalui, B. (1997). Teaching physical education in Botswana. In M. Marope & D. Chapman (Eds.), *Research in Education: Teaching and Teacher Education in Botswana.* Gaborone, Botswana: Lentswe la Lesedi (pty) Ltd.

Owolabi, E. O., & Keetile, L. (2007, September). *Overweight, obesity, and metabolic syndrome in Botswana.* Paper presented at the 8th International Institute of Health Promotion Biennial Congress, Institute for Sports and Sports Science of the University of Heidelberg, Germany.

Owolabi, E. O., & Mogotsi, I. (1999). *Combatting HIV/AIDS among university students in Botswana: Need for a change of strategy?* Paper presented at the 5th International Institute of Health Promotion Biennial Congress, American University, Washington D.C.

Owolabi, E. O., & Shaibu, S. (1999). Country profile: Botswana, an African success story. *Health Promotion: Global Perspectives, 2*(3), 6.

Ramatlala, M. S. (2002). *Recreational patterns and preferences among the University of Botswana male students.* Gaborone, Botswana: University of Botswana.

Republic of Botswana. (2007, December). *Government of Botswana country national response to the UNGASS Declaration of Commitment on HIV/AIDS.* To United Nations General Assembly Special Session on HIV/AIDS. Gaborone, Botswana: NACA.

Residents welcome home based care programme for AIDS victims. (2000, August). *Botswana Daily News.*

SADC. (1998). *SADC regional human development report.* Harare, Zimbabwe: SAPES Books.

UNAIDS. (2006). *Report on the global AIDS epidemic.* Gaborone, Botswana: UNAIDS/WHO.

UNAIDS. (2008). *Botswana: Epidemiological country profile on HIV/AIDS.* Gaborone, Botswana: UNAIDS/WHO.

UNDP (1999). *Human development report 1997.* New York, NY: UNDP.

World Health Organization. (2006). World health statistics: 2006. Retrieved June 4, 2010, from http://www.who.int/whosis/whostat2006/en

Chapter 3

# Brazil

Ricardo De Marchi

After reading this chapter you should be able to:

- Identify core strategies that are the focus of Brazilian workplace health promotion efforts
- Describe Brazil's historical evolution of workplace health promotion
- Explain the different approaches employed by corporate health promotion efforts throughout Brazil
- Review the central disease states and health issues driving Brazil's health promotion needs
- Name the components of, and the associated funding sources for, Brazil's healthcare system
- Discuss the impact of culture on Brazil's health status and health promotion efforts

Table 3-1 **Select Key Demographic and Economic Indicators**

| | |
|---|---|
| Nationality | Noun: Brazilian(s)<br>Adjective: Brazilian |
| Ethnic groups | White 53.7%, mulatto (mixed white and black) 38.5%, black 6.2%, other (includes Japanese, Arab, Amerindian) 0.9%, unspecified 0.7% (2000 census) |
| Religion | Roman Catholic (nominal) 73.6%, Protestant 15.4%, Spiritualist 1.3%, Bantu/voodoo 0.3%, other 1.8%, unspecified 0.2%, none 7.4% (2000 census) |
| Language | Portuguese (official and most widely spoken language); note—less common languages include Spanish (border areas and schools), German, Italian, Japanese, English, and a large number of minor Amerindian languages |
| Literacy | Definition: age 15 and over can read and write<br>Total population: 88.6%<br>Male: 88.4%<br>Female: 88.8% (2004 est.) |
| Education expenditure | 4% of GDP (2004)<br>Country comparison to the world: 105 |

*continued*

Table 3-1 **Select Key Demographic and Economic Indicators,** *continued*

| | |
|---|---|
| Government type | Federal republic |
| Environment | Deforestation in Amazon Basin destroys the habitat and endangers a multitude of plant and animal species indigenous to the area; there is a lucrative illegal wildlife trade; air and water pollution in Rio de Janeiro, São Paulo, and several other large cities; land degradation and water pollution caused by improper mining activities; wetland degradation; severe oil spills |
| Country mass | Total: 8,514,877 sq km<br>Country comparison to the world: 5<br>Land: 8,459,417 sq km<br>Water: 55,460 sq km<br>*Note:* includes Arquipelago de Fernando de Noronha, Atol das Rocas, Ilha da Trindade, Ilhas Martin Vaz, and Penedos de São Pedro e Sao Paulo |
| Population | 201,103,330<br>Country comparison to the world: 5 |
| Age structure | 0–14 years: 26.5% (male 27,170.378/female 26,134,844)<br>15–64 years: 66.9% (male 66,667,099/female 67,932,910)<br>65 years and over: 6.6% (male 5,578,397/female 7,619,702)<br>(2010 est.) |
| Median age | Total: 28.9 years<br>Male: 28.1 years<br>Female: 29.7 years (2010 est.) |
| Population growth rate | 1.166% (2010 est.)<br>Country comparison to the world: 109 |
| Birth rate | 18.11 births/1,000 population (2010 est.)<br>Country comparison to the world: 107 |
| Death rate | 6.35 deaths/1,000 population (July 2010 est.)<br>Country comparison to the world: 156 |
| Net migration rate | -0.09 migrant(s)/1,000 population (2010 est.)<br>Country comparison to the world: 93 |
| Urbanization | Urban population: 86% of total population (2008)<br>Rate of urbanization: 1.8% annual rate of change (2005–2010 est.) |
| Gender ratio | At birth: 1.05 male(s)/female under 15 years: 1.04 male(s)/female<br>15–64 years: 0.98 male(s)/female<br>65 years and over: 0.73 male(s)/female<br>Total population: 0.98 male(s)/female (2009 est.) |
| Infant mortality rate | Total: 22.86 deaths/1,000 live births<br>Country comparison to the world: 94<br>Male: 25.39 deaths/1,000 live births<br>Female: 18.15 deaths/1,000 live births (2010 est.) |

*continued*

| Table 3-1 **Select Key Demographic and Economic Indicators,** *continued* | |
|---|---|
| Life expectancy | Total population: 72.26 years<br>Country comparison to the world: 124<br>Male: 68.7 years<br>Female: 76years (2010 est.) |
| Total fertility rate | 2.19 children born/woman (2010 est.)<br>Country comparison to the world: 112 |
| GDP—purchasing power parity | $2.025 trillion (2009 est.)<br>Country comparison to the world: 10 |
| GDP—per capita (PPP) | $10,200 (2009 est.)<br>Country comparison to the world: 103 |
| GDP—composition by sector | Agriculture: 6.1%<br>Industry: 25.4%<br>Services: 68.5% (2009 est.) |
| Agriculture—products | Coffee, soybeans, wheat, rice, corn, sugarcane, cocoa, citrus, beef |
| Industries | Textiles, shoes, chemicals, cement, lumber, iron ore, tin, steel, aircraft, motor vehicles and parts, other machinery and equipment |
| Labor force participation | 101.7 million (2009 est.)<br>Country comparison to the world: 6 |
| Unemployment rate | 8.1% (2009 est.)<br>Country comparison to the world: 90 |
| Industrial production growth rate | -7% (2009 est.)<br>Country comparison to the world: 126 |
| Distribution of family income (GINI index) | 56.7 (2005)<br>Country comparison to the world: 10 |
| Investment (gross fixed) | 16.7% of GDP (2009 est.)<br>Country comparison to the world: 125 |
| Public debt | 60% of GDP (2009 est.)<br>Country comparison to the world: 54 |
| Market value of publicly traded shares | $589.4 billion (December 31, 2008)<br>Country comparison to the world: 12 |
| Current account balance | $-24.3 billion (2009 est.)<br>Country comparison to the world: 181 |
| Debt (external) | $216.1 billion (December 31, 2009 est.)<br>Country comparison to the world: 26 |
| Debt as a % of GDP | ——— |

*continued*

| Table 3-1 Select Key Demographic and Economic Indicators, *continued* | |
|---|---|
| Exports | $153 billion (2009 est.)<br>Country comparison to the world: 23 |
| Exports—commodities | Transport equipment, iron ore, soybeans, footwear, coffee, autos |
| Export—partners | China 12.5%, U.S. 10%, Argentina 8.4%, Netherlands 5.3%, Germany 4% (2009) |
| Imports | $127 billion (2009 est.)<br>Country comparison to the world: 26 |
| Import—commodities | Machinery, electrical and transport equipment, chemical products, oil, automotive parts, electronics |
| Import—partners | U.S. 16.1%, China 12.6%, Argentina 8.8%, Germany 7.7% (2009) |
| Stock of direct foreign investment at | |
| Home | $319.9 billion (December 31, 2009 est.)<br>Country comparison to the world: 13 |
| Abroad | $117.4 billion (December 31, 2009 est.)<br>Country comparison to the world: 24 |

Source: CIA. (2010). *The world factbook*. Retrieved December 16, 2010, from https://www.cia.gov/library/publications/the-world-factbook/

# Introduction

Health is a human right and a duty of the state, and it should be seen as an important issue for well-being, disease prevention, and quality of life. Moreover, it is a significant segment of any business; comprising the second-largest expense in a company's costs, it ranks just behind payroll and above costs associated with food. Thus, health promotion demands comparable effort from private sector companies in order to handle the complexity and responsibility of dealing with health issues.

To resolve this binomial health-versus-disease discussion, historically, countries have combined different types of action, as well as public and private campaigns, with varying degrees of success. Nevertheless, the concern with the issue of health has increased greatly, because health-related costs are on the rise. Everyone is trying to save money and cut costs, usually by placing the onus on the beneficiaries of the health system. Nonetheless, administrators and governments feel exacerbated by the escalation of costs associated with changing medical technology coupled with the media's focus on the acquisition and use of such medical innovations. This pattern continues to occur while the longevity and aging of the population changes. This is a worldwide phenomenon, which is due in large part to the medical advances and the decrease in growth and birth rates in many countries.

## Prevailing Health Issues and Risk Behaviors

The predominant Brazilian health issues include physical health (nutrition, sedentary lifestyles, smoking, etc.) and emotional issues (stress, depression), although there are other pressing topics such as managing personal health, the balance between personal and professional life, and healthy relationships.

The Brazilian corporate environment has a high level of physical inactivity (up to 65%), overweight (more than 50%) and stress (42%). These figures are results of a survey conducted by CPH Health, a consulting company of products and services in the area of corporate health, since the beginning of the 21st century, with more than 200 companies and among a population of more than 100,000 participants.

Since the beginning of the 21st century, CPH has evaluated the lifestyle of a corporate population made up of 194,600 individuals (61.9% men and 38.1% women). Table 3-2 illustrates the research data.

| Table 3-2 **CPH Study of Corporate Lifestyle** | |
|---|---|
| Weight changes (overweight or obese) | 45.1% |
| Low nutritional quality | 56.2% |
| Inadequate breakfast | 75.4% |
| Allergies | 24.3% |
| Asthma | 4.5% |
| High cholesterol | 13.8% |
| Diabetes | 1.4% |
| Migraines | 15.3% |
| High blood pressure | 6.7% |
| Backaches | 11.5% |
| High intake of alcoholic beverages | 5.6% |
| High intake of caffeine | 24.2% |
| Smoking | 12.5% |
| Insufficient physical activity | 76.1% |
| Work sitting most of the time | 68.0% |
| Significant level of stress | 49.2% |
| Anxiety | 48.3% |
| Low balance between personal and professional life | 41.4% |

Source: CPH study (2010).

Clearly, these results show that health has been damaged by an unhealthy lifestyle, which is also a great opportunity to take action in health promotion.

## Healthcare System

Brazil, with 200 million inhabitants, has its health system divided into two categories:

1. Unified Health System (SUS)—almost 160 million users;
2. Private Health System (Supplementary Health System)—41,500 million users.

The health system should actually be called *the disease system,* as it is concentrated in the hands of a small number of companies that provide nothing except medical assistance. This system basically provides just treatment of symptomatic patients, with costs prepaid or postpaid. There is little or no component of sharing health information and virtually no health-related integration, meaning no support or services, with the healthy population. The individual is monitored only from the moment he *enters* the system; and practically speaking, interaction with the asymptomatic population is nonexistent. This model makes it unappealing for health service providers to take preventive measures because they receive payment only for the treatments that they perform. Moreover, it causes uneasiness for both providers and consumers, as the consumer pays a relatively high cost and would like to receive better health care, and the seller makes a small profit and would like to be better paid. In recent decades, this model with its main goal of controlling costs has prevailed, resulting in the reduction in quality of care and limiting action in health promotion. There have been but few new initiatives on the part of healthcare providers, and although all actors in the sector share this perception, little has been done to change the status quo.

In Brazil, the healthcare issues are exacerbated by the peculiar contradictions of a country with continental dimensions but immense social inequality, a high degree of economic exclusion, and very little public investment in the healthcare sector. However, in certain cities there are centers of excellence in medicine that feature some of the most modern and advanced medical and hospital care systems in the world, both in technology and training. In fact, some of these medical and health experts travel abroad to share their expertise with other developed countries.

With respect to health care itself, it could be said that Brazil has a medical condition that alternates quality and insufficiency, creating a health system of marked contrasts. There is high-quality care, available to only a small portion of the population, and the poor and handicapped care offered to those most lacking quality insurance options.

In Brazil, the market segment of supplementary health care is about 30 billion *reais* per year, or 2.7% of the GNP, and guarantees coverage to almost 42 million people (26.8% of the population). However, the other 73% of the population who are not included in this market depend on scanty and insufficient public attention provided by the SUS, which faces chronic problems in financing, infrastructure, and services (Guiraldelli & Benz, 2009).

A Brazilian citizen spends much less than a U.S. citizen on health insurance, with his use of health services often equivalent, yet one cannot say that he spends a small amount on health because his purchasing power has eroded down from an annual increase of 7.32% in 2008 to only 0.89% in 2009 (Index Mundi, 2010). In addition, although he pays taxes toward health services, he receives an inadequate and unreliable public health service. Furthermore, some citizens must also pay private health insurance fees, which in turn are taxed to fund public services and care for the population that uses those services.

In Brazil, the government has invested little in health compared to other countries of Latin America and the world. There is dissatisfaction with the private system; health care costs are steadily increasing, and consumer dissatisfaction is prevalent. As medical science advances, the care system is failing to keep pace, creating an equation difficult to solve and crucial to well-being. Furthermore, the population is gleaning medical and technical knowledge from the web rather than from physicians, which increasingly undermines and discredits the doctor-patient relationship.

In the 1980s, Brazil's social and economic crises intensified, highlighting the deficiencies of the healthcare system. Brazil's global health policy remained focused on immediate care and curative medicine (instead of prevention) and also failed to reduce infant mortality or extend services to those not affiliated with Social Security. At the end of the decade, the Constitution of 1988 established health as a human right and a duty of the state. In this context, the SUS was created in 1988; health policy became a responsibility of the Ministry of Health, and Social Security continued to have a reduced role, acting only in the transfer of a portion of the tax revenues. The role of SUS was defined in 1990. Its mission was to bring together various public health services—centers and service centers, hospitals, laboratories, blood centers, foundations, and research institutes. However, most private offices, laboratories, and hospitals have continued noncontracted to SUS.

Prior to the creation of SUS, health was not considered a social right. Until then, the old model of health divided the population into three categories: (1) those who could afford private health care; (2) those who were entitled to public health because they were insured by the social welfare (workers with formal jobs); and (3) those who had no right to health care. Thus, SUS was designed to provide equal treatment and care and promote health for the entire population.

The SUS is one of the largest public health systems in the world, providing care to more than 180 million Brazilians. It ranges from simple outpatient care to organ transplants; ensuring full access, universal and free for the entire population of the country. In addition to offering consultations, examinations, and admissions, the system also promotes vaccination campaigns and prevention and health monitoring—such as monitoring food and drug regulation—and reaches the lives of all Brazilians. Thus, SUS is a unique social project that manifests itself through promotion, prevention, and health care for every Brazilian.

In June 2004, the private healthcare system had 38.2 million members in private health plans, of which 33.5 million were on health insurance plans, predominantly women (54%) compared to men (46%). The distribution of different population groups by age and place of residence (by federal unit) is presented in Figure 3-1.

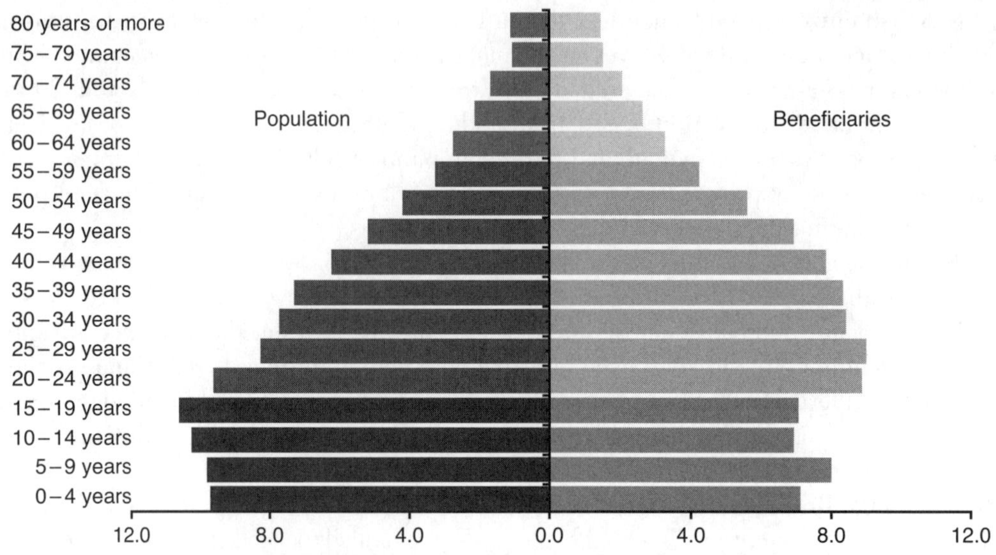


Figure 3-1 Pyramid related to age (population × beneficiaries) – Brazil, 2004.

Source: Instituto Brasileiro de Geografia e Estatística

The first age group (people up to 20 years) has a significantly lower rate of those receiving benefits than other age groups. The ratio of beneficiaries to total population is somewhat more equal among adults (20 to 59 years). There is a higher rate of beneficiaries within the elderly (60 years or more). The population pyramid shows that the population of beneficiaries is greater than the Brazilian population in that many individuals receive multiple payouts.

Another striking feature is the concentration of beneficiaries in the southeast and urban centers, particularly in capitals, reflecting the distribution of health centers and employers (Figure 3-2).

According to data from the national household sample survey, Pesquisa Nacional por Amostra de Domicilios, in 1998 and 2003, the rate of health insurance coverage was higher in social strata with higher income. Thus, more than half of the population that had private insurance plans were among the 20% richest Brazilians, as shown in Figures 3-3 and 3-4.

Several studies have shown the importance of socioeconomic factors on the health of the population and the outcomes of the health-disease process, such as mortality. Inequalities in health and the use of health services are reflections of large-scale inequalities in education, income, housing, and other characteristics of the household (e.g., sanitation/sewerage and water supply, etc.).

The Supplementary Health System is basically concentrated in the corporate environment and is the largest private health system in the world after that of the United States. Throughout history, Brazilian supplementary health companies (HMOs) survived all sorts of difficulties—clumsy economic plans; chronic shortages of resources; default; state indifference and inefficiency; corruption and inertia in public administration and political system; insensitivity of regulator organization to the demands of the industry; globalization; unemployment; and economic stagnation and instability. During these stormy scenarios, they sought some way for

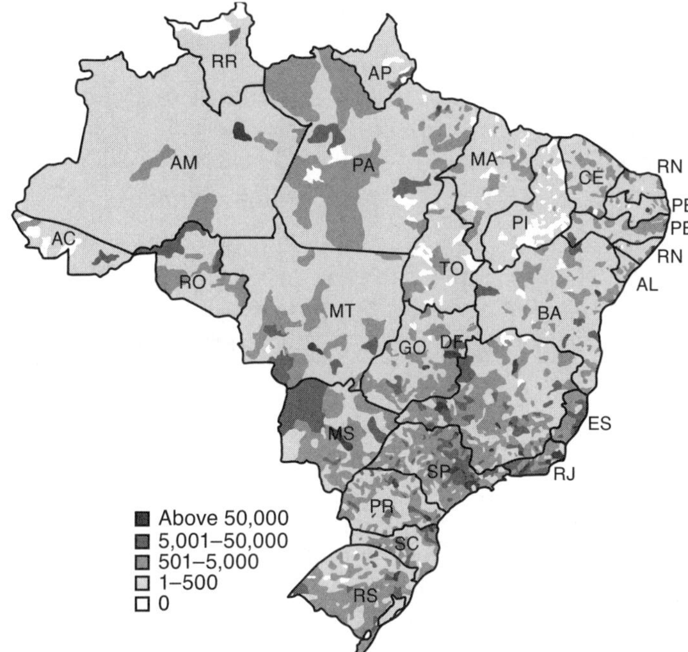


Figure 3-2 The population of beneficiaries per city.

Source: Agencia Nacional de Saúde

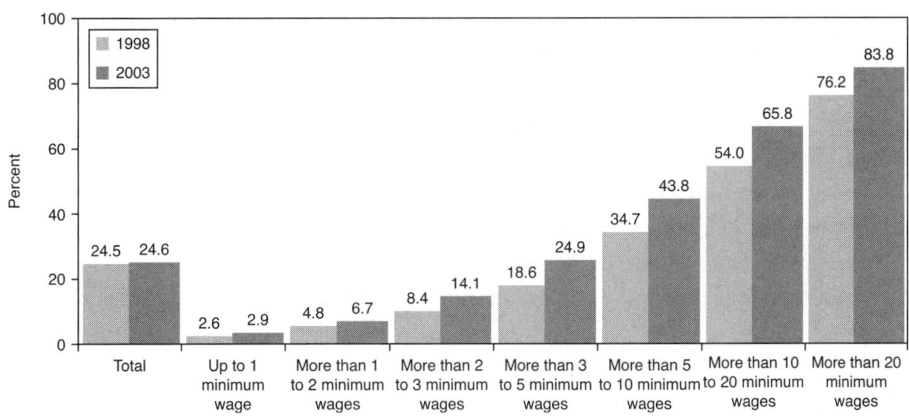


Figure 3-3 Coverage rate per health plan, according to income – Brazil, 1998 and 2003.

Source: Banco de Dados do Sistema Único de Saúde (SUS)

the business to survive financially with assurance of minimum profitability conditions for all players. The challenges are still great, and there is a need to start now to adapt to the new demographic and epidemiologic reality of chronic disease. Currently, supplementary companies need to expand the provision of health care and create educational and health promotion efforts, while maintaining economic viability.

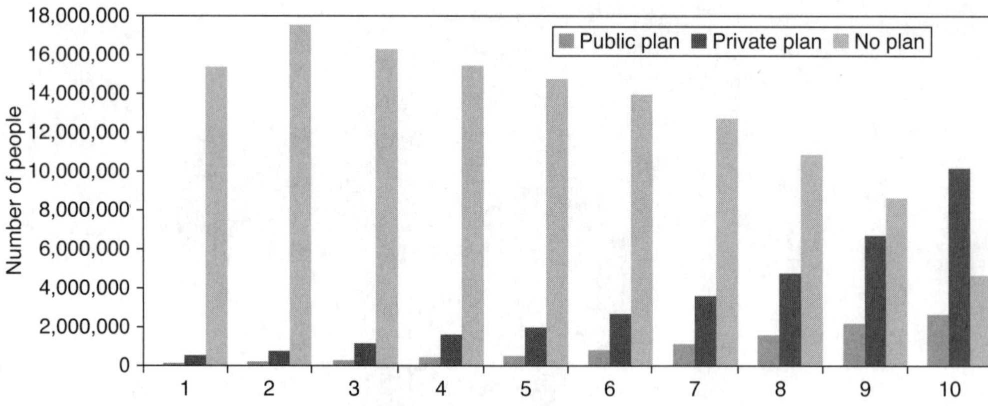


Figure 3-4 Brazilian population's distribution according to health plan × domestic income – Brazil, 2003.

Source: Pesquisa Nacional por Amostragem de Domicílios

Supplementary health care grew from the second half of the 20th century. HMOs have emerged in hospitals and clinics throughout the country as an alternative to private health care, out of the reach of most of the population, and to the unsatisfactory public service. From the 1980s, private medicine became more professional with respect to administrative and financial management, which attracted large investors such as large insurers, who contributed their best practices in managing and finance and an emphasis on the prevention of incidents.

Currently 1,122 private healthcare companies offer their services to corporations and individuals. The Brazilian National Health Agency has implemented regulations for the private healthcare sector in order to make it an area of health promotion, such that operators can become managers of health and beneficiaries can become conscious consumers of health care.

Health promotion is influenced by cultural idiosyncrasies and the particular characteristics of Brazil. Besides accounting for risk management, health promotion considers the welfare of the individual from physical, emotional, social, cultural, spiritual, and environmental perspectives.

Historically, health care in Brazil has invested in the formulation, implementation, and delivery of policies to promote the protection and recovery of health. Therefore, great effort has been put into building a model of health care that prioritizes quality of life and risk reduction and its determinants (e.g., lifestyle, working conditions, environment, education, leisure, and culture). Beginning in 2002, the Brazilian government, in collaboration with Pan American Health Organization, evaluated the impact of a newly established national health promotion policy and developed indicators of health promotion into the national data collection system for primary care practitioners. Activities that disseminate and implement the national health promotion policy have ranked as high priorities; for example, healthy nutrition, physical activity, prevention of smoking and tobacco control, and reduction of morbidity and mortality due to abuse of alcohol and other drugs.

## Influence of Culture and Mentality

The habits of Brazilians living in urban centers, especially in the more developed cities, contribute to the erosion of their health. Urban employees face heavy traffic, poor transportation systems and mobility difficulties, polluted air, and a generally inadequate environment. Typically, the Brazilian corporate employee:

- works hard and is under pressure
- is predominantly sedentary
- has very little time to relax
- has a hectic schedule
- eats an unhealthy diet
- gives more attention to professional life than to personal issues
- has a virtually nonexistent social life
- displays tiredness and fatigue at the end of the day
- has very short or infrequent vacations

Even in the more economically developed southeast and south regions, the majority of the companies do not seek health promotion as a useful tool for containing costs and increasing productivity. Many companies desire to implement practices that would improve the workplace ambiance, without any concern for the effectiveness of programs and the ability to monitor them. They do not target results that would reduce costs, return on their investment, improve health, or create an awareness of employee self-responsibility for health and lifestyle changes. In addition, the following behaviors characteristically determine the focus of workplace health promotion:

- When the human resources department leads the program, the focus is mainly on the management of people and in most cases there is not a focus on developing a well-structured health promotion program.
- Well-managed investments in promoting health are still somewhat rare, and few companies are prepared and willing to invest in proper health promotion efforts. Companies usually invest little but want to maximize program visibility. They often lack the commitment of managers; thus, their programs end up being little valued by their employees.
- The employees do not see personal benefits from the program and consequently their involvement is compromised.

Companies that desire to offer programs in health promotion could offer a variety of programs, such as physical activity programs; gym discounts; walking programs; a gymnasium in the workplace; nutrition counseling; intranet sites; call centers (proactive or responsive); low caloric, nutritional meals in cafeterias; assistance and counseling for problems related to alcohol and drugs; antistress monitoring; etc. However, it is rare to find companies that offer many of these items.

Well-structured educational programs truly exist, but alone, they do not lead to changes in personal habits. It is necessary that the culture and the environment are able to provide strong support to help employees adopt healthier behaviors.

## Drivers of Workplace Health Promotion

The demand for health promotion in the corporate environment has increased in the 21st century and the perception of this need has become clearer, mainly because the areas of human resources and occupational health have improved knowledge on the subject and show increasing interest in this area. However, because corporate health care is fragmented and human resources professionals do not yet have sufficient technical knowledge in the implementation of such programs, often the lowest price becomes the only consideration in the contracting process, thus devaluing the whole concept.

An important matter in workplace health promotion (WHP) is determining who will pay for health promotion. In Brazil, it currently is the employer who finances health promotion, and, most certainly, the employer will continue to pay for it in the future. Healthcare insurance policies provide a better structured health promotion package to their customers; however, they are still rudimentary as they don't relate to accidents, casualties, or medical costs.

The goal should be to build a program that promotes health outcomes, but this goal is often absent from the proposed models. The buyer profile is a company with more than a thousand employees, mostly multinational corporations (e.g., the headquarters) that purchase inconsistent products and services. This reality can ultimately cause great risk to the concept of health promotion.

The interest in health promotion and the purpose of health promotion vary from company to company—mainly big companies—as reflected in the following sections.

### Ambiance

Ambiance, perhaps the main driving force of WHP, is a concept already enshrined in human resources' planning: investing in something that will improve the whole atmosphere in the workplace is attractive to human resources, and many programs are implemented with this purpose. When employees acknowledge that they are taken care of, they commit themselves much more to the company and to the employer. It is a very interesting strategy that shows the success of human resource policies.

### Job Satisfaction

Job satisfaction is an important factor in "winning the game." Most Brazilian companies, especially those with more than 1,000 employees, focus on activities that promote job satisfaction. They emphasize that health is an important benefit; therefore, they provide more attractive health insurance policies, healthier meals, and other benefits that show the company is a good place to work.

## Absenteeism

Absenteeism is an important topic, but it usually is not dealt with or managed efficiently. Certainly management programs that reduce absenteeism by seeking reinstatement and improvement of the functional capacity of the employee will be one of the WHP topics included in the near term.

## Productivity

Very little has been done to evaluate, within a formal structure, the relationship between health and productivity. Monitoring systems in general, and monitoring productivity in particular, are still inefficient.

## Disease Management

Disease management is an important issue within the focus of health promotion. Disease is linked to workplace accidents and lost productivity. Effective disease management requires the monitoring of both patients and at-risk individuals. It has been part of most well-structured programs of health promotion.

## Attraction

Attraction is always a factor when discussing the reason for implementing WHP programs. Companies want to be good places to work, and this kind of benefit helps to improve the image of the employer.

## Managers' Commitment

The commitment of company managers to WHP is always emphasized as critical to the success of programs. Despite the importance of getting the support of managers, especially senior executives, there is some resistance to this approach. Some people disagree and propose that if the largest population of the company, the employee group, does not buy into the program, success becomes elusive. In theory, it makes sense; however, we know that if the program is not driven from top down, the chances of success are much smaller.

The managers' role is to translate the vision and the value of health concretely and sustain it over time. This is difficult to achieve in the health field, since it is complicated to demonstrate the real benefits that result from health promotion, especially in terms of economics and financial matters.

These drivers of WHP, of course, are the subject of discussion and focal areas when companies propose why and how they should have a WHP program. In addition, another very important reason still remains: the decrease of medical costs.

## Programs and Good Practices

As the corporate culture in Brazil is very complex, and specifically because of the extent of the diversity found in this country, the culture of health and well-being is even more diverse.

Programs to promote health and quality of life represent one of the best investments that an employer can make. Few companies are entirely aware of the gains they might get from implementing programs that focus on the promotion of health and quality of life; therefore, unfortunately, most of these programs are not designed to achieve this goal.

Successful programs in Brazil—those evaluated favorably by the Brazilian Association of Quality of Life and the recipients of the National Award for Quality of Life—have been guided by this principle, and are focused on achieving business results. Therefore, their components include interventions and attractive improvements in the physical work environment in addition to regular monitoring.

The National Award for Quality of Life, despite being national, has higher participation from companies located in the southeast region (88%). The companies who have received the award range in size from 200 to more than 50,000 employees. The characteristics of the winning programs are: (1) they are more than 2 years old and are usually managed by the human resources department (60%); and (2) most of them (69%) include family and dependents.

Interventions range from activities in terms of nutrition (85%); physical activity (66.7%); social integration (70.4%); and health programs (70.4%) including vaccinations, annual check-ups, prevention of prostate, breast, and cervical cancers, periodic screenings, monitoring of chronic cases, etc.

Companies of different sizes and various business sectors have implemented programs for over 5 years, and many have won the National Award for Quality of Life. Some companies that represent good practices are discussed in the following sections.

### Dow Chemical

Dow Chemical is among the best places to work in Brazil, and it is recognized for best practices in the areas of benefits, education, and health. With approximately 3,000 employees, it has a real emphasis on good management of the workforce. In late 1992, Dow Chemical established a multidisciplinary regional board for the purpose of defining actions and developing strategies to promote health and quality of life. From this board emerged the idea of implementing a program to promote health and quality of life. The program aims to be a catalyst for changes in behavior, strengthening the whole concept of health.

Dow Chemical implemented various practices such as:

- Healthy nutrition
- Gyms in the majority of its operational sites
- Employee assistance programs
- Health check-ups for the executive team
- Programs to relieve stress
- Programs to control smoking

## Accor

Accor, a company in the hotel, tourism, and services industry, has invested effectively in the area of protecting the health of its 13,000 employees in Brazil. Accor developed a strong focus on health promotion through managing benefits; the company has an organizational structure composed of different professionals (doctors, nurses, psychologists, physiotherapists, nutritionists, etc.) that acts to minimize risks and increase employees' personal responsibility in managing their own health.

In addition to its goals of establishing a good work environment and maximizing conditions for the well-being of employees in the workplace, the company seeks to develop effective management for its healthcare plan, aiming to reduce the accident rate.

The practices that have been developed at Accor include the following:

- Annual assessments of health profiles and lifestyles of its population
- Personalized services focused on emotional health
- Multidisciplinary team care for employees
- Programs to prevent breast, uterine, and prostate cancers
- Programs to manage chronic diseases
- Campaigns to stimulate physical activity
- Assessments to monitor executives' lifestyle
- Programs to control smoking
- Pharmaceutical benefit management

## VIVO

VIVO, a company in the mobile telephone industry, has a health management program that is considered one of the best in Brazil. VIVO has a workforce of approximately 12,000 employees. The corporation maintains its own health management, with a group of doctors trained in monitoring cases of illness and hospitalization. Health is strongly valued by the company and considered integral for the business results; therefore, it has a specific board for health and quality of life.

### CHESF

CHESF, a power company in the northeast region of the country, won the National Award for Quality of Life in 2008 because of its high commitment to the concept.

### Serasa/Experian

Serasa/Experian, a financial information company with approximately 3,000 employees, sustains a valuable process of managing people. Each year, risk and lifestyle profiles of its entire population are completed. The area of human resources is supported by the commitment of all the other management areas to move the program forward.

## Others

Other large companies that have developed good programs include Petrobras, Roche, Philips, Johnson & Johnson, Pfizer, Siemens, Alcoa, Caterpillar, Nestlé, TRF, Motorola, and Votorantim.

# Outcomes and Indicators

Although WHP has been in existence for more than 20 years, the results still fall short. Little has been done in terms of thorough analysis and monitoring the indicators. The evaluation of the process, its results, and impact are conducted in a superficial way; no doubt there is a great need for more investment in this area.

Participation in the program is always an informative indicator for human resources managers, because it shows the level of employees' awareness, the quality of communication, and whether or not the program is attractive. The average participation in Brazil in such programs is around 40% of the population. Because participation is not mandatory, the rate remains low, even with the introduction of incentives. From the author's point of view, in order to achieve good results, programs to promote health and quality of life must be a component of the business strategy requiring significant investment, and hence, they should be compulsory. Health and promotion programs are analogous to technical training programs and they should be similar. The company develops training programs in order to have quality products and competitive costs; employees should be trained to better manage personal health and lifestyle, which leads to the same goal—improving the performance and results of the business.

Indicators should be directly linked to company goals, and objectives should be monitored, including the following:

- Health insurance expenses
- Number of medical claims
- Proper use of the health insurance

- Participations in screenings
- Health indicators: nutritional quality, weight, BMI, physical activity level, etc.
- Sleep quality
- Absenteeism rate
- Physical inactivity/sedentary lifestyle
- Effective participation in integrated programs
- Smoking
- Reported stress level
- Balance between personal and professional life
- Level of risk
- Compliance in the treatment of chronic diseases

Tangible results are still rare, especially in reducing costs of health care, despite the development of systems able to assess this area more accurately. Brazil does not yet have a very effective management system; coordination among the various actors (occupational health, health care, human resources, benefits consulting, etc.) is still lacking, and investments are insufficient to raise the effectiveness of the process.

## Existing Research

Very little research has been done on WHP efforts in Brazil. Data on risk profiles are the most common, which reveals the needs and interests of corporations. Some universities have developed research primarily on assessing economic results and best practices to achieve good results. The Federal University of São Paulo, the Federal University of Santa Catarina, and the State University of São Paulo—academically renowned institutions—have very active nuclei in the field of health promotion and quality of life. The Brazilian Association of Quality of Life has advanced information concerning best practices and results through surveys.

The Social Service of the Industry is a national organization very active in the areas of sports, health, leisure, culture, and education of employees who work in the industrial sector. Social Service of the Industry has invested significantly in developing and promoting the concept of healthy industry and encouraging enterprises to adopt this philosophy.

## Conclusion

It is still very difficult to demonstrate strong financial results in established WHP programs, but the concept of WHP has solidified in recent years. Demand is high at the moment, and buyers are better informed in purchasing products and services appropriate to their needs.

Vendors in health and lifestyle promotion have become increasingly sophisticated and are currently seeking to create innovative products that can make a positive difference for their customers.

Many corporate events focusing on health promotion, such as bringing experienced professionals and international speakers to exchange information, have been added to programs. Benchmarking programs are held annually around the world, and the interest in this type of event has grown visibly.

The Brazilian National Agency of Health is promoting the concept of WHP and has even included health promotion as a requirement in qualifying those who want to provide medical assistance.

A good starting point to promote health is the regular annual medical examination, which in Brazil is compulsory by law and must be provided by every company. This is a fantastic opportunity for the employee to be evaluated by the occupational physician, informed about the importance of a healthy lifestyle, and encouraged to assume personal responsibility in the management of one's own health.

## Summary

Currently, there is a strong movement in Brazil toward new health approaches. The healthcare insurance policies offer improved structured health promotion packages for their customers; however, these packages are still rudimentary.

The current situation shows that health has been damaged by an unhealthy lifestyle, which is also a great opportunity for action in health promotion.

Currently, the health system provides only medical assistance. There is no integration of health promotion services, which causes uneasiness for both sides: the buyer and the seller. It can be said that Brazil has a medical condition that alternates between quality and insufficiency.

The segment of supplementary health care is about 30 billion *reais* per year and guarantees coverage to 42 million people (26.8% of the population). Public care is provided by the Unified Health System (SUS), which covers 160 million people, but SUS has chronic problems with financing, infrastructure, and services. The Supplementary Health System, which is basically concentrated in the corporate environment, is the largest private health system in the world after that of the United States. Currently, 1,122 private healthcare companies offer their products to corporations and individuals.

The culture and mentality contribute to the erosion of Brazilian worker health. Companies are trying to change some of these behaviors, investing in actions to better manage the work environment, job satisfaction, absenteeism, productivity, disease management, and managers' commitment to health-promotion efforts. Investments in well-managed health promotion programs are still somewhat rare, and few companies are prepared for this investment. Demand for WHP is high, and the buyers are now better informed to purchase products and services appropriate to their needs. Vendors in the health promotion market have become increasingly sophisticated and are currently seeking to create innovative products that can make a positive difference for their customers. The Brazilian National Agency of Health is promoting the concept of WHP and has even included health promotion as a requirement in qualifying those who want to provide medical assistance.

The chapter outlined the current challenges, barriers, mental and cultural influences, opportunities, and perspectives on this industry that is committed to substantial transformations.

## Review Questions

1. What do health issues and risk behaviors reveal about the corporate population of Brazil?
2. Explain the two categories of the Brazilian healthcare system and the purpose of each.
3. How does the Brazilian corporate culture help or hinder workplace health promotion efforts?
4. Identify and describe three challenges faced by Brazilian workplace health promotion efforts.
5. In order to qualify for the National Award for Quality of Life, what must a workplace health promotion program address?
6. List five outcome indicators for workplace health promotion programs and why they are necessary considerations.

## References

Brasil. Ministério da Saúde. (2008). Diretrizes e recomendações cuidado integral de doenças crônicas não-transmissíveis. *Promoção da saúde, vigilância, prevenção, e assistência.* Brasília: Ministério da Saúde.

Brasil. Ministério da Saúde. Secretaria Executiva. DataSUS. (2003, November). *A construção da política nacional de informação e informática em saúde.* Brasília: Ministério da Saúde.

Brasil. Ministério da Saúde. Secretaria de Vigilância em Saúde. Departamento de Análise de Situação de Saúde. (2005). *Saúde Brasil 2005—Uma análise da situação de saúde.* Brasília: Ministério da Saúde.

Brasil. Ministério da Saúde. Secretaria de Vigilância em Saúde. Departamento de Análise de Situação em Saúde. (2008). *Saúde Brasil 2007: Uma análise da situação de saúde no Brasil.* Brasília: Ministério da Saúde.

Brasil. Ministério da Saúde. Secretaria de Vigilância em Saúde. Secretaria de Gestão Estratégica e Participativa. (2009). *Vigitel Brasil 2008: Vigilância de fatores de risco e proteção para doenças crônicas por inquérito telefônico.* Brasília: Ministério da Saúde.

CPH Health. (2010). Homepage. Retrieved December 8, 2010, from http://www.cph.com.br/

Dias, Da Silva, M. A., & De Marchi, R. (1997). *Saúde e Qualidade de Vida no Trabalho.* São Paulo, Brazil: Editora Best Seller.

Evans, R. G., & Stoddart, G. L. (1994). *Why are some people healthy and others not? The determinants of health of populations.* New York, NY: Aldine de Gruyter.

Gomes, C. (2009). *Lazer na America Latina.* Belo Horizonte, Brazil: UFMG.

Instituto Brasileiro de Geografia e Estatística (IBGE). DataSUS. SE/MS. (2004). *Pyramid related to age (population × beneficiaries)—Brazil 2004.* Retrieved September 30, 2009 from http://ibge.gov.br

Guiraldelli, M. F., & Benz, A. (2009, March). A healthcare debate: Does the Brazilian healthcare model offer a guide to the U.S.? *Foreign Policy Digest.* Retrieved December 9, 2010, from http://www.foreignpolicydigest.org

Index Mundi. (2010). Brazil GDP. Retrieved from http://www.Indexmundi.com/brazil/gdp_(purchasing_power_parity).html

Kropf, A. J., Tafla, C., Souza, P. M. S. Furlan, V., Cardosa, P., Santos, S. R., & Vianna, D. (2009). *O sistema de saúde brasileiro sob a perspectiva da competição baseada em valor.* Brazil: Amil.

Malta, D. C., Moura, E. C., Castro, A. M., Cruz, K. A. D., de Morais Neto, O. L., & Monteiro, C. A. (2006). *Padrão de atividade física em adultos brasileiros.* Brasília, Brazil: DF.

Nahas, M. V. (2006). *Atividade Física, Saúde, e Qualidade de Vida.* (4th ed.). Londrina, Brazil: Midiograf.

Ogata, A., & De Marchi, R. (2007). *Wellness—Guia de Bem Estar e Qualidade de Vida.* Editora Campus: Elsevier.

Organizaçã Pan-Americana da Saúde. (2003). Doenças crônico-degenerativas e obesidade: Estratégia mundial sobre alimentação saudável, atividade física, e saúde. In *Estratégia Global para Doenças Crônicas e Obesidade.* Brasília, Brazil: Organizaçã Pan-Americana da Saúde.

Remington, P. L., Smith, M. Y., Williamson, D. F., Anda, R. F., Gentry, E. M., & Hogelin, G. C. (1988). Design, characteristics, and usefulness of state-based behavioral risk factor surveillance: 1981–87. *Public Health Rep, 103*, 366–375.

World Health Organization. (2002). Reducing risks, promoting healthy life. *World Health Report.* Geneva, Switzerland: WHO.

# Acknowledgments

I would like to thank the corporate health professionals and organizations who collaborated in helping me develop this chapter. They were willing to give testimonials and share their insights with me. I especially thank doctors Michel Daud, Luiz Monteiro, Paulo Marcos, Claudio Tafla, Catarina Jacob, Paulo Hirai, Alberto Ogata, and Flavia Kfouri. My sincere appreciation goes out to them!

Contributing organizations included Accor, Amil, ABQV, E-Pharma, and SESI.

Chapter 4

# Chile

Volney Vasquez Henríquez and Cinthia Ortiz Leiteiro

After reading this chapter you should be able to:

- Identify core strategies that are the focus of workplace health promotion efforts in Chile
- Describe the historical evolution of Chilean workplace health promotion efforts
- Explain the different approaches employed by corporate health promotion efforts throughout Chile
- Review the central disease states and health issues driving the health promotion needs of Chilean workplaces
- Name the components of, and the associated funding sources for, the Chilean healthcare system
- Discuss the impact of culture on the health status and health promotion efforts within Chilean workplaces

Table 4-1 **Select Key Demographic and Economic Indicators**

| | |
|---|---|
| Nationality | Noun: Chilean(s)<br>Adjective: Chilean |
| Ethnic groups | White and white-Amerindian 95.4%, Mapuche 4%,<br>Other indigenous groups 0.6% (2002 census) |
| Religion | Roman Catholic 70%, Evangelical 15.1%, Jehovah's Witness 1.1%, other Christian 1%, other 4.6%, none 8.3% (2002 census) |
| Language | Spanish (official), Mapudungun, German, English |
| Literacy | Definition: age 15 and over can read and write<br>Total population: 95.7%<br>Male: 95.8%<br>Female: 95.6% (2002 census) |
| Education expenditure | 3.2% of GDP (2006)<br>Country comparison to the world: 141 |
| Government type | Republic |

*continued*

| Table 4-1 **Select Key Demographic and Economic Indicators** *continued* | |
|---|---|
| Environment | Widespread deforestation and mining threaten natural resources; air pollution from industrial and vehicle emissions; water pollution from raw sewage |
| Country mass | Total: 756,102 sq km<br>Country comparison to the world: 38<br>Land: 743,812 sq km<br>Water: 12,290 sq km<br>*Note:* includes Easter Island (Isla de Pascua) and Isla Sala y Gomez |
| Population | 16,601,707 (July 2010 est.)<br>Country comparison to the world: 61 |
| Age structure | 0–14 years: 23.2% (male 1,966,017/female 1,877,963)<br>15–64 years: 67.8% (male 5,625,963/female 5,628,146)<br>65 years and over: 9.1% (male 627,746/female 875,872) (2010 est.) |
| Median age | Total: 31.7 years<br>Male: 30.7 years<br>Female: 32.8 years (2010 est.) |
| Population growth rate | 0.881% (2009 est.)<br>Country comparison to the world: 138 |
| Birth rate | 14.64 births/1,000 population (2010 est.)<br>Country comparison to the world: 143 |
| Death rate | 5.84 deaths/1,000 population (July 2009 est.)<br>Country comparison to the world: 167 |
| Net migration rate | NA (2009 est.) |
| Urbanization | Urban population: 88% of total population (2008)<br>Rate of urbanization: 1.3% annual rate of change (2005–2010 est.) |
| Gender ratio | At birth: 1.05 male(s)/female<br>Under 15 years: 1.05 male(s)/female<br>15–64 years: 1 male(s)/female<br>65 years and over: 0.72 male(s)/female<br>Total population: 0.98 male(s)/female (2010 est.) |
| Infant mortality rate | Total: 7.71 deaths/1,000 live births<br>Country comparison to the world: 165<br>Male: 8.49 deaths/1,000 live births<br>Female: 6.88 deaths/1,000 live births (2010 est.) |

*continued*

| Table 4-1 **Select Key Demographic and Economic Indicators** *continued* | |
|---|---|
| Life expectancy | Total population: 77.34 years<br>Country comparison to the world: 56<br>Male: 74.07 years<br>Female: 80.77 years (2010 est.) |
| Total fertility rate | 1.92 children born/woman (2010 est.)<br>Country comparison to the world: 142 |
| GDP—purchasing power parity | $242.2 billion (2009 est.)<br>Country comparison to the world: 47 |
| GDP—per capita | $14,600 (2009 est.)<br>Country comparison to the world: 76 |
| GDP—composition by sector | Agriculture: 4.8%<br>Industry: 50.5%<br>Services: 44.7% (2009 est.) |
| Agriculture—products | Grapes, apples, pears, onions, wheat, corn, oats, peaches, garlic, asparagus, beans, beef, poultry, wool, fish, timber |
| Industries | Copper, other minerals, foodstuffs, fish processing, iron and steel, wood and wood products, transport equipment, cement, textiles |
| Labor force participation | 7.42 million (2009 est.)<br>Country comparison to the world: 60 |
| Unemployment rate | 9.6 % (2009 est.)<br>Country comparison to the world: 115 |
| Industrial production growth rate | -3% (2009 est.)<br>Country comparison to the world: 94 |
| Distribution of family income (GINI index) | 54.9 (2003)<br>Country comparison to the world: 15 |
| Investment (gross fixed) | 20.5% of GDP (2009 est.)<br>Country comparison to the world: 87 |
| Public debt | 6.1% of GDP (2009 est.)<br>Country comparison to the world: 123 |
| Market value of publicly traded shares | $103.7 billion (December 31, 2009)<br>Country comparison to the world: 30 |
| Current account balance | $4.217 billion (2009 est.)<br>Country comparison to the world: 31 |
| Debt (external) | $60.9 billion (December 31, 2009 est.)<br>Country comparison to the world: 43 |

*continued*

| Table 4-1 Select Key Demographic and Economic Indicators *continued* | |
|---|---|
| Debt as a % of GDP | ——— |
| Exports | $53.74 billion (2009 est.)<br>Country comparison to the world: 44 |
| Exports—commodities | Copper, fruit, fish products, paper and pulp, chemicals, wine |
| Exports—partners | China 14.1%, United States 11.3%, Japan 10.4%, Brazil 5.9%, South Korea 5.7%, Netherlands 5.2%, Italy 4.4% (2008) |
| Imports | $39.75 billion (2009 est.)<br>Country comparison to the world: 50 |
| Imports—commodities | Petroleum and petroleum products, chemicals, electrical and telecommunications equipment, industrial machinery, vehicles, natural gas |
| Imports—partners | United States 21.77%, China 12.76%, Brazil 6.46%, Argentina 9.55%, South Korea 5.35 (2009) |
| Stock of direct foreign investment at | |
| Home | $116.5 billion (December 31, 2009 est.)<br>Country comparison to the world: 30 |
| Abroad | $33.68 billion (December 31, 2009 est.)<br>Country comparison to the world: 34 |

Source: CIA. (2010). *The world factbook.* Retrieved August 1, 2010, from www.cia.gov

# Introduction

Chile is located in the southwest area of South America, between the Pacific Ocean and the Andes Mountains, and borders Peru, Argentina, and Bolivia. Chile, a country well known for its long and narrow shape, has an area of 2,006,096 square kilometers. It is divided into 15 regions, including the Metropolitan Region, where the capital city of Santiago is located (University Selection Test—PSU, n.d.).

According to the 2002 census, the Chilean population comprises 15,116,435 inhabitants (Health Ministry & National Statistics Institute, 2002). Compared to the data collected in the year 1992, the country showed an average annual growth rate of 1.2%, which was a decrease compared to 1.6% growth rate during the period from 1982 to 1992, as shown in Figure 4-1.

It is evident from the decrease in the population growth rate that Chile places among the four countries with the lowest growth rates in Latin America. With regard to gender distribution, there is a higher percentage of women, 50.7% of the population, compared to 49.3% men. Geographically the largest percentage of the population, 86.6%, is concentrated in urban areas, compared to 13.4% in the rural areas (Encyclopedia of the Nations, 2010).

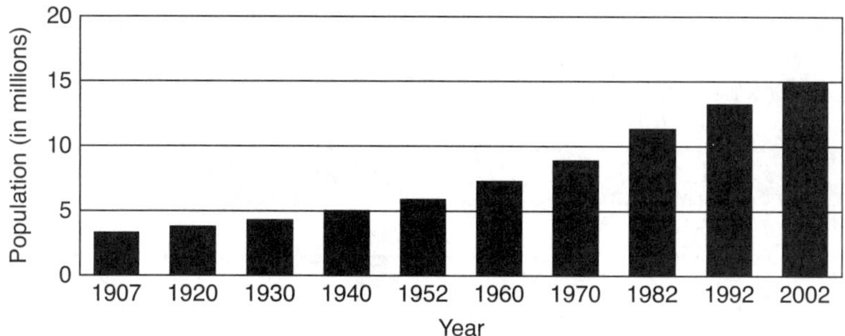


Figure 4-1 Evolution of total population.

Source: Ministerio de Salud. Instituto Nacional de Estadística

The indigenous population of Chile comprises 4.6% of the country's total population according to *Censo* (Health Ministry & National Statistics Institute, 2002). The Mapuche Indians, "people of the earth" who originated in the central-southern part of Chile, represent a majority of the indigenous population at 87.3%, followed by Aimara with 7.0%, and thirdly, the Atacamenian with 3.0%. The Araucanìa region, in southern Chile, contains the majority of the ethnic groups with 23.5%.

In economic terms, Chile is considered one of the most developed countries in Latin America. It is the most important producer of copper in the world, and mining is the main economic sector (Chilean Copper Commission, n.d.). The Corporación del Cobre de Chile, known as Codelco, is a state-owned company that is considered to be the main copper producer in the world. Another state-owned copper company is the Empresa Nacional de Minería. The rest of the copper producers are private companies according to the data from the Chilean Copper Commission (Chilean Copper Commission, n.d.). As shown in Table 4-2, Chile's mining production has grown to over one third of the world's production of copper.

Table 4-2 **Copper Production in Chile and Worldwide, Percentage and Tonnage**

| Year | World mine production | Chile mine production | Chile's share in world production % |
|---|---|---|---|
| | (Thousand metric tons) | (Thousand metric tons) | |
| 1998 | 12,272.7 | 3,686.90 | 30.0% |
| 1999 | 12,749.4 | 4,391.20 | 34.4% |
| 2000 | 13,426.5 | 4,602.0 | 34.7% |
| 2001 | 13,756.7 | 4,739.0 | 34.4% |
| 2002 | 13,565.4 | 4,580.6 | 33.8% |

*continued*

Table 4-2 **Copper Production in Chile and Worldwide, Percentage and Tonnage,** *continued*

| | | | |
|---|---|---|---|
| 2003 | 13,696.1 | 4,904.2 | 35.8% |
| 2004 | 14,721.1 | 5,412.5 | 36.8% |
| 2005 | 15,188.3 | 5,320.5 | 35.0% |
| 2006 | 15,210.4 | 5,360.8 | 35.2% |
| 2007 | 15,649.9 | 5,557.0 | 35.5% |
| 2008 | 15,588.6 | 5,327.9 | 34.20% |

Source: Data obtained from the Chilean Copper Commission, from the World Bureau of Metal Statistics, World Production.

According to data obtained from *Censo* (Health Ministry & National Statistics Institute, 2002), participation in the workforce of Chileans 15 years of age and older reached 52.4% out of a possible 11,226,309 persons. It is noted that men represent approximately 70% and women approximately 35.6% of the labor force of 5,085,885 working people. In addition, 791,264 people are classified as unemployed or looking for work for the first time. It is important to note that the female participation in the labor market increased 7.5% between 1992 and 2002. However, in 2009 due to the global crisis, Chile was among the countries most affected by unemployment, as evidenced by the increase in the unemployment rate. In March of 2009, the unemployment index reached 12.8%. Labor Minister Claudia Serrano, in an interview given to the online newspaper, *Diario Financiero* in 2009, said that the current figures have not been seen since 2003, and the government is ready to fight unemployment ("Concern of government with unemployment figures," 2009). The Central Bank of Chile estimated the loss in gross domestic product (GDP) reached 4.5% in 2009 ("Chile's GDP decreases," 2009). Table 4-3 shows the national GDP per economic activity.

Table 4-3 **Gross Domestic Product per Type of Economic Activity According to Constant Prices in 2003**

| | **2003** | **2004** | **2005** | **2006** | **2007** | **2008** |
|---|---|---|---|---|---|---|
| Agriculture, livestock, forestry | 1,842,431 | 1,994,734 | 2,179,569 | 2,323,865 | 2,333,853 | 2,404,128 |
| Fisheries | 627,436 | 747,248 | 754,244 | 727,576 | 768,203 | 762,779 |
| Mining | 4,321,571 | 4,585,327 | 4,406,826 | 4,436,557 | 4,575,427 | 4,344,725 |
| Copper mining | 3,599,969 | 3,811,802 | 3,624,227 | 3,633,949 | 3,761,566 | 3,544,191 |

*continued*

Table 4-3 **Gross Domestic Product per Type of Economic Activity According to Constant Prices in 2003,** *continued*

| | | | | | | |
|---|---|---|---|---|---|---|
| Other mining | 721.601 | 773.526 | 782.601 | 802.608 | 813.861 | 800,533 |
| Manufacturing | 8,398,990 | 8,985,620 | 9,520,422 | 8,896,183 | 10,200,157 | 10,200,496 |
| Electricity, gas and water | 1,461,211 | 1,501,678 | 1,547,224 | 1,664,079 | 1,185,538 | 1,138,643 |
| Construction | 3,531,382 | 3,645,945 | 4,014,703 | 4,173,722 | 4,401,103 | 4,829,432 |
| Commerce, hotels and restaurants | 4,950,884 | 5,313,188 | 5,764,234 | 6,161,216 | 6,534,117 | 6,781,007 |
| Transport | 3,540,881 | 3,696,506 | 3,945,681 | 4,240,162 | 4,488,016 | 4,713,877 |
| Communications | 1,170,555 | 1,274,305 | 1,367,858 | 1,441,490 | 1,653,202 | 1,824,618 |
| Financial services (1) | 7,650,975 | 8,252,215 | 8,946,350 | 9,352,007 | 10,232,481 | 10,855,502 |
| Home ownership | 2,977,723 | 3,055,12 | 3,156,331 | 3,258,423 | 3,378,072 | 3,508,859 |
| Personal services (2) | 5,911,639 | 6,112,124 | 6,315,977 | 6,549,766 | 6,862,876 | 7,007,882 |
| Public administration | 2,214,718 | 2,264,252 | 2,349,883 | 2,427,451 | 2,514,293 | 2,582,357 |
| SUBTOTAL | 48,600,393 | 51,428,264 | 54,269,302 | 56,652,494 | 59,127,340 | 60,954,305 |
| | | | | | | |
| Less: Bank charges | 1,740,067 | 1,925,667 | 2,225,221 | 2,361,718 | 2,733,927 | 3,004,893 |
| Plus: Net VAI revenue | 3,770,274 | 4,091,626 | 4,422,326 | 4,714,226 | 5,115,528 | 5,435,901 |
| Plus: Import duties | 525.814 | 652.596 | 796.236 | 885.969 | 1,185,142 | 1,291,704 |
| | | | | | | |
| Gross domestic product | 51,156,416 | 54,246,819 | 57,262,645 | 59,890,971 | 62,694,084 | 64,677,016 |

Notes:
(1) Includes financial services, insurance, property rentals, and B2B services.
(2) Includes education, health care, and other services.

Source: Banco Central, dado obtenidos en la Comisión Chilena del Cobre.

Chile has a high level of literacy, equivalent to 95.8% of the population 10 years of age or higher, a number equally distributed between men and women. Comparisons between the census data gathered in 1992 and 2002 indicate that the percent of the population with some higher education increased from 9% to 16% (Health Ministry & National Statistics Institute, 2002).

## Health Promotion in Chile

The Ministry of Health has defined the promotion of health as follows: "the transversal axis of Public Health and inter-sector pro-development action, it is the basis of action intended to get a better quality of life in the country" (Nuñez et al., 2008, p. 94).

In Chile, the concept of health promotion started with the 1997 Program Reform, which had the objective of promoting health by means of preventive actions. One year later the Health Ministry (MINSAL) created the Health Promotion Department. The focus of the Health Promotion Department is to achieve changes in lifestyle and the creation of a healthy environment, actively involving all Chilean society. Its approach is characterized by a participative and decentralized method of assessing and adapting programs according to the reality and needs of every region. The Health Promotion Department has the proper legal framework and funding to transcend government administrations and a solid foundation of agreed-upon goals to look after well-being. It also proposes to actively involve the population in seeking health and quality of life. In 1999, led by MINSAL and with the participation of 28 integrated institutions, the National Council for Health Promotion, also known as Vida Chile, was established. Health policies were elaborated and addressed by the National Council for Health Promotion to meet the needs of the population. In this context, in 1998 the First Chilean Congress of Health Promotion presented the slogan "For a healthy country." Through these government actions, promotion of Chilean health came to be established as a national policy financially supported by the government (Nuñez et al., 2008).

As an innovative strategy, MINSAL conducted the First National Life Quality and Health Survey in 2000 (Health Ministry & National Statistics Institute, 2000), in order to establish conditions, assess impact of actions to compare results achieved, and generate inputs for the formulation of sanitary objectives for the decade (2000–2010). In 2006, this survey was conducted for a second time (Health Ministry & National Statistics Institute, 2006). The most important goals were the discernment of the economic, social, and cultural factors related to Chileans' quality of health and life conditions and the development of a facilitating tool for the identification of health conditions in the country. The National Health Survey became a key element for the planning and assessment of health programs for the Chilean population. The significance of chronic diseases became apparent as the main element responsible for death and incapacity.

## Prevailing Health Issues and Risk Behaviors

Chile is in a prestigious position regarding life expectancy, according to the research prepared by the National Statistics Institute (INE) (Health Ministry & National Statistics Institute, 2002). The life expectancy is 80.4 years for women and 74.4 years for men, with an overall average of 77.4 years. There are similar results in Costa Rica and Cuba, with 77.3 and 76.7 years for women and men respectively, thus ranking Chile among the three countries with the highest life expectancy in Latin America. Chile's Coquimbo region holds the highest index with 78.43 years followed by Santiago with 77.86 years; Antofagasta with 75.3 years and Magallanes with 75.7 have the lowest indexes. However, there is no significant variation among the regions. Infant mortality showed a decrease of 41% in the last decade; however, while significant progress has been made in this area, the infant mortality rate remains 8.5 per 1,000 live births.

According to the World Health Organization (WHO), there have been several demographic and sanitary changes in the Chilean population during the last century. During the last 50 years there was a decrease on infant and mother mortality, malnutrition has almost disappeared, and there was also a reduction of infectious diseases; however, there were new challenges in the elderly population, and therefore an increase in nontransmissible chronic diseases. The last national survey for Quality of Life and Health (Health Ministry National Statistics Institute, 2006), showed that nontransmissible chronic disease affects 25% of the Chilean adult population and that more than 50% of the elderly population has high cardiovascular risk, with a significant rate of high blood pressure, dyslipidemia, predominantly unhealthy lifestyles, and an increase in smoking, sedentary lifestyles, and obesity. These statistics are shown in Figure 4-2.

Concerned with the National Plan of Health Promotion, Vida Chile, in agreement with WHO, proposed strategies according to the population needs and epidemiology profile and established four disease groups: cardiovascular (the main cause of death in Chile), mental problems, accidents, and cancer. In addition, five conditioning factors were established: eating habits, tobacco, physical activities, psychological-social protection factors, and environmental factors (Health Ministry National Statistics Institute, 2003).

In 2000, MINSAL and Vida Chile set goals for 2010, established objectives to stop the increase of risk factors, and developed health, psychological-social, and environmental protection factors, fostering citizen participation and strengthening social networks. At the same time, they reinforced the state's responsibility in overseeing the conditioning factors of health and creating public health policies and life quality, thereby creating a great challenge for the country (Crovetto & Vio del Rio, 2009). Results determining whether these targets have been met were to be assessed at the end of 2010.

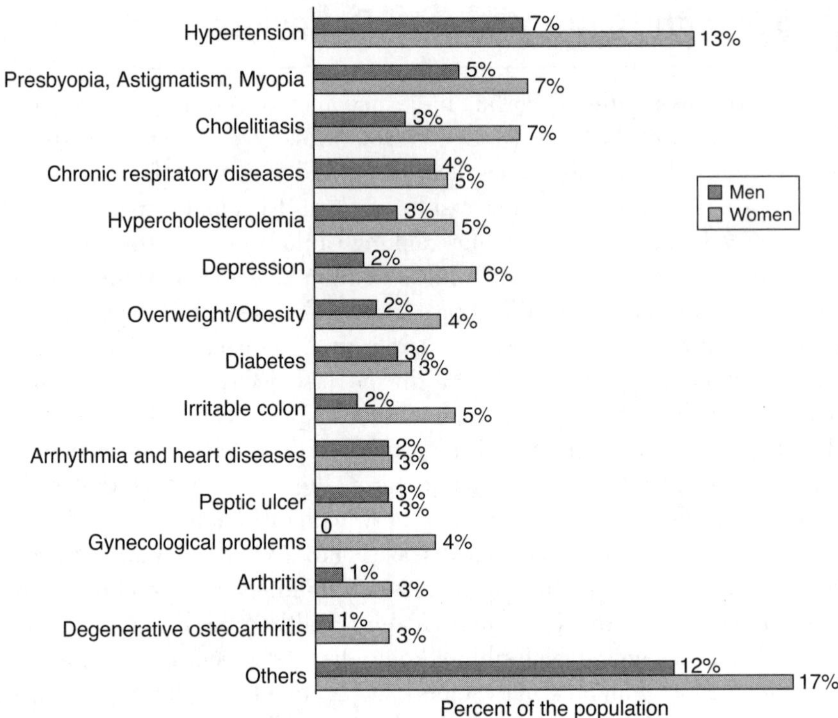


Figure 4-2 Declared morbidity – prevailing chronic diseases according to gender.
Source: Ministerio de Salud. Instituto Nacional de Estadística

# Healthcare System

Health is a basic right for all citizens, as declared in the Chilean constitution (Montes & Ugas, 2008). The indicators of the population's health status places Chile among the best on the continent and very close to developed countries; nonetheless, Chile has been heavily criticized for its public health system. For Gambi (2005), there is an association between the effects of health and poverty; every time a person gets sick, he/she faces increasing difficulties to work and make an income. Thus, failing health affects the level of poverty.

In Chile, the insurance companies are responsible for providing health coverage and are divided into two groups: public, known as National Health Fund (FONASA) and private insurance companies (ISAPRE). Each worker contributes 7% from his or her salary, and is responsible for choosing one system (Health Ministry, 2009).

## National Health Fund

The National Health Fund (FONASA) provides health services at public clinics or hospitals, and depending upon the member's income, the complementary payment varies from 25 to

50% of the value. Under the free choice system, the user can choose a private health service registered at FONASA, but the complementary payment is higher and will depend upon the price assigned by the health provider. FONASA also takes care of those who lack funds through direct government support (Health Ministry, 1985)

Law 18.469, known as FONASA Law (Health Ministry, 1985) reflects the constitutional right to health protection and creates a special regime of health coverage. It establishes in Article 1, "The constitutional right to health protection involves free and equal access to the promotion, protection, and health recovery actions and to those focused on the rehabilitation of individuals, as well as freedom to choose the state or private health system to which any person would like to adhere to" (Health Ministry, 1985).

FONASA provides insurance to four groups of people classified according to their income level (Health Ministry, 1985; Health Ministry, 2009) as listed below:

- *Group A:* Indigent or poor people who benefit from family welfare and pensions. People with no income belong to this group.
- *Group B:* Members whose monthly income does not exceed the minimum monthly salary (less or equivalent to 165,000 Chilean pesos), applicable to workers more than 18 years old and younger than 65.
- *Group C:* Members whose salary is higher than minimum monthly salary (higher than 165,000 Chilean pesos), applicable to workers between 18 and 65 years old who do not exceed 1.46 times the minimum salary (in other words, who earn less than or equal to 240,900 Chilean pesos per month), except when benefits include three or more dependants; in such case they will be in Group B.
- *Group D:* Members whose monthly income is higher than 1.46 times the minimum monthly salary (higher than 240,900 Chilean pesos), applicable to workers between 18 and 65 years old, provided they have no more than two dependants. If dependants benefited are three or more, they will be included in Group C.

Persons under Groups C and D have the option to use private health providers.

## Private Health Insurance

Persons within Groups C and D can pay an additional amount to increase the variety of services or to lower the complementary payments.

Schwartzmann (2003) describes the 1990s as characterized by an increase in technological advances, family problems, loss of motivation, stress, and other factors, yet on the other hand, an increase in longevity, but not necessarily improvement in life quality. Starting from that point, the health-related concept of life quality began to be used to assess results in health. It is valid, reliable, and scientifically based, and associates results to quantitative indicators such as mortality, morbidity, expectations, and costs, without excluding the perception of users.

The research performed by FONASA, published by Director Hernán Monasterio in the online newspaper *Crónica Digital* (2003) estimated that approximately 1 million Chilean citizens, equivalent to 7.3% of the population, must pay their health costs on their own, lacking health coverage, regardless of their socioeconomic position ("One Million Chileans," 2003).

### AUGE Plan

The Universal Access for Comprehensive Attention and Explicit Health Guarantees, or the AUGE-GES Plan, is a comprehensive health system that benefits all Chilean people, regardless of age, gender, socioeconomic condition, or health system to which they adhere. The Health Ministry, by means of a sanitary regulation instrument, the Health Guarantee Regime, accounts for this plan. The AUGE includes highly complex diseases that are costly and that present high impact on health. Covering all stages of illness, it guarantees access to quality health attention. The first stage began by providing guaranteed access coverage for three health problems in the year 2002 and increased coverage for a total of 56 illnesses in 2007. Persons who receive benefits must be insured by FONASA or a private ISAPRE. In the year 2005, the AUGE law was approved and established, guaranteeing health benefits, prompt access, quality care, and financial protection to all Chileans (Health Ministry, n.d. b).

## Influence of Culture and Mentality

Chile has a cultural, social, and economic dynamic that fosters unhealthy lifestyles. It is a country with increasing technological and environmental changes, which cause favorable results in the increase of life expectancy, as well as sanitary improvements, reduction of infectious diseases, and so on; however, there have been negative impacts on the lifestyle of the population. The economic factors trigger a high consumption of fast food, rich in fat, saturated fat, calories, and high sodium content, along with easy access to the purchase of goods such as cars, televisions, and computers that directly relate to reduction of physical activity. Thus, obesity rates are increasing and becoming a great challenge for Chilean public health. A research study performed among students from the Pontificia Universidad Católica de Valparaíso (Macmillan, 2007), led to the conclusion that there is low consumption of fruits, vegetables, dairy products, and fish by most of the population. On the contrary, there is much sedentary behavior and excessive consumption of sugar and fat. This is reflected in the high levels of overweight classification in the college population, which are similar to the rates in other social groups such as children and workers.

Another important factor in Chilean culture is lack of time, expressed by high indexes of required hours or overtime at the workplace compared to developed countries, equivalent to over 100 overtime days a year. According to Diaz and Figueroa (2008), overtime is justified to counteract the high level of debts, for social promotion, or to complement insufficient income.

However, the impact of extended work hours must be examined as it relates to quality of life, and, in particular, the close link between extended work hours and the quality of family life, especially in regards to women's participation in the labor market. According to the last census (Health Ministry & National Statistics Institute, 2002), female participation in the labor market increased 7.5% compared to the census in 1992, and male participation had a decrease of 1.5% in the same period. Due to this change, the potential for conflict between family and work is higher. Considering that family and work are the main sources of well-being and satisfaction of people, they are the fundamental pillars of the life quality assessment. However, there are company actions that foster these negative conditions.

## Drivers of Workplace Health Promotion

Within the stage of human development known as the economically active age, Chilean individuals take part in production and go into the labor force. This corresponds to half of the life span of humans, and generally they spend one third of the day doing work-related activities. Considering the importance of work–life balance in the promotion of health, in 2002 the government introduced the concept of health promotion in the workplaces through the National Council for Promotion of Health, Vida Chile. *Healthy Life in the Company: Practical Guide for Companies* (Calderon, Salinas, & Vio, 2004) was created, with the assistance from the Ministry of Health, the Nutrition and Technology Institute of Food (INTA–Universidad de Chile), the Fundación Acción Empresarial, and other experts. The guide was prepared in a participative manner and written in a didactic style, highlighting concepts, methodology, and recommendations for interventions to promote health and healthier lifestyles within the working environment.

In 2005, the regional sanitary authorities incorporated the implementation of the concept health-promoting workplaces to approximately 100 public and private companies. The main objectives were to reduce smoking, obesity, and sedentary behavior; train employers and employees in the implementation of health policies; create a health sector within the work environment; foster support networks; and identify risk and protection factors. Of course these programs brought improvements to workers' health, but the results for companies were even better, as expressed by a better corporate image, decrease of health expenses, decrease of absence, better work climate, improved motivation and commitment from employees to the company, and positive results in production.

The Chilean government, through the National Service of Training and Employment, supported by Law 19967, under Ministry of Work and Social Prevention (2004), fosters the use of tax exemption as a tool to incentivize companies to invest in training for their workers. Therefore, there is a discount in the amount payable to the Internal Revenue Service, that will depend on payroll (Table 4-4) and the training executed by a technical training organization (Labor Secretary, 1998).

Table 4-4 **Payroll and Tax Exemption for Training Workers**

| Annual payroll | Amount to be discounted |
|---|---|
| From 0 to 34.99 UTM | 0 UTM |
| From 35.00 to 44.99 UTM | 7 UTM |
| From 45.00 to 900 UTM | 9 UTM |
| From 900.01 UTM | 1% of annual payroll |

1 UTM=30,825 Chilean pesos

Another benefit established for Chilean workers is the obligation of social security against work accidents and occupational illnesses, supported by Law 16.744 approved in 1968 (Labor and Social Security Ministry, 2005). This benefit is administered by entities in charge of managing the social security for work accidents: Mutual de Seguridad de la Cámara Chilena de la Construcción, Asociación Chilena de Seguridad e Instituto de Seguridad del Trabajo (private institutions) and by the public system managed by the Instituto de Normalización Previsional. Payment of this benefit is performed by the employer, and it is independent from the health insurance system (ISAPRE or FONASA).

The Chilean government acknowledges the importance of implementation of health policies for workers within workplaces. However, there has been little development in this area.

## Programs and Good Practices

The Vida Chile program was launched with the challenge to create a state policy for health promotion. Its main characteristic was to be an intersector and participative model with the main objective of achieving positive changes in lifestyle and healthy work environments, actively involving the Chilean society. The program has a proper legal framework and funding and transcends government administrations. It started from agreed-upon goals for the search of common well-being, assuming the task of actively involving the population with quality of life and health issues and emphasizing healthier eating habits and a more active lifestyle. The National Plan for the Promotion of Health and Vida Chile launched the Communication Campaign, "Building a Healthier Country."

## Public Policies for Health Promotion in Chile

### Vida Chile

As mentioned previously, Vida Chile has developed a health promotion policy and some important programs. These include:

- Programs for the accreditation of healthy schools, implemented by the Junta Nacional de Jardines Infantiles, Junta Nacional de Auxilio Escolar y Becas, and Fundación INTEGRA (focused on the comprehensive development of children who live in poverty), with the support of the Education Ministry.
- Promotion of physical activity, including guidelines for active life that were created and developed in conjunction with Chile Deportes and the Instituto de Nutrición y Tecnología de Alimentos de la Universidad de Chile.
- Creation of tobacco-free environments with the Chilean Society of Respiratory Diseases and the health network.
- Recovery of public spaces performed by the Housing Ministry.
- Citizen participation performed by the Government General Secretary Ministry through the Social Organizations Division.
- Training of human resources through nongovernmental organizations and universities.

### Global Strategy Against Obesity

Obesity is a relevant subject not only in Chile, but the WHO is also concerned with the increase in the obesity rate worldwide, and has proposed strategies for healthy eating habits and physical activity. The Global Strategy Against Obesity program (Health Ministry, 2005) was developed in Chile in July 2006. It aims to decrease the prevailing obesity in all stages of life, taking into account social and cultural determining factors and fostering healthy eating habits and physical activity. The program is an initiative to provide new strategies and actions to control the problem.

### Antitobacco Law

Law 19.419, known as the antitobacco or antivice law, was established in 1995 (Public Health Ministry, Law 19.419 of 1995), although the WHO recommended more strict actions than those legally established in Chile. Chile has a light legislation that is not respected by the population and is not enforced by the authorities. One example is that Chile has the highest consumption of tobacco among teenagers in the world, with a consumption index close to 70% at the age of 15, despite legal prohibitions against tobacco advertisements located less than 300 meters from schools and against selling tobacco to people under 18 (Health Ministry, n.d. a). There is also a law that regulates the tobacco consumption in public places such as companies, restaurants, entertainment facilities, etc.

### Preventive Medicine Test

The Preventive Medicine Test was developed in 2005, and it is already included in the AUGE Plan (Health Ministry, n.d. b) with free and voluntary coverage for all members of FONASA and ISAPRE. The objective is the prevention and early detection of diseases and reduction and control of the morbidity and mortality rates. It covers lab tests, physical evaluations, and questionnaires and establishes protocols and definitions for the most frequent diseases in each stage of life (Health Ministry, n.d. a).

## Companies and Quality of Life

Some companies concerned with the health of workers developed programs that focused on fostering quality of life and healthy habits of their employees. Starting from qualitative exploratory research (as described in the *Guideline for Healthy Policies at the Work Place* developed by the Health Ministry), companies selected health promotion practices to evaluate, taking into account knowledge of the successful implementation of health promotion programs at workplaces. They also considered the objectives of the National Promotion Plan, which are to reduce obesity rates, sedentary lifestyle, and smoking, and to foster protection factors. The research was performed in the year 2005; however, compliance with regulations was not considered. Five companies were selected: two from the private sector (Compañía Minera Cerro Colorado and Banco de Chile) and three public companies (Empresa Nacional del Petróleo, Centro de Atención Primaria de Salud Municipal, and Hospital Público) (Salinas, 2005).

### Company 1: Compañía Minera Cerro Colorado (Private Level)

Minera Cerro Colorado, located in the first region of Chile, Región de Tarapacá, has developed the program "Living Healthy" due to the increase of overweight and obesity of its employees. The company wants to improve quality of life and promote healthy lifestyles to avoid or decrease influence of nontransmissible chronic diseases on 1,200 employees and families. The program started with the restructuring of company food services, then the implementation of a gymnasium, an occupational health assessment program focused on the detection and prevention of nontransmissible chronic diseases, and control of smoking. All programs follow objectives set by the Chile Vida Council. The company has an executive committee formed by health and safety managers, environment and community managers, human resources, and mine managers, as well as a technical committee.

Other psychological and social activities have been performed, such as an education and scholarship program for sons and daughters of employees; current information on health topics by means of the monthly magazine, intranet, and bulletin boards; and funding of environmental projects.

### *Healthy Eating Habits Program*

In order to provide healthy food in the company's cafeteria, an initial assessment is performed, where each employee can choose foods based on his/her preference and caloric requirements in accordance with the Food Pyramid recommendations. Also, there are periodic education campaigns through workshops and publications.

### *Physical Activity Program*

With the objective of reducing sedentary lifestyle, the company built a gymnasium including a tennis court, soccer field, and trekking circuit. The gym also offers different training classes and the annual Mining Olympics. All activities have free access and the gym has a permanent team of instructors and trainers.

### *Tobacco, Alcohol, and Drugs Program*

Creating a tobacco-free environment was signed as a company policy in 2004. In addition, there were education campaigns, the creation of smoking spaces, and free treatment for those trying to quit smoking.

### *Preventive Tests Program*

Preventive health tests are conducted every 2 years. These tests are aimed at both the early diagnosis of individual risk factors and to prepare an analysis of the company's profile of cardiovascular risk.

## Company 2: Empresa Nacional de Petróleo (Public Level)

Empresa Nacional de Petróleo, located in Punta Arenas, extracts and refines oil. Its approximately 1,200 employees show high overweight and obesity rates, and 35% of the staff has smoking habits. In 1999, the program known as "Healthy Lifestyle Policy" was started due to company concern for improving the biologic, psychologic, and social well-being of the workers. Thus, based on the public health policy, a two-pronged approach was established. The first prong focused on preventive medicine, and the second focused on health promotion—both associated with risk and protection factors.

### *Cardiovascular Risk Prevention Program*

As part of a prevention program, the employee undertakes a preventive health test to diagnose cardiovascular risk, detect other existing risk factors, and determine individual and family education actions regarding healthy food and physical activity.

### *Activation and Pause Gymnastics*

Specialized occupational gymnastics programs are provided; different activities have different objectives. Activation gymnastics starts at the beginning of the work shift and prepares workers' muscles for work activities. It also provides social interaction with other members in the group. As a result, this gymnastics program creates a better work environment, better posture for participants, and improved quality of rest. These gymnastic activities are executed in short pauses during work hours.

***Program for Promotion of Tobacco-Free Environments***

This program is part of the company policy established by the Hygiene and Safety Joint Committee; it presents educational activities to sensitize employees and families to health risks of alcohol, tobacco, and other drugs. Preoccupational tests are performed to detect drugs and alcohol. In addition, random tests are given in cases of accidents that are under suspicion of substance abuse or at the request of the human resources department. Should it be necessary to put a worker under treatment and rehabilitation, this is paid for by the company for a period up to 2 years.

### Company 3: Promondo Capacitación LTDA

With the mission of improving the health quality and quality of life of workers, Promondo founder and current executive director Volney Vasquez began the development of health promotion programs in different companies throughout the country in 1990. These programs have a team of physical education teachers as well as a health team. The program is divided into three main areas: physical, mental, and social.

1. *Physical:* Develops physical activity programs such as occupational gymnastics, exercises and nutrition assistance, chiro-massage, implementation of corporate gymnasium, ergonomics programs, medical assessment (preventive medicine), and assistance to the company restaurant and monitoring of risk group.
2. *Mental:* Programs for management of work stress and prevention of addictions.
3. *Social:* Recreational programs such as winter and summer camps, adventure sports, corporate Olympics, events, parties, etc.

Promondo, as a pioneer of quality of life in Chile, created software called Organizational Health Administrator (also known as ASO system), which is an innovative tool in the domestic market. Employees and companies registered as Promondo members have access to information including historical body mass index measurements, attendance records, and control of nontransmissible chronic diseases; and resources such as the assessment of physical conditions and flexibility, etc. This tool provides a fundamental support for workers' health management and quality of life.

## Outcomes and Indicators

Indicators for measuring the impact of health promotion programs have become an extremely relevant issue, and professionals have started debating and discussing this issue at length.

Although there is no evaluation scale to follow in Chile, there have been some studies about work absence and work accident rates; however, a study for presenteeism was not found. Some companies are trying to measure the impact using the return on investment (ROI) model.

## Work Absence

In Chile, the cost of work absence does not represent a direct cost for companies; it is garnished from the worker's wages, except for the death of son/daughter or spouse (7 days in a row), infant mortality during pregnancy, or the death of a parent of the worker (3 working days of leave). These exceptions are considered paid leave included in the Labor Code, article 66 of law 20.137, published in the Official Journal dated on December 16, 2006. However, we cannot say that the cost of work absence is totally absorbed by the health system, as it only pays for the lost day of the worker. We must consider the company point of view that the indirect costs must also be considered, i.e. the temporary replacement of worker for the time of absence.

A research study published in the *Chile Medical Magazine* (2004) shows a review analysis of papers concerning the last 30 years of work absence in Chile, collected from 14 theses and scientific papers. A universally accepted methodology was used to analyze absenteeism and medical leave, including the frequency, duration, and the causes. The article emphasizes the big challenge for the country in terms of possible changes to the medical leave system. Currently, payment comes from the health system from the 4th day on, and the first 3 days are not covered by the system. However, the cause of the medical leave determines who will fund it, who will pay it, and who will supervise it, as can be seen in Table 4-5.

Table 4-5 **Types, Funding Entities, Paying Entities, and Regulatory Entities of Medical Leaves**

| Type of medical leave | Funding | Paying organization | Supervising organization |
|---|---|---|---|
| Prenatal and postnatal leave | State through the Unique Fund of Family Attention | Employer ISAPRE COMPIN* Indemnity Fund | ISAPRE COMPIN |
| Leave for sick child less than 1 year old | State through the Unique Fund of Family Attention | Employer ISAPRE COMPIN Indemnity Fund | ISAPRE COMPIN |
| Leave due to common disease or healing leave | ISAPRE FONASA | Employer ISAPRE COMPIN Indemnity Fund | ISAPRE COMPIN |

*Medical Comission for Prevention and Disability

** Institute for Provisional Normalization

Source: Mesa, F., & Kaempffer, A. (2004). 30 years of study about work absence in Chile: A perspective per type of company. *Chile Medical Magazine, 132(9)*, 1100–1108.

Mesa and Kaempffer (2004) concluded that the hospital sector had the largest number of studies about the subject of medical leave and represented the highest rates of leave in the sector. However, as there was only one documented study in the industrial sector, there is no way to compare the data found. Nonetheless, it can be asserted that mining had the greatest rates of work absence compared to other industrial sectors. Included in the study was information about the most frequent pathologies across all sectors studied, and in most cases it was confirmed that respiratory, osteomuscular, and trauma diseases prevail.

Chile had a national incapacity rate of 5 days per worker in 1999, reflecting an increase of 16% in 9 years compared to 1990 when the rate was 4.3 days; however, it is still a low indicator compared to other countries. Table 4-6 shows the results obtained per each sector studied. Incapacity rate (TI) corresponds to the average number of days absent per worker due to medical leave; the frequency rate (TF) is defined as the average number of days of healing medical leave presented by a worker during 1 year, and the severity rate (TS) corresponds to the average duration of medical leaves analyzed in a work population (Mesa & Kaempffer, 2004).

Table 4-6 **Incapacity, Frequency, and Severity Rates Classified per Sector**

| Sector | Number of studies performed | Publication year(s) | Average TI | Average TF | Average TS |
|---|---|---|---|---|---|
| Hospital | 6 | 1989/1996/1996/1992/1998 | 14.3 | 1.3 | 10.6 |
| Mining | 3 | 1993/1989/2001 | 12 | 1.3 | 8.7 |
| Industrial | 1 | 1987 | 7.1 | 0.6 | 8.2 |
| Universities and research centers | 3 | 1989/1991/1998 | 6.2 | 0.7 | 8.2 |

Source: Data obtained from Mesa, F., & Kaempffer, A. (2004). 30 years of study about work absence in Chile: A perspective per type of company. *Chile Medical Magazine, 132(9),* 1100–1108.

## Work Accidents

Work accidents and occupational illnesses in Chile recently account for approximately 7% a year, corresponding to 3,223,388 work days in 2005; this represents significant data compared to results obtained in the last century, with a rate of 32%. Men account for 80% of all lost days from work due to work accidents, with the majority being allocated to construction, agriculture, and the manufacturing industry (Guzmán, 2006).

The government, along with other representatives, signed the National Agreement of Work Accidents Prevention (2005–2010), which established strategies aimed to introduce cultural changes and internalize the concept of work safety across economic sectors. In addition, in

1997, the International Labor Organization established a project with the purpose of creating policies and programs along with the labor ministry. The agreement has been effective, mainly with the elaboration of Law 16.744 and the extension of accident surveillance (Guzmán, 2006).

According to Guzmán (2006), drug and alcohol consumption is an important issue that corresponds to 25% of accidents reported. Drug and alcohol consumption is directly related to reduced productivity, especially as a factor in the increase of accidents, as well as the increase of medical leave (absence). However, little is being done to address these problems; only 5% of Chilean companies have specific programs related to this issue.

## Existing Research

Several cost-benefit studies have been developed in Chile, mainly addressing the medical sector, cancer dissemination, and vesicle and other diseases; however, little has been done in health promotion. An experimental case study (the first in the country) was designed and implemented between 1990 and 1999 to address the concern of unhealthy lifestyles among the Chilean population. The survey was conducted by the department of the Universidad Católica de Chile that created the Mírame program, which presents health promotion strategies intended to promote healthy habits in the students and their families. The study was conducted in the Metropolitan Region, represented by five communities, with students from the fifth and sixth grade levels. Measurements were conducted comparing pre- and postintervention results with the program cost at $11.7 per student, which is a very low cost for prevention compared to the high cost of treating addictions. According to the survey done by Universidad Católica de Chile, treatment costs for 2 years are approximately U.S. $2,750,000 for alcohol, U.S. $3,350,000 for drugs, and U.S. $1,000,000 for tobacco. It should also be noted that the emotional, psychological, and family factors were not measured; however, these are important aspects to be considered in a future study (Berríos, Bedregal, & Guzmán, 2004).

## Conclusion

It is urgent to create a culture that strongly promotes healthy lifestyles, not only in Chile but in other countries as well. There is no doubt there are difficulties in obtaining positive results because of the economic model of the country, the idiosyncrasies of its population, and the expectations and needs of the citizens. Both the state and private sector should play a more active role in taking responsibility for promoting health and quality of life. The duration of work hours must be reviewed in light of work–family relationships, health benefits, and well-being in the job position and work environment. Finally, tax benefits from the government to educate the population on health issues must also be reviewed and analyzed.

## Summary

Chile is considered one of the most developed countries in Latin America. Chile is well known for its economic stability and is the most important copper producer in the world. Chile has a high literacy rate, has shown significant improvement in the reduction of infant mortality and malnutrition, and has made numerous technological advances that have been favorable for national development. However, in spite of these positive changes, Chile has shown some negative trends, including a decrease in the growth rate of the population. Its people have been attracted to fast food (junk food), and they lack personal time. Due to extended working hours—considered one of the longest work shifts in the world—there have been many changes in people's eating patterns, as well as a high rate of sedentary habits, overweight and obesity issues, and a significant increase of nontransmissible chronic diseases among children and adults. Organizations concerned by these changes determined that health priorities should be a goal for the period 2000–2010, with a primary focus on preventing and treating cardiovascular diseases, the main cause of death.

The challenge of promoting health in Chile is no longer a concern only for the public health sector; today, private companies concerned by productivity and reduction of medical costs have implemented health policies for their employees.

## Review Questions

1. What is the main economic sector of Chile and what impact (if any) does it have on health?
2. Describe the focus of the Health Promotion Department within the Health Ministry of Chile.
3. Explain the initial purpose and ultimate outcome of the First National Life Quality and Health Survey.
4. List the prevailing health issues and risk behaviors that are the focus of MINSAL and Vida Chile.
5. Describe the two groups responsible for providing health coverage in Chile.
6. How does the Chilean culture affect population health and workplace health promotion efforts?
7. Explain the Global Strategy Against Obesity program.
8. What is the name of the evaluation scale used for measuring the impact of health promotion programs in Chile?

# References


Berríos, M., Bedregal, P., & Guzmán, B. (2004). Cost-effectiveness of health promotion in Chile: Experience of the "MIRAME!" program. *Revista Médica de Chile, 132,* 361–370. Retrieved October 2009 from http://www.scielo.cl/pdf/rmc/v132n3/art13.pdf

Calderón, B., Salinas, J., & Vio, F. (Eds.). (2004). *Healthy life in the company: Practical guide for companies*. Santiago, Chile: Health Ministry, INTA Universidad de Chile, Consejo Nacional Vida Chile, & Acción RSE.

Chilean Copper Commission. (n.d.). *Main mining companies.* Retrieved September 2009 from http://www.cochilco.cl/atencion_usuario/prin_empresas.asp

Chile's GDP decreases 4.5% in second quarter. (2009, August 18). *América Economía: Finance*. Retrieved August 2009 from http://www.americaeconomia.com/322308-PIB-de-Chile-cae-45-en-segundo- trimestre.note.aspx

Concern of government with unemployment figures. (2009, April 23). *Diario Financiero Online: Economics*. Retrieved August 2009 from http://df.cl/portal2/content/df/ediciones/20090423/cont_110822.html

Crovetto, M. M., & Vio del Rio, F. (2009). International and national background of health promotion in Chile: Lessons learned and future projections. *Rev Chi Nutr, 36*(1), 32–45.

Diaz, E., & Figueroa, A. (2008). Work factors of balance between work and family. *Rev. Universum, 23*(1), 116–133. Retrieved September 2009 from http://www.scielo.cl/pdf/universum/v23n1/art07.pdf

Encyclopedia of the Nations. (2010). Retrieved August 2009 from http://www.nationsencyclopedia.com/economies/Americas/Chile.html

Gambi, M. (2005). Access to health in Chile. *Bioethics Act, 11*(1), 47–64. Retrieved August 2009 from http://www.scielo.cl/scielo.php?script=sci_arttext&pid=S1726-569X2005000100006&lng=es&nrm=iso

Guzmán L. (2006). Work accidents in Chile: 3 million days lost. *Ciencia y Trabajo, 19*, A20–A24. Retrieved September 2009 from http://www.cienciaytrabajo.cl/pdfs/19/pagina%20a20.pdf

Health Ministry. (1985, November 23). Ley Fonasa Nº 18.469 de 1985. Retrieved September 2009 from http://www.supersalud.cl/normativa/571/article-556.html#h2_2

Health Ministry. (2005, December). *Global strategies against obesity (EGO—Chile)* [Work Document].

Health Ministry. (2009). *National Health Fund. (FONASA).* Retrieved August 2009 from http://www.fonasa.cl/prontus_fonasa/antialone.html?page=http://www.fonasa.cl/prontusfonasa/site/artic/20041219/pags/20041219235847.html

Health Ministry. (n.d. a). *Clinical guideline for preventive medicine test.* Retrieved September 2009 from http://www.supersalud.cl/568/articles-974_guia.pdf

Health Ministry. (n.d. b). *Universal access for comprehensive attention and explicit health guarantee: Plan AUGE.* Retrieved September 2009 from http://www.enredsalud.cl/?idcategoria=400

Health Ministry National Statistics Institute. (2003). *Main death causes in Chile* by region. Retrieved August 2009 from http://www.ine.cl/canales/chile_estadistico/demografia_y_vitales/estadisticas_vitales/pdf/causas_de_muerte_regiones%202003.pdf

Health Ministry & National Statistics Institute. (2000). *First national survey of quality of life and health*. Retrieved August 2009 from http://www.ine.cl/canales/chile_estadistico/calidad_de_vida_y_salud/calidadvida/informefamiliar.pdf

Health Ministry & National Statistics Institute. (2002). *Censo.* Retrieved August 2009 from http://www.ine.cl/cd2002/sintesiscensal.pdf

Health Ministry & National Statistics Institute. (2006). *Second national survey of quality of life and health.* Retrieved September 2009 from http://epi.minsal.cl/epi/html/sdesalud/calidaddevida2006/Informe%20Final%2 Encuesta%20de%20Calidad%20de%20Vida%20y%20Salud%202006.pdf

Labor Secretary. (1998). National Service of Training and Employment (SENCE): Ley Nº 19.518 de 1998. Retrieved September 2009 from http://www.mesadiscapacidad.cl/leyes/Ley_Nro_19518_SENCE.pdf

Labor and Social Security Ministry. (2005). Social Security Against Work Accidents and Occupational Illnesses. Law 16744 of 2005. Retrieved September 2009 from http://www.sinteci.cl/laboral/legislacion/Ley_16744.pdf

Macmillan, N. (2007). Valorization of eating habits, physical activities, and nutritional conditions in students at the Pontificia Universidad Católica de Valparaíso. *Rev Chil Nutr, 4*, 330–336. Retrieved September 2009 from http://www.scielo.cl/scielo.php?script=sci_arttext&pid=S07177518 2007000400006

Mesa, F., & Kaempffer, A. (2004). 30 years of study about work absence in Chile: A perspective per type of company. *Rev Méd Chile, 132*(9), 1100–1108. Retrieved September 2009 from http://www.scielo.cl/scielo.php?script=sci_arttext&pid=S0034-98872004000900012&lang=pt

Montes, C., & Ugas, A. (2008). Principle of justice and health in Chile. *Bioethics Act, 14*(2), 206–211. Retrieved September 2009 from http://www.scielo.cl/scielo.php?pid=S1726569X2008000200011&script=sci_arttext

Nuñez, G. et al. (2008). *Quality of life and health in Chile: Challenges for health promotion*. Santiago, Chile: Government of Chile.

One million Chileans do not have health coverage. (2003, August 6). *Santiago de Chile (Crónica Digital)*. Retrieved August 2009 from http://www.cronicadigital.cl/modules.php?name=News&file=article&sid=4827

Public Health Ministry. (1995). Regulation of Activities Related to Tobacco. Law 19419 of 1995. Retrieved September 2009 from http://www.minsal.cl/ici/tabaco/LEY_19419.doc

Salinas, J. (Ed.). (2005). *Building policies at the work place: Contribution from 5 experiences.* Santiago. Health Ministry, MINSAL/Consejo Nacional Vida Chile.

Schwartzmann, L. (2003). Life quality related to health: Concept aspects. *Ciencia y Enfermería, 9* (2), 9–21. Retrieved September 2009 from http://www.scielo.cl/scielo.php?script=sci_arttext&pid=S0717-95532003000200002&lang=pt

University Selection Test—PSU. (n.d.). *History and social sciences.* Retrieved August 2009 from http://www.saladehistoria.com/Preu/GM802.pdf

Chapter 5

# China

Jian Li and Wei-Qing Chen

After reading this chapter you should be able to:

- Identify core strategies that are the focus of mainland China's workplace health promotion efforts
- Describe the historical evolution of workplace health promotion efforts on mainland China
- Explain the different approaches employed by corporate health promotion throughout mainland China
- Review the central disease states and health issues driving mainland China's health promotion needs
- Name the components of, and the associated funding sources for, the Chinese healthcare system
- Discuss the impact of Chinese culture on mainland China's health status and health promotion efforts

Table 5-1 **Select Key Demographic and Economic Indicators**

| | |
|---|---|
| Nationality | Noun: Chinese (singular and plural)<br>Adjective: Chinese |
| Ethnic groups | Han Chinese 91.5%, Zhuang, Manchu, Hui, Miao, Uyghur, Tujia, Yi, Mongol, Tibetan, Buyi, Dong, Yao, Korean, and other nationalities 8.5% (2000 census) |
| Religion | Daoist (Taoist), Buddhist, Christian 3%–4%, Muslim 1%–2%<br>*Note:* officially atheist (2002 est.) |
| Language | Standard Chinese or Mandarin (Putonghua, based on the Beijing dialect), Yue (Cantonese), Wu (Shanghainese), Minbei (Fuzhou), Minnan (Hokkien-Taiwanese), Xiang, Gan, Hakka dialects, minority languages (see Ethnic groups entry) |
| Literacy | Definition: age 15 and over can read and write<br>Total population: 91.6%<br>Male: 95.7%<br>Female: 87.6% (2007 census) |

*continued*

| Table 5-1 Select Key Demographic and Economic Indicators, *continued* | |
|---|---|
| Education expenditure | 1.9% of GDP (1999). Country comparison to the world: 169 |
| Government type | Communist state |
| Environment | Air pollution (greenhouse gases, sulfur dioxide particulates) from reliance on coal produces acid rain; water shortages, particularly in the north; water pollution from untreated wastes; deforestation; estimated loss of one fifth of agricultural land since 1949 to soil erosion and economic development; desertification; trade in endangered species |
| Country mass | Total: 9,596,961 sq km<br>Country comparison to the world: 4<br>Land: 9,569,901 sq km<br>Water: 27,060 sq km |
| Population | 1,338,612,968 (July 2010 est.)<br>Country comparison to the world: 1 |
| Age structure | 0–14 years: 19.8% (male 140,877,745/female 124,290,090)<br>15–64 years: 72.1% (male 495,724,889/female 469,182,087)<br>65 years and over: 8.1% (male 51,774,115/female 56,764,042)<br>(2010 est.) |
| Median age | Total: 35.2 years<br>Male: 34.5 years<br>Female: 35.8 years (2010 est.) |
| Population growth rate | 0.655% (2009 est.)<br>Country comparison to the world: 148 |
| Birth rate | 14 births/1,000 population (2010 est.)<br>Country comparison to the world: 148 |
| Death rate | 7.06 deaths/1,000 population (July 2010 est.)<br>Country comparison to the world: 129 |
| Net migration rate | -0.39 migrant(s)/1,000 population (2010 est.)<br>Country comparison to the world: 101 |
| Urbanization | Urban population: 43% of total population (2008)<br>Rate of urbanization: 2.7% annual rate of change (2005–2010 est.) |
| Gender ratio | At birth: 1.104 male(s)/female<br>Under 15 years: 1.17 male(s)/female<br>15–64 years: 1.06 male(s)/female<br>65 years and over: 0.93 male(s)/female<br>Total population: 1.06 male(s)/female (2010 est.) |

*continued*

**Table 5-1 Select Key Demographic and Economic Indicators, *continued***

| | |
|---|---|
| Infant mortality rate | Total: 20.25 deaths/1,000 live births<br>Country comparison to the world: 103<br>Male: 18.87 deaths/1,000 live births<br>Female: 21.77 deaths/1,000 live births (2010 est.) |
| Life expectancy | Total population: 73.47 years<br>Country comparison to the world: 108<br>Male: 71.61 years<br>Female: 75.52 years (2010 est.) |
| Total fertility rate | 1.54 children born/woman (2010 est.)<br>Country comparison to the world: 160 |
| GDP—purchasing power parity | $8.748 trillion (2009 est.)<br>Country comparison to the world: 3 |
| GDP—per capita | $6,600 (2009 est.)<br>Country comparison to the world: 128 |
| GDP—composition by sector | Agriculture: 10.6%<br>Industry: 46.8%<br>Services: 42.6% (2009 est.) |
| Agriculture—products | Rice, wheat, potatoes, corn, peanuts, tea, millet, barley, apples, cotton, oilseed, pork, fish |
| Industries | Mining and ore processing, iron, steel, aluminum, and other metals, coal; machine building; armaments; textiles and apparel; petroleum; cement; chemicals; fertilizers; consumer products, including footwear, toys, and electronics; food processing; transportation equipment, including automobiles, rail cars and locomotives, ships, and aircraft; telecommunications equipment, commercial space launch vehicles, satellites |
| Labor force participation | 813.5 million (2009 est.)<br>Country comparison to the world: 1 |
| Unemployment rate | 4.3% (September 2009 est.)<br>Country comparison to the world: 37 |
| Industrial production growth rate | 9.5% (2009 est.)<br>Country comparison to the world: 5 |
| Distribution of family income (GINI index) | 41.5 (2007)<br>Country comparison to the world: 54 |
| Investment (gross fixed) | 45.2% of GDP (2009 est.)<br>Country comparison to the world: 3 |
| Public debt | 16.9% of GDP (2009 est.)<br>Country comparison to the world: 109 |

*continued*

| Table 5-1 Select Key Demographic and Economic Indicators, *continued* | |
|---|---|
| Market value of publicly traded shares | $5.011 trillion (December 31, 2009 est)<br>Country comparison to the world: 4 |
| Current account balance | $297.1 billion (2009 est.)<br>Country comparison to the world: 1 |
| Debt (external) | $347.1 billion (December 31, 2009 est.)<br>Country comparison to the world: 22 |
| Debt as a % of GDP | ——— |
| Exports | $1.204 trillion (2009 est.)<br>Country comparison to the world: 2 |
| Exports—commodities | Electrical and other machinery, including data processing equipment, apparel, textiles, iron and steel, optical and medical equipment |
| Exports—partners | United States 20.03%, Hong Kong 12.03%, Japan 8.32%, South Korea 4.55%, Germany 4.27% (2009) |
| Imports | $954.3 billion (2009 est.)<br>Country comparison to the world: 4 |
| Imports—commodities | Electrical and other machinery, oil and mineral fuels, optical and medical equipment, metal ores, plastics, organic chemicals |
| Imports—partners | Japan 12.27%, Hong Kong 10.06%, South Korea 9.04%, Taiwan 6.84%, United States 7.66%, Germany 5.54% (2009) |
| Stock of direct foreign investment at | |
| Home | $576.1 billion (December 31, 2009 est.)<br>Country comparison to the world: 9 |
| Abroad | $227.3 billion (December 31, 2009 est.)<br>Country comparison to the world: 15 |

Source: CIA. (2010). *The world factbook*. Retrieved December 16, 2010, from https://www.cia.gov/library/publications/the-world-factbook/

# Introduction

China is located in eastern Asia with an area of 9.6 million square kilometers, bordering the East China Sea, Korea Bay, Yellow Sea, and South China Sea. China's main neighbors include Russia, Mongolia, North Korea, Vietnam, India, and Pakistan (CIA, 2009).

China has the largest population in the world, exceeding 1.3 billion people comprising 56 ethnic groups (91.59% are Han Chinese). There are a total of 4 municipalities, 22 provinces, 5 autonomous regions, and 2 special administrative regions, namely Hong Kong and Macau. In this chapter, we will only focus on mainland China.

## Demographic, Economic, Employment, and Work Status

The dramatic demographic, economic, and social changes that occurred since 1990 in China are unprecedented in human history (Table 5-2). No country has ever industrialized as fast as China, faced as many new types of industries and hazards in such a short time, or experienced such a rapid transition from rural agricultural to urban industrial living (Table 5-3). This industrialization is just now beginning to create substantial challenges in terms of its impact on many aspects of employment and people's well-being, in particular, on occupational health.

**Table 5-2 Demographic Transition**

| | 1990 | 1995 | 2000 | 2005 | 2008 |
|---|---|---|---|---|---|
| Total population ($\times 10^4$) | 114,333 | 121,121 | 126,743 | 130,756 | 132,802 |
| Urban vs. rural population ($\times 10^4$) | | | | | |
| Urban | 23,887 | 28,563 | 32,499 | 41,128 | 44,643 |
| Rural | 90,446 | 92,558 | 94,244 | 89,628 | 88,159 |
| Gender ($\times 10^4$) | | | | | |
| Male | 58,904 | 61,808 | 65,437 | 67,375 | 68,357 |
| Female | 55,429 | 59,313 | 61,306 | 63,381 | 64,445 |
| Age distribution (%) | | | | | |
| 0–14 years | 27.7 | 26.6 | 22.9 | 20.3 | 19.0 |
| 15–64 years | 66.7 | 67.2 | 70.1 | 72.0 | 72.7 |
| 65 years and over | 5.6 | 6.2 | 7.0 | 7.7 | 8.3 |
| Education distribution (%) | | | | | |
| Primary school | 37.2 | 38.4 | 35.7 | 31.2 | 29.3 |
| Middle school | 23.3 | 27.3 | 34.0 | 35.8 | 38.4 |
| High school | 8.0 | 8.3 | 11.1 | 11.5 | 12.9 |
| University and higher | 1.4 | 2.0 | 3.6 | 5.2 | 6.3 |

Source: Data from *China Health Statistical Yearbook*, 2009.

**Table 5-3 Economic Trends**

| | 1990 | 1995 | 2000 | 2005 | 2008 |
|---|---|---|---|---|---|
| Gross domestic product (GDP) ($\times 10^8$ yuan) | 18,667.8 | 60,793.7 | 99,214.6 | 183,217.5 | 300,670.0 |
| Indices of GDP | 3.8% | 10.9% | 8.4% | 10.4% | 9.0% |
| GDP per capita (yuan) | 1,644 | 5,046 | 7,858 | 14,053 | 22,698 |

Source: Data from *China Health Statistical Yearbook*, 2009.

The employment structure in China has changed profoundly. The employment percentages in primary industry (agriculture, forestry, stock raising, and fishing) have dropped markedly, while percentages for secondary industry (machinery manufacture) and tertiary industry (services) have risen rapidly (Table 5-4).

**Table 5-4 Employment Status**

| | 1990 | 1995 | 2000 | 2005 | 2007 |
|---|---|---|---|---|---|
| Working population ($\times 10^4$) | 64,749 | 68,065 | 72,085 | 75,825 | 77,480 |
| Primary industry | 38,914 | 35,530 | 36,043 | 33,918 | 30,654 |
| Secondary industry | 13,856 | 15,655 | 16,219 | 18,092 | 21,109 |
| Tertiary industry | 11,979 | 16,880 | 19,823 | 23,815 | 25,717 |

Source: Data from *China Health Statistical Yearbook*, 2009.

Compared to other countries in the world, the unemployment rate is still relatively low in China, but increasing trends may cause alarm in China's labor market. The rate climbed from 2.5% to 4.2% between 1990 and 2008 (Table 5-5).

**Table 5-5 Registered Unemployment Rate in Urban Areas (%)**

| 1990 | 1992 | 1994 | 1996 | 1998 | 2000 | 2002 | 2004 | 2006 | 2008 |
|---|---|---|---|---|---|---|---|---|---|
| 2.5 | 2.3 | 2.8 | 3.0 | 3.1 | 3.1 | 4.0 | 4.2 | 4.1 | 4.2 |

Source: Data from *China Population and Employment Statistical Yearbook*, 2008.

Another critical issue is the number of working hours. Although working hours tend to be shorter than in the past, Chinese people still have the longer work hours than people in many other countries (Table 5-6).

Table 5-6 **Weekly Working Hours of Urban Employed Persons**

| 2003 | 2004 | 2005 | 2006 | 2007 |
|---|---|---|---|---|
| 45.4 | 45.5 | 47.8 | 47.3 | 45.5 |

Source: Data from *China Population and Employment Statistical Yearbook*, 2008.

## Role of Workplace Health Promotion in Society

It has been pointed out clearly by the *Workers' Health: Global Plan of Action* (WHO, 2007), that "workers represent half the world's population and are the major contributors to economic and social development. Their health is determined not only by workplace hazards but also by social and individual factors and access to health services." Thus, the Objective 2 of the *Global Plan* is "to protect and promote health at the workplace" (WHO, 2007).

The workplace is one of the most important settings that affect the health of workers, which subsequently affects the health of their families, communities, and society. The workplace also offers an ideal setting to support the promotion of health of a large population. By improving workers' knowledge and skills in managing their health and by establishing an environment conducive to health inside and outside the workplace, the workers, their families, and the workplace itself benefit (Chu et al., 2000).

In recent years, the concept of workplace health promotion (WHP) has become more integrative, focusing on both the organizational level (mechanical, physical, chemical, biological, and psychosocial risks in the working environment) and the individual level (health risk behaviors). Therefore, workplace health promotion involves both workers and management collectively changing the workplace into a healthy setting. With the rapid process of globalization, more and more organizations are increasingly aware that a healthy, qualified, and motivated workforce is essential in order to be successful in the modern world. A healthy workplace can ensure a dynamic balance between the organization's goal of profits and workers' need for health and personal development. At the national level, a healthy workplace is a prerequisite for sustainable social and economic development (Harris, Lichiello, & Hannon, 2009; Song, Chang, &Yu, 2003).

# Prevailing Health Issues and Risk Behaviors

## Life Expectancy

Since 1982, the life expectancy rate in China has increased, with the life expectancy of males at 70 years and of females, 74 years in 2005 (Table 5-7). As a developing country, China has a relatively high life expectancy.

Table 5-7 **Life Expectancy (Years) in China, 1982, 1990, 2000, and 2005**

| | 1982 | 1990 | 2000 | 2005 |
|---|---|---|---|---|
| Total population | 67.8 | 68.6 | 71.4 | 73.0 |
| Male | 66.3 | 66.8 | 69.6 | 70.0 |
| Female | 69.3 | 70.5 | 73.3 | 74.0 |

Source: Data from *China Health Statistical Yearbook*, 2009.

## Disease Trends: Mortality and Morbidity Ranking

Mortality and morbidity indicators have been improved dramatically in China over the past years. Like much of the world, China's health problems are now shifting from infectious diseases to chronic diseases. For example, the five leading causes of death in urban areas are malignant tumors, heart diseases, cerebrovascular diseases, respiratory diseases, and injuries and poisonings; in rural areas, the leading causes of death are the same but with different rankings (malignant tumors, cerebrovascular diseases, respiratory diseases, heart diseases, and injuries and poisonings) (Tables 5-8, 5-9, and 5-10).

Table 5-8 **Standardized Mortality Rates ($1/10^4$) in the Urban Population**

| | 1990 | 1995 | 2000 | 2005 | 2008 |
|---|---|---|---|---|---|
| Malignant tumors | 96.69 | 88.05 | 90.24 | 76.85 | 153.60 |
| Cerebrovascular diseases | 88.29 | 83.70 | 70.74 | 61.38 | 112.28 |
| Heart diseases | 66.21 | 59.01 | 58.01 | 53.42 | 114.36 |
| Respiratory diseases | 68.37 | 56.79 | 41.86 | 36.14 | 69.87 |
| Injuries and poisonings | 34.98 | 32.82 | 27.02 | 34.40 | 30.14 |

Source: Data from *China Health Statistical Yearbook*, 2009.

Table 5-9 **Standardized Mortality Rates ($1/10^4$) in the Rural Population**

| | 1990 | 1995 | 2000 | 2005 | 2008 |
|---|---|---|---|---|---|
| Respiratory diseases | 123.52 | 123.19 | 98.97 | 91.82 | 140.57 |
| Malignant tumors | 92.97 | 88.29 | 87.33 | 80.05 | 189.81 |
| Cerebrovascular diseases | 76.41 | 74.97 | 78.18 | 80.97 | 175.53 |
| Heart diseases | 51.48 | 43.79 | 49.40 | 44.46 | 116.31 |
| Injuries and poisonings | 63.47 | 66.25 | 57.16 | 38.68 | 59.98 |

Source: Data from *China Health Statistical Yearbook*, 2009.

Table 5-10 **Morbidity Rates ($1/10^3$) of Diseases**

| | 1993 | 1998 | 2003 | 2008 |
|---|---|---|---|---|
| Two-week morbidity rate | 140.1 | 149.8 | 143.0 | 188.6 |
| Morbidity rates of chronic diseases | | | | |
| Hypertension | 11.9 | 15.8 | 26.2 | 54.9 |
| Heart diseases | 13.1 | 14.2 | 14.3 | 17.6 |
| Diabetes | 1.9 | 3.2 | 5.6 | 10.7 |
| Cerebrovascular diseases | 4.0 | 5.9 | 6.6 | 9.7 |
| Elderly chronic bronchitis | 13.8 | 12.9 | 7.5 | 6.9 |
| Malignant tumors | 1.0 | 1.2 | 1.3 | 2.0 |

Source: Data from *China Health Statistical Yearbook*, 2009.

## Health Risk Behaviors

When looking at the data of health risk behaviors, it shows that the prevalence of smoking has declined year by year (Table 5-11); however, more than half of Chinese men are still currently smokers, and the increase in the amount of smoking is notable.

Most Chinese are inactive with respect to physical exercise, and the percentage of men actively engaged in exercise has actually declined from 1997 to 2006 (Table 5-12). In addition, with the sufficient food supply and popularity of fast food, the body mass index (BMI) has increased for both women and men. The BMI for Chinese men has increased almost 1 unit over the past 10 years, while the increase of BMI in women is about 0.8 unit. Thus, it is not surprising that the morbidity rates of hypertension and diabetes have sharply climbed from 11.9% in 1993 to 54.9% in 2008 and from 1.9% in 1993 to 10.7% in 2008.

Table 5-11 **Smoking**

| | 1997 | 2000 | 2004 | 2006 |
|---|---|---|---|---|
| Men | | | | |
| Current smoking (%) | 58.45 | 56.28 | 56.04 | 53.54 |
| Age of starting smoking | 21.50 | 21.33 | 21.61 | 21.63 |
| Cigarettes per day | 16.19 | 16.17 | 16.45 | 16.78 |
| Women | | | | |
| Current smoking (%) | 4.74 | 4.51 | 4.02 | 3.55 |
| Age of starting smoking | 26.46 | 26.78 | 27.47 | 27.57 |
| Cigarettes per day | 12.82 | 12.00 | 11.04 | 11.79 |

Source: Data from China Health and Nutrition Survey, 1997–2006.

Table 5-12 **Regular Physical Exercise and Body Mass Index (BMI)**

| | 1997 | 2000 | 2004 | 2006 |
|---|---|---|---|---|
| Men | | | | |
| Regular physical exercise (%) | 15.79 | 13.39 | 11.89 | 12.55 |
| BMI (kg/m$^2$) | 22.16 | 22.70 | 22.97 | 23.14 |

*continued*

| Table 5-12 **Regular Physical Exercise and Body Mass Index (BMI),** *continued* | | | | |
|---|---|---|---|---|
| Women | | | | |
| Regular physical exercise (%) | 7.62 | 5.92 | 7.82 | 8.59 |
| BMI (kg/m²) | 22.45 | 22.98 | 23.23 | 23.26 |

Source: Data from China Health and Nutrition Survey, 1997–2006.

## Occupational Diseases and Accidents

With regard to the occupational diseases, pneumoconiosis accounts for two thirds or more of all cases, even as recently as 2007 (Table 5-13). Physical hazards (dust) and chemical poisonings remain the dominant occupational hazards (He, 1998; Liang & Xiang, 2004). Even though work stress-related diseases are currently not legally recognized occupational diseases on the compensation list, psychosocial hazards in the workplace in China have been recognized as emerging occupational health problems (Li & Jin, 2007) (Table 5-14).

Table 5-13 **Statistics of Reported Cases of Occupational Diseases (1994–2007)**

| | 1994 | 1997 | 2000 | 2003 | 2007 |
|---|---|---|---|---|---|
| Pneumoconiosis | 10,830 | 7,418 | 9,100 | 8,364 | 10,963 |
| Chronic poisonings | 2,016 | 1,313 | 1,196 | 882 | 1,638 |
| Acute poisonings | 1,087 | 598 | 785 | 504 | 600 |
| Others | 1,388 | 899 | 637 | 717 | 1,095 |
| Total Cases | 15,321 | 10,228 | 11,718 | 10,467 | 14,296 |

Source: Data from China annual statistics of occupational diseases, 1994–2007.

Table 5-14 **Statistics of Reported Occupational Accidents (2002–2008)**

| | 2002 | 2004 | 2006 | 2008 |
|---|---|---|---|---|
| Cases of occupational accidents | 1,073,434 | 803,573 | 627,158 | 413,752 |
| Cases of death due to occupational accidents | 139,393 | 136,755 | 112,822 | 91,172 |

Source: Data from annual statistics of work safety, 2002–2008.

## Major Challenges Now and for the Future

With regard to China's health problems—the major shift from infectious diseases to chronic diseases; the inactivity of the population and the subsequent increase in BMI for both males and females; the prevalence of smoking, and thus, the increasing morbidity rates of hypertension and diabetes—there are major challenges for China both now and for the future.

Major challenges include:

- reducing health risk behaviors and obtaining a healthy lifestyle
- preventing chronic diseases, particular cardiovascular diseases, and diabetes
- promoting occupational health and safety

# Healthcare System

## Healthcare Organization and Structure

The current healthcare system in China is comprised of hospitals, centers for disease control and prevention, and institutes of health inspection at different administrative levels: province, city, and county. Since 2002, centers for disease control and prevention and institutes of health inspection have been established based on the existing structure (at different administrative levels: province, city, and county) of epidemic prevention stations with the function of conducting health surveillance at its own level and reporting to the upper-level stations. Generally, hospitals are responsible for disease diagnosis and treatment; centers for disease control and prevention are responsible for public health issues; while institutes of health inspection are the executive and legal body to enforce a set of health standards and to apply health-related laws and regulations into practice (Liu, 2004).

### *Healthcare Spending, Resources, and Insurance*

China's total health expenditure as a percentage of GDP increased from 4.00% in 1990 to 4.52% in 2008, but the overall government spending on health as a share of total health expenditure decreased from 25.1% in 1990 to 20.4% in 2008. In contrast, individual out-of-pocket spending as a share of total health expenditure increased from 35.7% to 45.2% during the same period (Table 5-15). Even though 85.32% of Chinese people were covered by the three main types of medical insurance in China in 2008, the costs of medical care in both urban and rural areas have increased year by year (in urban areas, accounting for 1.69% of total annual income in 1990 and increasing to 4.61% in 2008, and in rural areas increasing from 1.92% to 3.67% in the same time period) (Liu, Rao, Wu, & Gakidou, 2008) (Tables 5-16 and 5-17). The numbers of healthcare facilities and people in the workforce have changed significantly during the past 20 years (Table 5-18). However, it is surprising that a shortage of nurses is a serious problem in China. According to the *World Health Report* (WHO, 2006), the average density of nurses per 1,000 people throughout the world is 4.06, whereas the density of nurses per 1,000 people in China is only 1.25 (Li et al., 2009).

Table 5-15 **Healthcare Spending**

| | 1990 | 1995 | 2000 | 2005 | 2007 |
|---|---|---|---|---|---|
| Total health expenditure ($\times 10^8$ yuan) | 747.39 | 2,155.13 | 4,586.63 | 8,659.91 | 11,289.50 |
| % of GDP spent on health | 4.00 | 3.54 | 4.62 | 4.73 | 4.52 |
| % of total expenditure on health funded by the government | 25.1 | 18.0 | 15.5 | 17.9 | 20.4 |
| % of total expenditure on health funded by individuals | 35.7 | 46.4 | 59.0 | 52.2 | 45.2 |

Source: Data from *China Health Statistical Yearbook*, 2009.

Table 5-16 **Costs of Medical Care and Coverage of Health Insurance (Yuan)**

| | 1990 | 1995 | 2000 | 2005 | 2008 |
|---|---|---|---|---|---|
| Urban areas | | | | | |
| Average annual income per capita | 1,522.8 | 4,288.1 | 6,316.8 | 11,320.8 | 17,067.8 |
| Costs of medical care | 25.7 | 110.1 | 318.1 | 600.9 | 786.2 |
| Rural areas | | | | | |
| Average annual income per capita | 990.4 | 2,337.9 | 3,146.2 | 4,631.2 | 6,700.7 |
| Costs of medical care | 19.0 | 42.5 | 87.6 | 168.1 | 246.0 |

Source: Data from *China Health Statistical Yearbook*, 2009.

Table 5-17 **Coverage of Medical Insurance**

| | 2004 | 2005 | 2006 | 2007 | 2008 |
|---|---|---|---|---|---|
| Basic medical insurance for urban residents (×10⁸) | | | | 0.43 | 1.18 |
| Basic medical insurance for urban employees (×10⁸) | 1.24 | 1.38 | 1.57 | 1.80 | 2.00 |
| New rural cooperatives medical care (×10⁸) | 0.80 | 1.79 | 4.10 | 7.26 | 8.15 |

Source: Data from *China Health Statistical Yearbook*, 2009.

Table 5-18 **Healthcare Resources**

| | 1990 | 1995 | 2000 | 2005 | 2008 |
|---|---|---|---|---|---|
| Health institutions | 208,734 | 190,057 | 324,771 | 298,997 | 278,337 |
| Hospitals | 14,377 | 15,663 | 16,318 | 18,703 | 19,712 |
| Centers for disease control and prevention | 3,618 | 3,729 | 3,741 | 3,585 | 3,534 |
| Institutes of health inspection | | | 571 (2002) | 1,702 | 2,675 |
| Beds in health institutions (×10⁴) (total) | 292.54 | 314.06 | 317.70 | 336.75 | 403.87 |
| Beds per thousand people | 2.32 | 2.39 | 2.38 | 2.45 | 2.84 |
| Licensed physicians (total) | 1,302,997 | 1,454,926 | 1,603,266 | 1,555,658 | 1,714,670 |
| Licensed physicians per thousand people | 1.15 | 1.23 | 1.30 | 1.22 | 1.30 |
| Registered nurses (total) | 974,541 | 1,125,661 | 1,266,838 | 1,349,589 | 1,653,297 |
| Registered nurses per thousand people | 0.86 | 0.95 | 1.02 | 1.06 | 1.25 |

Source: Data from *China Health Statistical Yearbook*, 2009.

## *Development of Health Education and Promotion in China*

In the early 1950s, the main policy driver in the area of health education and promotion was health propaganda emphasizing prevention of communicable diseases and basic hygiene. During the 1960s, the health propaganda activities started to decline due to the Cultural

Revolution. In the 1970s, the health policy movement emphasized health education, networking, training of professionals and development of settings, and a population approach to promote health. From late 1980s onward, the policy directive continued to move away from the health propaganda approach to a health education approach. In 1984, the Chinese Health Education Association was established, and by 1986, there were Institutes of Health Education at different levels in 26 provinces and over 150 cities. Starting in the mid-1980s, new health education guidelines were established for health departments at national, provincial, city, and county levels. In addition, to better coordinate and support such programs, appropriate infrastructure was developed by the Institute of Health Education. Beginning in the 1990s, health promotion has been enhanced by developing many programs such as school health education, worksite health education, community-based health education for chronic illnesses, and prevention of noncommunicable diseases in many provinces and cities. Meanwhile, there was a significant change in conducting health promotion from risk factor orientation to setting approach, and from expert lead approach to participatory and problem-based approach (Lee, Fu, & Chenyi, 2007).

## Influence of Culture

The health and health-related attitudes of Chinese people are influenced by their cultural values. First, the teachings of Confucius are principles for social interaction and have a great influence on Chinese behaviors. *Jen* (benevolence), *yi* (righteousness), *chung* (loyalty), *hsia* (filial piety), and *te* (virtue) are five characteristics of and important concepts in Confucianism. Harmony with all others and a lack of self-centeredness, respect for parents, and loyalty to family are the main teachings of Confucianism. Chinese people believe that being respected by family members, friends, and colleagues is essential for their happiness and health.

A second major Chinese religion or tradition is Taoism. *Tao* or *the way* is the major idea of Taoism: "Man models himself on earth, earth on heaven, heaven on the way, and the way on that which is naturally so." Taoism teaches that human beings should be in harmony with nature, that is, with the Tao. To achieve health, an individual would need to modify himself to fit into the natural rhythms of the universe.

A third belief is in the idea of *yin* and *yang*. As this concept is an extension of Taoism, yin and yang have been long dominated traditional Chinese thinking with respect to health and illness. In Chinese medicine, health is viewed as the harmony between the forces of yin and yang within the body and between the body and its environment. Illness, in contrast, is viewed as an imbalance of these powerful forces. The combined force of yin and yang is called *qi* (vital energy), which is the source of life and manifests as the energy circulating in one's body. The study of human qi relates to health and longevity. This system of qi forms the basis for the diagnosis and treatment of illness, as well as for promoting health and preventing illness.

A fourth major religious tradition in China is Buddhism. Mercy, thriftiness, and humility are the three treasures of Buddhism. *Inn* and *ko* (cause and effect) are the principles that encourage people to do good and do right, which will result in receiving good in return. Therefore, always doing good for others and being a good person are of great importance in this philosophy of life. When people are aware of their behavior and are morally good, they would have little or no guilt and would be in a peaceful state; thus awareness and goodness will promote their health (Graham, 1990).

Traditional Chinese medicine grows from the prevailing culture and has served the people for thousands of years. It mainly includes herbal treatments, acupuncture, and diet therapy. In China, people value traditional Chinese medicine as well as western medicine. Modern Chinese medicine constitutes an attempt to merge the traditional and Western medical practices. The foundation of Chinese cultural tradition, in combination with Western science, will perhaps prove important to the future advancement of health care, benefiting China and the world.

# Drivers of Workplace Health Promotion

## Relevant Laws and Regulations

### *The Law of the People's Republic of China on Occupational Disease Prevention and Control*

The Occupational Disease Control Law, adopted by the Standing Committee of the National People's Congress on May 1, 2002, defines the occupational health rights of workers, the obligations and duties of employers to protect the health of their employees, the responsibilities of the government at various levels, and trade unions' representation in workers' health protection. The law stipulates basic principles governing the prevention and control of occupational disease, protective measures, hazards monitoring and management in workplaces, diagnosis of occupational disease, health authority inspections, and the liabilities incurred by those violating the law (Pringle & Frost, 2003; Su, 2003).

According to this law, the workplace should meet the basic occupational health requirements, which include (Su, 2003):

- Control of the intensity or concentration of an occupational hazardous substance in compliance with the national occupational health standards
- Institution of appropriate occupational-disease–prevention facilities
- Rational production layout in compliance with the principle of separating harmful from harmless operations
- Deployment of appropriate sanitation facilities such as dressing rooms, bathhouses, and rest rooms for pregnant women
- Ensuring that equipment, tools, and appliances comply with requirements for protecting the well-being of workers

- Other requirements established by laws, regulations, and administrative rules related to workers' health protection published by the health authority under the state council

## The Law of the People's Republic of China on Work Safety

The Work Safety Law, adopted by the Standing Committee of the National People's Congress on November 1, 2002, has 97 provisions covering work units' safety measures, the rights and interests of workers, supervision and management of work safety, rescue work in times of accidents, accident investigation, and legal liabilities (Pringle & Frost, 2003; Su, 2003).

Some important basic systems and/or measures are stipulated by the law (Pringle & Frost, 2003):

- A production unit must meet all the relevant laws and regulation; otherwise it may not undertake production activities.
- An enterprise must appoint an individual who is responsible for all aspects of safety.
- An enterprise must also implement a safety management organization or individual.
- An enterprise must implement a system of education, training, and assessment of safety knowledge for occupational health and safety (OHS) directors (that is, personnel with overall responsibility), OHS managers, and workers.
- Enterprises must implement a system of three simultaneous OHS measures at all stages of all projects; that is, OHS measures should be evident at the planning stage, during construction (of the plant and so on), and when production is under way.
- Production units must register exceptionally dangerous hazards with the local safety inspectorate.
- Enterprises must implement a safety management system specifically addressing workplaces where explosives, working at heights, and other dangers are involved

Both the Occupational Disease Control Law and the Work Safety Law emphasize the employers' duties and the rights of workers.

Employers hold the primary responsibility for both the health and safety of their employees in workplaces, and for their occupational disease prevention and treatment. The law requires employers to establish a system to protect health and safety.

The chief duties of employing units are as follows:

- Employers should ensure the various managerial aspects of OHS, including planning, organization, directing, control, and coordination.
- An OHS responsibility system should be set up, based on the special characteristics of the company's sector. The person with overall responsibility for implementing the system in the company must also ensure that all departments are linked to and administer a reward-and-punishment system related to all aspects of OHS.
- Effective measures should be taken for hazard control and occupational disease prevention.

- Workers who are exposed to hazardous factors at workplaces should have regular health examinations.
- Employers have the responsibility to educate their workers.
- Those enterprises that have been informed to temporarily halt production in order to rectify OHS systems but fail to do so can be closed down and have their licenses revoked.

The rights of workers in the workplace are also clearly prescribed:

- to receive occupational health and safety education and training
- to access occupational health services (e.g., health examinations, occupational disease diagnosis, and rehabilitation)
- to know of the health effects of hazards and all dangers in the workplace, which includes the right to take active steps to prevent OHS hazards and dangers
- to request and receive claim improvement of working conditions and personal protective equipment that conforms to national standards
- to criticize and accuse perpetrators of malpractices that violate the laws and regulations with regard to any aspect of OHS
- to reject illegal orders and commands to undertake operations without appropriate safeguard measures
- to refuse to carry out instructions from management that violate laws and regulations
- to stop working in life-threatening situations
- to receive insurance compensation following an accident at work
- to participate in the democratic management of the employer's occupational health practice, and make comments and suggestions with regard to the occupational disease prevention practices of the employer

### *Interim Administrative Provision on Worksite Occupational Health Inspection*

The Provision on Worksite Occupational Health Inspection, which was issued by the State Administration of Work Safety on September 1, 2009, requires all employers to:

- honestly inform employees about any occupational hazards and their consequences
- provide training on occupational hazards prevention to employees
- establish an internal auditing/supervision department within the employing unit
- offer necessary health examination programs and establish health records for employees
- equip employees at hazardous jobs with qualified personal protection equipment
- conduct timely upgrades for manufacturing equipment and conduct the six simultaneous OHS measures mentioned at the bottom of p. 105 and the top of p. 106
- deliver all relevant documentation of the six OHS measures to local work safety authorities

- regularly report on occupational hazards monitoring and risk assessment to local work safety authorities; the frequency of the occupational hazards monitoring should be at least once per year, and the frequency of the occupational risk assessment should be at least once every 3 years

Any violation of the provision will be subject to administrative or economic punishment (State Administration of Work Safety, 2009).

It is important to be aware of the administrative changes in the implementation of occupational health inspection:

- 1949–1998: organized by Ministry of Labor
- 1999–2008: organized by Ministry of Health, implemented by epidemic prevention stations and institutes of health inspection
- 2009–present: organized by the State Administration of Work Safety

## History of Workplace Health Promotion in China

In China, a national network for workplace health promotion emerged out of a workshop facilitated by the Ministry of Health in 1993. In the workshop, it was suggested for the first time that workplace health promotion should be carried out in factories and enterprises as soon as possible. During the following years, the Committee on Health Education in the Workplace was developed, and it formalized in July 1996 under the leadership of the Chinese Association of Health Education. The Committee on Health Education in the Workplace is a national, academic, nongovernmental social organization for leaders of workplaces, health education workers, and other health workers in the fields of health education and workplace industrial health (Song et al., 2003).

In August 2000, the Notification on Implementation of Workplace Health Promotion was released from the Ministry of Health and the All-China Federation of Trade Unions jointly. It required that health bureaus, trade unions, factories, and enterprises at all levels conduct workplace health promotion activities based on local conditions (Zhang & Sun, 2005). Recently, the National Institute of Occupational Health and Poison Control has launched a nationwide program, Health Promoting Enterprises, to explore the effective models of health promotion for various enterprises in different industries.

## Occupational Health Inspection and Workplace Health Promotion

In China, occupational health inspection and workplace health promotion are usually integrated in working toward the goal of improving occupational health. The former focuses on more hard aspects of the workplace, while the latter focuses on soft aspects of the workplace, such as modification of health risk behaviors and stress management (Song et al., 2003; Su, 2003; Zhang & Sun, 2005).

The main tasks of occupational health inspection include:

- audit and approval of the preventive assessment of new construction, expansion, and the rebuilding of industrial premises; and technical innovation and reformation and import projects that might produce occupational hazards
- on-site inspection of enterprises/workplaces to ensure implementation of laws and hazard-control measures; and environmental monitoring, to ensure that concentrations of occupational hazards in workplaces meet national industrial hygienic standards
- monitoring whether the preplacement and periodic health examinations of workers exposed to occupational hazards are in compliance with national laws and regulations
- ensuring that workers suffering from occupational diseases are properly treated, have recovered, and are transferred to other jobs suitable for them in line with related regulations
- supervising occupational health record keeping and occupational disease reporting

# Programs and Good Practices

## State-Owned Enterprises

Shanghai is the largest industrial city in China, with a population of over 18.8 million people. In collaboration with WHO and supported by the government of the People's Republic of China, the Shanghai Municipal Health Bureau and the Shanghai Health Education Institute conducted a pilot workplace health promotion project from 1993 to 1995. The project involved 21,613 workers in 4 workplaces: Wujing Chemical Complex, Shanghai Hudong Shipyard, Shanghai No. 34 Cotton Mill and Shanghai Baoshan Steel Company (Gan, Gu, Zhang, & Sally, 1995; Liu, Gu, & Gan, 1996).

Based on data gathered through a baseline survey conducted in early 1993 and guided by members of the Shanghai Health Education Institute and an occupational health expert advisory reference group, each workplace developed, implemented, and evaluated workplace health promotion programs.

The project adopted an integrative model of workplace health promotion and sought to address identified organizational, environmental, and behavioral factors that were negatively impacting the health of the workers. Health promotion programs sought to develop healthy policies and regulations, create safe and supportive environments, strengthen preventive health services, facilitate workers' participation, and educate workers to promote healthy behaviors. Initiatives undertaken included the establishment of health education and health promotion committees, the drafting and implementation of workplace standards for identified occupational hazards, improved management of workplace sanitation and hygiene, and improved occupational health hazard monitoring and control (e.g., noise, dust, and chemical leakage). Other initiatives included the supply of nutritious foodstuffs and the reduction of salt in food in workplace canteens, planting trees and flowers, cigarette smoking and alcohol cessation programs, cervical screening and thorough follow-up treatments, improved preventive health services for workers, and greater worker participation in the identification and control of occupational hazards.

During the project, particular attention was given to such issues as staff mobilization and training; the establishing, coordinating and networking mechanisms; and regular consultation with workers, management, and expert reference groups. These measures ensured that all interested parties were involved in the planning of the project and that they were given opportunities to participate in its implementation. Furthermore, there was an emphasis on multisectoral involvement and the integration of health promotion into management practices.

The project was closely monitored, and an evaluation carried out in 1995 showed excellent measurable outcomes, for example:

- reduced incidence of work-related injuries by 10–20%
- reduced diseases and related healthcare costs (e.g., pharyngitis, from 16% to 10%)
- improved health and safety knowledge and practices (the use of safety devices or protective equipment increased from 20–30% to 70–90%)
- reduced risk behaviors (reduction of salt consumption, cigarette smoking)
- reduced levels of sick leave by 50%

Learning from this pilot project, the project team has since developed what they have proudly called the Shanghai model of workplace health promotion. The model's four distinctive features are: comprehensive, integrative, a system of management and multisectoral networks, and a multiplicity of intervention strategies. Since then, the Shanghai project team has developed draft Chinese language guidelines for workplace health promotion.

## Joint Ventures

More and more joint ventures (including Sino-foreign joint ventures, Sino-foreign cooperative enterprises, and multinational enterprises) have been established since 1985 in China. Some evidence shows that joint ventures could also play a critical role in supporting and even funding health promotion in the workplace in China. In general, foreign enterprises could open relatively free spaces for workers to participate in important factory decisions and could create mechanisms to respond to workers' complaints and concerns (O'Rourke & Brown, 2003).

A workplace health promotion project was conducted in 15 joint ventures (Ni, Wang, & Li, 2007). The highlight of this project was to include workers as well as managers. In total, there were 817 workers and 925 managers who participated the 2-year intervention. The major activities of intervention were to:

- set up OHS management networks and rules
- train managers and workers in occupational health
- clarify the responsibilities and operating manuals

- establish health records of employees
- fulfill the system of monitoring occupational hazards
- strengthen the surveillance of usage of personal protective equipment

The project was evaluated in 2006, and the results indicated that workplace health promotion is an effective way to improve the working conditions and workers' health in joint ventures. The main changes were:

- an increased awareness rate of the occupational disease control law in both managers and workers
- an acquired basic knowledge of occupational hazards and its health effects in both managers and workers
- an increased awareness rate of three simultaneous OHS measures in managers
- an improved participation rate of regular occupational health examinations, usage of personal protective equipment, and safety operating manuals in workers
- reduced health risk behaviors (cigarette smoking, alcohol drinking, and physical inactivity) in workers
- an increased pass rate of occupational hazards in the workplace to meet the national standards
- increased coverage of occupational health service to workers

# Existing Research

## The Earliest Workplace Health Intervention Program in China

Cardiovascular disease (CVD) has been a major cause of mortality, morbidity, and disability in China. The importance of prevention and control of cardiovascular disease in the population level is widely recognized. Therefore, a 24-year worksite-based intervention program (1974–1998) was implemented among 110,000 employees at Capital Iron and Steel Company of Beijing (CISC) focusing on primary prevention for CVD and control of hypertension.

> *Intervention components comprised of infrastructure setting-up, health education and health promotion, professional training, detection and management of hypertensive patients, and reasonably readjusting their diet structure focusing on salt intake reduction, reducing their overweight, quitting smoking, and restricting alcohol consumption in high-risk population. Changes in level of risk factors, incidence and mortality of stroke and coronary events and their trend were evaluated between the intervention group at CISC and eight simultaneously parallel reference groups in other provinces outside Beijing with population surveillance data. (Wu et al., 2003)*

The major risk factors for CVD, including blood pressure, body mass index and serum cholesterol level, were decreased relatively in the intervention population at CISC during 1974 to 1998, while those in the majority of eight parallel reference groups in different provinces of China were significantly increased at the same time. Systolic blood pressure was decreased 0.8 mmHg and 4 mmHg in average for men and women, respectively, and their diastolic blood pressure remained the same as baseline for both men and women at CISC; while systolic blood pressure was increased 2–11 mmHg and 6–8 mmHg in average for men and women in the reference groups, respectively, and diastolic blood pressure was increased 2–6 mmHg in average for men in five of eight reference groups, and 3–6 mmHg for women in four of eight reference groups. Serum level of cholesterol was decreased 0.26 mmol/L in women and slightly increased for men at CISC; while it was increased 0.35–0.97 mmol/L for men and 0.29–1.05 mmol/L for women in all reference groups. Prevalence of overweight was increased 51.7% for men and 11.3% for women at CISC; while it was increased 1–22 folds in eight reference groups. Awareness of health knowledge was improved significantly with an average net reduction of systolic blood pressure/diastolic blood pressure of 2.5/2.2 mmHg in the enforced intervention group at CISC than that in general intervention groups. Incidence and mortality rates of stroke were decreased 54.7% and 74.3%, respectively, in the intervention group at CISC, but those of coronary events were slowly increased with fluctuation.

These data show the worksite-based comprehensive intervention for CVD prevention and control was feasible and cost effective in decreasing risk factors for CVD and incidence and mortality rate of stroke in Chinese population.

## Work Stress and Workplace Health Promotion

A recent report from WHO indicated clearly that psychosocial stress in the workplace has been recognized as an emergent occupational hazard in China. According to an epidemiologic study among the general working population, the percentage of workers who reported that they had high or very high work stress was 37.3% in men and 27.5% in women (Li & Jin, 2007). It has been reported that work stress has a significant impact on both the individual (poor health) and the organization (productivity loss). The human and economic costs of work stress strongly suggest that it is in everybody's interest–employees, employers, and the community at large–that stress intervention initiatives are high on the agenda of workplace health promotion programs (Noblet & Lamontagne, 2006).

Generally, interventions of work stress are commonly classified into three levels: primary intervention (e.g. stressor reduction), secondary intervention (e.g. stress management), and tertiary intervention (e.g. employee assistance programs/workplace counseling). Thus, work stress interventions are rated in terms of the level of approach used.

> *A high rating is defined as both organizationally and individually focused, versus moderate (organizational only), and low (individual only). Studies using high-rated approaches represent a growing proportion of the work stress intervention. Individual-focused, low-rated approaches are effective at the individual level, favorably affecting*

*individual-level outcomes, but tend not to have favorable impacts at the organizational level. Organizationally focused high- and moderate-rated approaches are beneficial at both individual and organizational levels. (Lamontagne, Keegel, Louie, Ostry, Landsbergis, 2007)*

There was a work stress intervention study with 1-year follow-up available in China (Wu et al., 2006). The intervention group consisted of 459 middle school teachers and the control group consisted of 502 teachers. The integrated interventions were applied, including the following:

- organizational strategy: aiming to modify or diminish sources of stress inherent in the work environment (e.g., redesigning the task, establishing flexible work schedules and redesigning the work environment)
- individual intervention: aiming to improve the stress management skills of the individual through training and education activities, which taught teachers about impact of stress, and developed a range of techniques and skills to cope with occupational stress

The main results demonstrated that the scores with regard to occupational role and personal strain decreased significantly and the scores of personal resources and work ability increased significantly after intervening. This study suggested that interventions were efficient in reducing the teachers' work stressors, increasing their coping resources and improving their work ability.

# Conclusion

Workplace health promotion in China is still at the early stage, but its perspectives are brilliant due to the huge contribution of China to the world economy and to the world health development. There is growing interest in proposing implications for workplace health promotion in China in the near future.

## Differentiated Activities for Various Enterprises

China is a big country with a huge population, and there are enormous differences in socioeconomic status and working conditions because of unbalanced development in diverse areas, industries, and enterprises. As a result, it is suggested that the focus of workplace health promotion for the township enterprises should be on the spread of basic health knowledge and occupational hazards, particularly the prevention of occupational dusts and chemical poisoning; for the state-owned enterprises and joint ventures, the comprehensive programs could be implemented, combining the management of occupational health and safety, lifestyle modification, and disease prevention; for other enterprises, the feasible activities of workplace health promotion would be taken as they fit the local conditions.

## All Stakeholders' Participation

It is clear that the participation and cooperation of different stakeholders are critical to the success of workplace health promotion. In China, it is necessary to ensure that governments and stakeholders continue their support for workplace health promotion programs in order to develop an essential budget for relevant activities, to maintain enthusiasm among participating enterprises and occupational and health promotion professionals, and to encourage new work organizations to participate in developing healthy workplaces. Workers' participation is critical for improving working conditions as well. Meaningful workers' participation requires strengthening institutional protections, increasing opportunities for participation, and building worker capacities. Workers can benefit from training and technical assistance in areas such as identifying hazards, knowing their rights, and remediating problems. External assistance should thus also support longer term development of means for workers to represent themselves and negotiate for improvements in health and safety and other workplace conditions.

## Integration With Occupational Health Inspection

Occupational health inspection has legal implications in China. The inspection covers monitoring of the hazardous working environment, health screening of employees, and surveillance of occupational diseases. According to the Occupational Disease Control Law and the Work Safety Law, it is the employers' primary responsibility to ensure the health and safety of workers. It is strongly recommended that all comprehensive workplace health promotion programs in China should be integrated tightly with occupational health inspection in the future.

## More Attention to Migrant Workers and Precarious Employment

Nearly 70% of the Chinese population live in rural areas. However, there were fewer projects conducted in the primary industry with respect to the health and safety of working population in rural areas. Importantly, the notable phenomenon in the contemporary Chinese labor market has been observed as the rapid mobility of migrant workers, particularly those from rural areas to urban areas. Usually, they do the manual work with temporary contract and part-time job (so-called precarious employment) in cities, which contains more physical, chemical, biologic, and psychosocial hazards, due to their lack of education and skills. The future programs of workplace health promotion should pay more attention to the disadvantaged working population.

## Issues of Work Stress

With the development of globalization, rising competition, greater cross-national mobility, and changing employment relationships, stress at work has become an increasingly important occupational health problem and a significant cause of productivity loss in China. Though the work stress-related diseases (e.g., cardiovascular disease, mental illness, and musculoskeletal disorders) are not legal occupational diseases in the compensation list yet, governments, researchers, and the public have started to show increasing concerns about work stress and its adverse effects. The current framework of occupational health inspection does not include the psychosocial hazards at work, so that workplace health promotion may put a special emphasis on the relevant issues of work stress.

## Summary

As a developing country with rapid industrialization, China is undergoing dramatic economic and social transformation, which has a huge impact on labor market and workers' health. During the past decades, the working conditions and health status of the Chinese working population have been improved remarkably. However, the main health problems are now shifting from infectious diseases to behavior-related chronic diseases; and the occupational diseases and accidents are also threatening the health and safety of workers. The workplace health promotion has been regarded as a feasible and cost-effective way to improve the workers' health and organizations' well-being. This chapter describes the healthcare system and health trends and examines the history and development of workplace health promotion in current China. This is followed by legislative issues with respect to workplace health promotion and some good practices and research projects in this area. The authors conclude that, in China, all stakeholders' participation is crucial to implement a health promotion program in the workplace, and the concept of workplace health promotion should be comprehensive and integrative, focusing on both an organizational level and individual level, particularly working tightly with occupational health inspection.

## Review Questions

1. Why are the demographic, economic, and social changes occurring over the past 2 decades significant to mainland China's health status?
2. What are the components of the healthcare system on mainland China?
3. How do the four major Chinese religions affect population health and health promotion efforts?
4. What are the drivers of workplace health promotion programs for mainland China?
5. Describe the Shanghai model of workplace health promotion.

# References


Central Intelligence Agency (CIA). (2009). *The world factbook.* Retrieved December 16, 2010, from https://www.cia.gov/library/publications/the-world-factbook/index.html

China Health and Nutrition Survey 1997–2006. (n.d). The Carolina Population Center at the University of North Carolina at Chapel Hill and the National Institute of Nutrition and Food Safety at the Chinese Center for Disease Control and Prevention. Retrieved from http://www.cpc.unc.edu/projects/china

Chu, C., Breucker, G., Harris, N., Stitzel, A., Gan, X., Gu, X., & Dwyer, S. (2000). Health-promoting workplaces—international settings development. *Health Promotion International, 15*(2), 155–167.

Gan, X., Gu, X., Zhang, W., & Sally, R. (1995). Workplace health promotion in Shanghai: Needs assessment in four different industries. *Health Promotion International, 10*(1), 25–33.

Graham, A. C. (1990). *Studies in Chinese philosophy and philosophical literature.* Albany, NY: State University of New York Press.

Harris, J. R., Lichiello, P. A., & Hannon, P. A. (2009). Workplace health promotion in Washington state. *Preventing Chronic Disease, 6*(1), A29.

He, F. (1998). Occupational medicine in China. *International Archives of Occupational and Environmental Health, 71*(2), 79-84.

Lamontagne, A. D., Keegel, T., Louie, A. M., Ostry, A., & Landsbergis, P. A. (2007). A systematic review of the job-stress intervention evaluation literature, 1990–2005. *International Journal of Occupational and Environmental Health, 13*(3), 268–280.

Lee, A., Fu, H., & Chenyi, J. (2007). Health promotion activities in China from the Ottawa charter to the Bangkok charter: revolution to evolution. *Promotion & Education, 14*(4), 219–223.

Li, J., Fu, H., Hu, Y., Shang, L., Wu, Y. H., Kristensen, T. S., … Hasselhorn, H. M. (2010). Psychosocial work environment and intention to leave the nursing profession: Results from the longitudinal Chinese NEXT study. *Scandinavian Journal of Public Health, 38*(3 suppl), 69–80.

Li, J., & Jin, T. Y. (2007). Work stress and health—Current research activities and implications in China. *WHO Global Occupational Health Network (GOHNET) Newsletter* (Special), 25–28.

Liang, Y., & Xiang, Q. (2004). Occupational health services in PR China. *Toxicology, 198*(1–3), 45–54.

Liu, M., Gu, X., & Gan, X. (1996). Final evaluation report of WHO project of workplace health promotion in Shanghai industries [in Chinese]. *Shanghai Journal of Preventive Medicine, 8*(10), 433–443.

Liu, Y. (2004). China's public health-care system: Facing the challenges. *Bulletin of the World Health Organization, 82*(7), 532–538.

Liu, Y., Rao, K., Wu, J., & Gakidou, E. (2008). China's health system performance. *Lancet, 372*(9653), 1914–1923.

National Bureau of Statistics of China. (2008). *China population & employment statistical yearbook 2008* [in Chinese]. Edited by the Department of Population & Employment Statistics. Beijing, China: Statistics Press.

National Bureau of Statistics of China. (2009). *China health statistical yearbook 2009* [in Chinese]. Edited by the Ministry of Health. Peking, China: Union Medical College Press.

National Institute of Occupational Health and Poison Control. (n.d.) *Annual statistics of occupational diseases* [in Chinese]. Retrieved from http://www.niohp.net.cn

Ni, J. H., Wang, Y. M. & Li, J. L. (2007). Effect evaluation of health promotion at workplace in joint ventures [in Chinese]. *Chinese Journal of Health Education, 23*(9), 656–658.

Noblet, A., & Lamontagne, A. D. (2006). The role of workplace health promotion in addressing job stress. *Health Promotion International, 21*(4), 346–353.

O'Rourke, D., & Brown, G. D. (2003). Experiments in transforming the global workplace: Incentives for and impediments to improving workplace conditions in China. *International Journal of Occupational and Environmental Health, 9*(4), 378–385.

Pringle, T. E. & Frost, S. D. (2003). The absence of rigor and the failure of implementation: Occupational health and safety in China. *International Journal of Occupational and Environmental Health, 9*(4), 309–316.

Song, W., Chang, C., & Yu, D. (2003). Current status and perspectives of occupational health education and promotion in China [in Chinese]. *Chinese Journal of Industrial Medicine, 16*(6), 321–323.

State Administration of Work Safety, China. (2009, July 1). *Interim administrative provision on worksite occupational health inspection* [in Chinese]. Retrieved from http://www.chinasafety.gov.cn/newpage/Contents/Channel_5351/2009/0708/65936/content_65936.htm

State Administration of Work Safety, China. *Annual statistics of work safety* [in Chinese]. Retrieved from http://www.chinasafety.gov.cn

Su, Z. (2003). Occupational health and safety legislation and implementation in China. *International Journal of Occupational and Environmental Health, 9*(4), 302–308.

*The World Factbook 2009.* (2009). Washington, DC: Central Intelligence Agency. Retrieved August, 2009, from https://www.cia.gov/library/publications/the-world-factbook/index.html

World Health Organization (WHO). (2006). World health report. Working together for health. Geneva, Switzerland: WHO.

WHO. (2007, May 23). Workers' health: Global plan of action. The sixtieth world health assembly. WHA60.26. Retrieved from http://apps.who.int/gb/ebwha/pdf_files/WHA60/A60_R26-en.pdf

Wu, S. Y., Li, J., Wang, M. Z., Wang, Z. M., & Li, H. Y. (2006). Intervention on occupational stress among teachers in the middle schools in China. *Stress and Health, 22*(5), 329–336.

Wu, X., Gu, D., Wu, Y., Yu, X., Wang, S., Wang, N., … Liu, L. (2003). An evaluation on effectiveness of worksite-based intervention for cardiovascular disease during 1974–1998 in Capital Iron and Steel Company of Beijing [in Chinese]. *Chinese Journal of Preventive Medicine, 37*(2), 93–97.

Zhang, Z., & Sun, Q. (2005). Workplace health promotion and control of occupational hazards [in Chinese]. *Chinese Journal of Health Education, 21*(12), 966–969.

## Acknowledgment

This paper is partly supported by a Marie Curie International Incoming Fellowship within the 7th European Community Framework Programme (PIIF-GA-2008-220641) and a grant from the China Medical Board (CMB 08-924). The authors gratefully acknowledge Prof. Johannes Siegrist for his suggestions during the preparation of this paper. We also thank Vivian Ng for her assistance in English editing.

Chapter 6

# Czech Republic

Radim Šlachta and Vladimir Hobza

After reading this chapter you should be able to:

- Identify core strategies that are the focus of the Czech Republic's workplace health promotion efforts
- Describe the historical evolution of the Czech Republic's workplace health promotion efforts
- Explain the different approaches employed by corporate health promotion throughout the Czech Republic
- Review the central disease states and health issues driving workplace health promotion in the Czech Republic
- Name the components of, and the associated funding sources for, the Czech Republic healthcare system
- Discuss the impact of culture on the health status and health promotion efforts within the Czech Republic

Table 6-1 **Select Key Demographic and Economic Indicators**

| | |
|---|---|
| Nationality | Noun: Czech(s)<br>Adjective: Czech |
| Ethnic groups | Czech 90.4%, Moravian 3.7%, Slovak 1.9%, other 4% (2001 census) |
| Religion | Roman Catholic 26.8%, Protestant 2.1%, other 3.3%, unspecified 8.8%, unaffiliated 59% (2001 census) |
| Language | Czech 94.9%, Slovak 2%, other 2.3%, unidentified 0.8% (2001 census) |
| Literacy | Definition: NA<br>Total population: 99%<br>Male: 99%<br>Female: 99% (2003 est.) |
| Education expenditure | 4.4% of GDP (2004)<br>Country comparison to the world: 93 |

*continued*

**Table 6-1 Select Key Demographic and Economic Indicators, *continued***

| | |
|---|---|
| Government type | Parliamentary democracy |
| Environment | Air and water pollution in areas of northwest Bohemia and in northern Moravia around Ostrava present health risks; acid rain damaging forests; efforts to bring industry up to EU code should improve domestic pollution |
| Country mass | Total: 78,867 sq km<br>Country comparison to the world: 115<br>Land: 77,247 sq km<br>Water: 1,620 sq km |
| Population | 10,211,904 (July 2010 est.)<br>Country comparison to the world: 80 |
| Age structure | 0–14 years: 13.6% (male 712,045/female 673,657)<br>15–64 years: 71% (male 3,641,887/female 3,604,044)<br>65 years and over: 15.5% (male 623,882/female 956,389)<br>(2010 est.) |
| Median age | Total: 40.1 years<br>Male: 38.6 years<br>Female: 41.9 years (2009 est.) |
| Population growth rate | -0.094% (2009 est.)<br>Country comparison to the world: 212 |
| Birth rate | 8.83 births/1,000 population (2009 est.)<br>Country comparison to the world: 215 |
| Death rate | 10.74 deaths/1,000 population (July 2009 est.)<br>Country comparison to the world: 49 |
| Net migration rate | 0.97 migrant(s)/1,000 population (2009 est.)<br>Country comparison to the world: 56 |
| Urbanization | Urban population: 73% of total population (2008)<br>Rate of urbanization: 0% annual rate of change (2005–2010 est.) |
| Gender ratio | At birth: 1.06 male(s)/female<br>Under 15 years: 1.06 male(s)/female<br>15–64 years: 1.01 male(s)/female<br>65 years and over: 0.66 male(s)/female<br>Total population: 0.95 male(s)/female (2010 est.) |
| Infant mortality rate | Total: 3.79 deaths/1,000 live births<br>Country comparison to the world: 211<br>Male: 4.13 deaths/1,000 live births<br>Female: 3.43 deaths/1,000 live births (2010 est.) |

*continued*

Table 6-1 **Select Key Demographic and Economic Indicators,** *continued*

| | |
|---|---|
| Life expectancy | Total population: 76.81 years<br>Country comparison to the world: 61<br>Male: 73.54 years<br>Female: 80.28 years (2010 est.) |
| Total fertility rate | 1.25 children born/woman (2010 est.)<br>Country comparison to the world: 215 |
| GDP—purchasing power parity | $254.1 billion (2009 est.)<br>Country comparison to the world: 42 |
| GDP—per capita | $24,900 (2009 est.)<br>Country comparison to the world: 53 |
| GDP—composition by sector | Agriculture: 2.3%<br>Industry: 37.2%<br>Services: 60.5% (2009 est.) |
| Agriculture—products | Wheat, potatoes, sugar beets, hops, fruit, pigs, poultry |
| Industries | Motor vehicles, metallurgy, machinery and equipment, glass, armaments |
| Labor force participation | 5.401 million (2009 est.)<br>Country comparison to the world: 68 |
| Unemployment rate | 8.1% (2009 est.)<br>Country comparison to the world: 90 |
| Industrial production growth rate | -13.1% (2009 est.)<br>Country comparison to the world: 153 |
| Distribution of family income (GINI index) | 26 (2005)<br>Country comparison to the world: 131 |
| Investment (gross fixed) | 22.7% of GDP (2009 est.)<br>Country comparison to the world: 63 |
| Public debt | 34.1% of GDP (2009 est.)<br>Country comparison to the world: 76 |
| Market value of publicly traded shares | $54.48 billion (December 31, 2009)<br>Traded shares country comparison to the world: 53 |
| Current account balance | $-2.146 billion (2009 est.)<br>Country comparison to the world: 151 |
| Debt (external) | $76.83 billion (December 31, 2009 est.)<br>Country comparison to the world: 38 |
| Debt as a % of GDP | ——— |

*continued*

| Table 6-1 **Select Key Demographic and Economic Indicators,** *continued* | |
|---|---|
| Exports | $112.6 billion (2009 est.)<br>Country comparison to the world: 32 |
| Exports—commodities | Machinery and transport equipment 52%, raw materials and fuel 9%, chemicals 5% |
| Exports—partners | Germany 32.25%, Slovakia 9.02%, Poland 5.8%, France 5.62%, United Kingdom 4.93%, Austria 4.71%, Italy 4.38% (2009) |
| Imports | $103.1 billion (2009 est.)<br>Country comparison to the world: 30 |
| Imports—commodities | Machinery and transport equipment 46%, raw materials and fuels 15%, chemicals 10% |
| Imports—partners | Germany 30.67%, Poland 6.97%, Slovakia 6.6%, Netherlands 5.99%, China 5.7%, Austria 5.26%, Russia 4.93%, Italy 3.98% (2009) |
| Stock of direct foreign investment at | |
| Home | $117 billion (December 31, 2009 est.)<br>Country comparison to the world: 30 |
| Abroad | $11.2 billion (December 31, 2009 est.)<br>Country comparison to the world: 48 |

Source: CIA. (2010). *The world factbook*. Retrieved December 16, 2010, from https://www.cia.gov/library/publications/the-world-factbook/

# Introduction

The Czech Republic consists of 10.4 million inhabitants as of the end of 2008. The per capita gross domestic product (GDP) is $16,600 (2008 U.S. dollars), with an unemployment rate of 8.4%, and an inflation rate of 6.3% measured by consumer price index (CPI) (Český statistický úřad, 2009a). As a result of foreign migration, the Czech Republic has become a country with a growing share of foreigners. In 2007, 3.8% of the country's inhabitants did not have Czech citizenship. The aging of the population is characterized by a decreasing percentage of children in the population, with the present value at 14.2% (i.e., a decrease of 0.2% of population and an increasing percentage of persons aged 65 or older. The share of people in the productive age range remains unchanged, along with the index of economic burden (40.4 children and seniors per 100 people at productive age), but the age preference index has increased, as there are 102.4 seniors per 100 children (compared with only 100.2 in 2006).

The Central European countries formerly belonging to the Soviet Bloc are characterized by their socioeconomic traits, which cannot be omitted in research and must be considered when developing preventive measures. For example, one distinguishing characteristic is the equalization of wages; i.e., the earnings ratio of one fifth of the richest to one fifth of the poorest population is 4:1. The housing market is not well developed, and there is a relatively low willingness of inhabitants to change their residence (e.g., only 2.11% of inhabitants moved in 2004) (Český statistický úřad, 2005). In addition, the Czech Republic has low socioeconomic status compared to more developed countries. Only 8% of the population is classified as poor (Eurostat, 2008). Fewer persons have a university education (14.3% in 2008) and the number of work hours per week is generally high (43 hours) (Český statistický úřad, 2009b).

# Prevailing Health Issues

## Life Expectancy

The average life expectancy in evaluated regions is 73.67 years for men and 79.90 years for women in the period 2006–2007 (only available data) (Institute of Health Information and Statistics of the Czech Republic, 2007).

## Mortality Ranking

The most frequent causes of death, according to 2007 statistics, are diseases of the circulatory system, with 45.8% of total mortality in men and 51.5% of total mortality in women (Institute of Health Information and Statistics of the Czech Republic, 2007). The standardized death rate decreased for most diseases, except hypertension and chronic ischemic heart disease. The second most frequent cause of death is neoplasm (28.0% in men and 26.4% in women).

## Health Status (Morbidity Ranking)

The statistics from patients who are monitored for selected diseases show that about one fifth of the Czech population over 18 years suffers from hypertension, and the proportion grows with an increase in age, up to two fifths in persons at the age of 65 or older. The next most frequent diseases are ischemic heart diseases, which afflict 10% of the population over 18 years of age and about one third of people 65 years or older. Cerebrovascular diseases afflict around 3% of adult population and over 10% of the senior population (Institute of Health Information and Statistics of the Czech Republic, 2007).

A very serious and dreaded disease is malignant neoplasm. This disease causes every fourth death in the Czech population and shows a longstanding increasing trend. However, the trend of mortality from malignant neoplasm is fortunately decreasing. Diabetes is another common disease among the Czech population. Diabetology offices provided a total of 2,132,000 treatments of 755,000 patients in 2007. Annually, the number of treated diabetics rises slightly.

## Overweight and Obesity

Obesity affects approximately 25% of women and 22% of men and generally affects 50% of the middle-aged population. The rise in obesity occurrence was very strong in the last decade of the previous century (1990s). The same effect has been proven in the majority of developed countries (Institute of Health Information and Statistics of the Czech Republic, 2007).

## Health or Risk Behaviors

### *Alcohol*

The yearly alcohol consumption is around 10 liters of pure alcohol. Alcohol consumption rose significantly in the 1990s. The same unfavorable increase was also seen in alcohol consumption and drunkenness of youth and adolescents, as well as other significant indicators. This trend contrasts with developments in Western countries; for example, in Poland, alcohol consumption has dropped or at least stabilized.

### *Smoking*

The Czech Republic has a high prevalence of smokers, especially among the teenage population and young people up to 34 years of age (20% of 15-year-olds, including 22% of boys and 18% of girls, smoke at least one cigarette per week). There is a low level of protection for nonsmokers from secondhand smoke, leading to a higher prevalence of fatal and nonfatal consequences of smoking than in other countries, such as a higher mortality rate by smoke-related tumors (Sovinová, 2008).

### *Physical Activity*

More than one half of the Czech population does not comply with the recommended level of physical activity. The lack of moderate intensity physical activity causes frequent disorders in body structure and contributes to the development of chronic diseases such as obesity, cardiovascular diseases, diabetes, osteoporosis, etc. The resulting illnesses affect a significant number of people at productive age and are reasons for a long-term incapability for work (Ministry of Education, Youth, and Sports, 2002). Walking is still the most common physical activity (Frömel et al., 2003) and the most important component of total physical activity. Czech research findings show that men walk on average 75 minutes per day and women, 84 minutes per day. Generally 46.7% of men and 52.9% of women walk every day. Only 6.6% of men and 3.7% of women do not engage in any walking activity during a week. The most important issue is to sustain the habit of walking in children and teenagers, which increases the chances that they will engage in walking at older ages (Mitáš & Frömel, 2007). According to trends in walking activity monitored in the context of pedestrian environment, walking is the key preventive indicator of a healthy lifestyle of Czech citizens. The greatest danger regarding lifestyle is the anticipated drop in walking activity (Frömel et al., 2003).

### *Food*

The state of the health of the population is negatively affected by the inappropriate composition of food, especially due to the excessive prevalence and energetic intake of animal fat, sugar, and salt, and insufficient consummation of fiber, fruit, and vegetables. Even though the eating habits have improved over the last few years, the current state in the Czech Republic is unsatisfactory. The recommended daily amounts of grains are well kept, but the consumption of vegetables is about 60% of the recommended amount; fruit, 65%; and milk, 60%. The consumption of meat is about 20% above the recommended levels (Ministry of Education, Youth, and Sports, 2002).

## Healthcare System

The current healthcare system in the Czech Republic is characterized by the following traits:

- Direct management by the state
- Central planning and financing of healthcare services
- Unified system of healthcare facilities on every municipal and regional level
- The option of choosing one's own doctor is administratively complicated
- Access to health care is officially free of charge

The Ministry of Health has statutory authority as a specialized authority of the government. The ministry is responsible for the development of healthcare policies, the creation of legislative norms, and the coordination of the healthcare system (including health insurance and guarantee of solvency of the healthcare fund). The protection of public health is ensured by sanitary and hygienic stations. The ministry also controls medicines, healthcare equipment, technology, and investment policy in the healthcare sector. It supervises healthcare education and medical research.

The Ministry of Health manages and finances budgetary and allowance organizations. Budget organizations are those that are fully financed using the state budget. Allowance organizations are only partially financed with money from the state budget. At lower levels, the ministry manages the following public services:

- Health service trade unions in regional units, e.g., regional and municipal offices. They ensure coordination of activities within the law to provide public health care and provide support and financing of health care in unexpected events.
- Regional hygienic stations that provide supervision to assure the health of the population.

Other authorities, such as professional chambers, health insurance companies, and nongovernmental organizations contribute to managing the healthcare system.

Public health insurance plays an essential role in financing health service. It is based on the principle of solidarity between the poor and the rich. The public insurance is based on legislative acts pertaining to public health insurance, health insurance for general health care, and insurance company law. The public insurance is obligatory. Insurance companies are public companies and are bound to cover the expenses of medical facilities (hospitals and ambulances) for services provided in accordance with the law.

The healthcare insurance guarantees the right for a free healthcare service. Children, students, and seniors are free from paying insurance premiums unless they receive discretionary income. For those who are registered as unemployed, the state pays for health insurance. If the unemployed is willingly unemployed, according to a legislative act for the year 2009, she/he must pay a monthly insurance fee, which amounts to minimal 1,080 CZK (approximately 42 €). This measure ensures the statutory condition of standard health care.

Sickness insurance is guaranteed by the district administration of social security. This sickness insurance is not mandatory for the self-employed people.

## Influence of Culture and Mentality

Current care for health and the body is not significantly affected by any historic, regionally determined tradition, unlike, for example, in Asian cultures (yoga, tai chi) or Nordic cultures (survival in extreme conditions). The most important Czech tradition was the *Sokol* movement (established 1862), which emphasized strengthening of physical and mental health through physical exercise. Even though the movement still exists today, its positive social influence is small. In historical context, the care for health is negatively affected by the fact that public health care is provided for free and by the existence of a legal claim for free health care. Moreover, free health care was one of the key issues in propaganda during the Communist era. Unfortunately, the situation has not changed much since the revolution. For in the Czech Republic, there generally exists the notion that care for one's own health is not an issue of personal responsibility, but instead is the role of the national health system. Cost-cutting in health care primarily leads to the reduction of prevention campaigns that educate about healthy changes in lifestyle. Caring for one's own health and making lifestyle changes can be seen as unreasonably high standards, depending on the attitude of the individual.

The development of workplace health promotion (WHP) programs is therefore connected with the initiative of foreign companies in the Czech Republic; WPH is usually a part of their transnational corporate strategy. Even in such cases, the implementation of a program meets with little initiative in employees. It has been observed that the offer of programs alone does not guarantee the desired effect. Therefore, it is important to emphasize the motivation of employees and their long-term participation.

The Czech private sphere prefers employee benefits to complex WHP programs. In addition to pension insurance; luncheon vouchers; and company computer, mobile phone, and car, some of the benefits focus on improving lifestyle and health conditions. Some benefits provide memberships to fitness centers, swimming pools, relaxation centers, and the like. In most cases, there is no incentive to use the proposed benefits or to provide effective feedback on their effects. Therefore, it is not possible to choose an effective long-term strategy based on data.

## Drivers of Workplace Health Promotion

Activities focusing on workplace health promotion in the Czech Republic operate at three basic levels:

1. Programs initiated by companies and implemented by the company or an external organization
2. Initiatives of insurance companies in the field of WHP
3. Efforts by government and local administration (Hanuš Šlachta, & Hrabalik, 2002)

### The Role of Firms and Companies

Given that there are minimal outside incentives (advantages in sickness insurance, subsidies from health insurance companies, etc.), the implementation of WHP programs is mainly dependent on the internal incentives of companies. Especially in the case of international companies, the driver for WHP is often corporate culture and strategy. Foreign company owners, and often managers, have a better understanding that programs are efficient for reducing sick leave and increasing productivity. Entirely Czech companies, especially those with few employees, show very low incentive. This is reflected in the current extension and quality of WHP programs.

### The Role of Health Insurance Companies

In the Czech Republic, health insurance companies are classified as public corporations. They are bound to cover the expenses of medical facilities (hospitals and ambulances) for services provided in accordance with the law. Three percent of the budget of insurance companies can be used for preventive health programs. Especially in the preventive health area, health insurance companies can differentiate themselves by the range of services offered. Therefore, the preventive health programs generally serve as a tool to attract new clients. Only 3 health insurance companies out of 10 offer WHP-oriented programs. The quality of programs varies significantly. A unified complex program is offered by only 1 health insurance company, Metal-Aliance. It focuses on complex health goals and specific interventions in lifestyle. The stated objective of the program is the reduction of occurrence of illnesses and the prevention of injuries caused by the work environment, lifestyle, and natural environment. The true objective for the insurance company is the motivation of management and employees to register with the health insurance company.

The health insurance company Škoda, which is a part of an automobile manufacturing holding, has a specific position in the field of WHP for the care of its employees in the Czech Republic.

## The Role of State and Regional Authorities

A political document titled, *Long Term Program for Promoting Health of Czech Citizens—Health 21*, details important activities of state administration, including the field of WHP. The following is one of the key objectives: to commit at least 10% of big- and middle-sized companies to the concept of a healthy company/firm (Ministry of Education, Youth, and Sports, 2002).

The most visible activity is the competition, "A Company Promoting Health," which is run by the National Institute of Public Health (an entity founded by the Ministry of Health for the protection of public health). As part of beneficial programs for the public, the document announces grants for the local level (regions, municipalities) and program Health 21 to support a healthy lifestyle of the local population. This promotion is not reflected in WHP, however, and municipalities are not informed about the existence of these programs.

It is currently difficult to predict the progress that will take place in the future. The situation can be described as a stage with sufficient information about the importance and principles of WHP. The scale of practical use and complex implementation does not reach the level of other developed countries, however. We can only speculate about the main causes of the current situation. This could be due to the current financial situation, a health and social system with little incentives, and societal attitudes concerning individual health and preferred lifestyle. A positive sign is the progress in private businesses that are able to offer complete WHP programs and implement them.

# Programs and Good Practices

In the Czech Republic, there is a whole range of programs and activities that can be categorized in the field of WHP. Their characteristics depend on who initiates and implements the programs.

Government documents, the National Institute of Public Health, and health insurance companies promote and declare support for complex programs. These include, in addition to prevention of workplace injuries, important activities that focus on changing key lifestyle factors. The currently implemented programs in firms and companies usually consist of advanced preventive medical care, which consists of preventive check-ups, vaccinations, and spa therapy. These programs focus less on the detection of specific health-related risks (cardiovascular, oncologic, osteoporosis, etc.) than on recommendation of proper measures. At the level of companies, there are only a few complex programs that offer not only preventive medical health care and healthcare consulting, but also their practical implementation at the workplace or in direct connection to the workplace.

Each year, only a few companies in the Czech Republic reach the National Institute of Public Health's criteria to be called "a company promoting health" (see the "Outcomes and Indicators" section). Between the years 2005 and 2008, it was 6–8 companies a year, and the number dropped in 2009. Since 2007, a new category was created for small and middle-sized companies. Only a few organizations received the award—mainly schools and government offices. Therefore, it can be concluded that small businesses show minimal interest in WHP programs (Kožená, 2008).

As examples of best practices, the following WHP programs of companies and firms placed at leading positions in the National Institute of Public Health's evaluation.

## Government Initiative

### *Competition: "A Company Promoting Health"*

The winner of the "A Company Promoting Health" competition, which has been in existence in the Czech Republic since the year 2005, is officially announced by the chief hygienist officer. While protection of health at the workplace is legislatively regulated, promotion of health at a workplace is not based on legislative requirements. The competition therefore follows the criteria, "Quality Criteria of Workplace Health Promotion," from the European Network for Worksite Health Promotion.

This competition provides an incentive for companies and informs them in a pleasant way about the principles and importance of WHP. The following health areas are targeted:

- Preference for healthy food
- Physical activity
- Incentives for smokers to quit smoking
- Stress management

According to the contest rules, the organizers (National Institute of Public Health) publish the results annually in newspapers and on the web. Nonetheless, the results are not very visible from a public point of view.

## Health Insurance Companies

The program "Healthy Company," created by Metal-Aliance, includes health promotion, care of employees' health, and their safety at work. At the same time, the program aims to create a coordinated system of managing and educating employers, employees, and medical workers in the WHP field.

The main program goals are:

- Creation of a healthy and safe work environment
- Healthy meals

- Higher rate of physical activity outside work
- Education for health and healthy lifestyle
- Health measures in the sphere of companies

The concrete conditions of cooperation between insurance and company are arranged individually (based on the size of the company, number of employees insured, etc.). This kind of information is not publicly available. The scale of implementation, support, and organization of the health insurance company and their actual programs are therefore not known.

## Private Sector

### Česká Rafinérská, a.s. (ČeR)

Česká rafinérská is the biggest manufacturer of crude oil and oil products in the Czech Republic. It currently employs 700 employees. The company is certified in ISO 9001 and ISO 14001 (ISO is an international organization for standardization). It can also use the label Secure Company and Responsible Care, indicating a responsible business in the chemistry industry, and the title "Company Promoting Health 2005."

The company's health promotion program is divided into four basic groups:

1. Lifestyle and positive changes
2. Support of physical activities
3. Special prevention of specific diseases
4. Other supportive actions

The following are examples of implementation of the health support program in Česká rafinérská:

***Groups 1 and 2***

(These projects last a year or longer.)

- *Health and safety in the office.* Administrative workers have access to an educational program on the company's intranet. The program contains important information about health aspects of work in an office (sitting, exercises during breaks at work, arrangement of a workplace, positioning of computers, prevention of injuries, interpersonal relationships, and communication).
- *PROBETA—Environment without tobacco (PROstředí BEz Tabáku).* This project provides basic information about smoking and addiction and ways to quit smoking (series of articles in the company magazine, *ECHO*, posters, information on the intranet). This also includes motivational competition "Stop and Win" with lottery-drawn prizes.
- *NEVA—Do not hesitate with weight (NEváhej nad Váhou).* The project includes a series of information about the causes of obesity and reasonable ways to lose weight (articles in *ECHO* magazine, posters, and information on the intranet). A motivational competition is

regularly organized. As a part of the project, people select courses to reduce their weight according to a popular method in the Czech Republic. The participants receive partial reimbursement for the courses.

- *Handling of psychological stress and its minimization—antistress program.* The program includes training in self-knowledge and self-evaluation, building a positive relationship to oneself and others, identification of stress, and building effective personal resiliency for stress situations.
- *AKTIVITALITA—promotion of exercise and well-being.* This project provides support for a year of sports activities, including at least one sports afternoon for employees, divisional and sectional competitions, and the organization of 9–10 company-wide sports competitions and tournaments. In addition, there is a series of articles, "Trips to Yourself," in the company's magazine. These articles cover stress identification, the influence of social environment, and principles of prevention. Psychological testing is provided for identifying habits, patterns of thinking, and personal character. Finally, AKTIVITALITA include a 2-day course about psychological health and relaxation techniques.

### *Group 3: Special Prevention of Specific Diseases*

- *Osteoporosis screening for seniors.* The examination of bone density in employees at preretirement age provides information about how much a person is likely to suffer from osteoporosis, whether it is necessary to start intensive treatment to minimize risk, and whether it is necessary to continue monitoring bone density.
- *Stress ECG in managers.* Managers are a key human resource and their education and growth costs a lot of money. The prosperity of a company depends on their decisions for many years. Usually a high workload prevents them from keeping a healthy lifestyle, and they are exposed to a higher level of stress. The examination of stress ECG (bicycle ergometry) enables them to identify serious cardiovascular diseases sooner.

### *Group 4: Other Supportive Actions*

As examples:

- Medical advisory center for employees (reducing overweight, smoking)
- Offering Juwim products (Czech-patented preparation with immunomodulative effects) is included in program offerings
- Vaccination against flu (optional benefit)
- Massages

## Škoda Auto a.s.

The company Škoda Auto is an example of a company in the Czech Republic that is taking the most complex approach to WHP programs. Its approach covers of four basic fields:

1. *Protection of health of employees in the company Škoda Auto a.s.* This is a key priority in the field of complex health care for employees. The company is abundantly active in the field of work-related care, beyond the legislative requirements.
2. *Special preventive programs.* These programs encourage early recognition of risk factors and prevention of diseases. The programs consist of:
   - *Cardiovascular program*
     - Revealing the risks of heart and venous diseases, which are a cause of death for more than 50% of the population in the Czech Republic
     - Recommendations of regimen and therapeutic measures for elimination of risks
   - *Oncologic prevention program*
     - Early detection of tumorous diseases
     - Prevention of the most prevalent forms of cancer
   - *Prevention of osteoporosis in women after menopause with cooperation with external professionals*
     - To detect the thinning of bones from the lack of calcium
   - *Program to quit smoking with cooperation of external experts*
     - Employees can enroll for one of three programs to quit smoking, organized by Škoda Auto with cooperation with trade unions
   - *Psychosocial care program with cooperation of external specialists*
     - Discovering and eliminating psychological problems to prevent formation of other serious diseases
3. Other preventive programs for the promotion and maintenance of health.
   - Inoculation against flu
   - Supplementation with vitamin C before the winter
   - Inoculation and consultations for employees travelling to epidemiologically risky areas
   - Rehabilitation programs
   - Relaxation and reconditioning stays at treatment facilities
   - Preventive programs for students of Škoda Auto schools
4. *Health facilities in Škoda Auto a.s.* The company runs a private health facility, Poliklinika Škoda, which is located for easy access directly in the factory area in Mladá Boleslav. The health center building houses examination rooms for some doctors,

while other doctors work directly at the production facilities. This company's health facility provides work-related health care, rehabilitation, and first aid for all employees (Vavřinová, 2007).

The complexity of the above-standard care for employees is indicated by the existence of the company's own health insurance company, Zdravotní pojišťovna Škoda.

As a part of the physical fitness-oriented arm, the company cooperates directly with a specialized fitness center (Medispo s.r.o.) that focuses on healthy and preventive physical activity. In its "Report About Sustainable Development in 2007/2008," Škoda Auto a.s. maintained that its health care and health promotion programs are very successful, documented by the low levels of sick leave, which amount to about half of the average Czech rate.

## Outcomes and Indicators

The National Institute of Public Health is the institution that evaluates WHP programs on a broader scale, comparing program quality across different companies.

The *protection of health at work* is legislatively regulated in the Czech Republic, but *health promotion in the workplace* has no legislative requirements. Therefore, the tool, "Quality Criteria of Workplace Health Promotion, European Network for Workplace Health Promotion" is used for the assessment of effectiveness and quality of WHP programs (Komarek et al., 2005).

The criteria are divided into six sections, which together make a more complex picture of quality of health promotion at a workplace:

1. Worksite and factory health promotion
2. Human resources and workplace organization
3. Health promotion planning
4. Social responsibility
5. Applying health promotion at a workplace
6. The results of worksite health promotion

These indicators are used in the Czech Republic mainly in the competition for "A Company Promoting Health."

Indicators for the quality of worksite health promotion created in the Czech Republic are used by the National Institute of Public Health for small- and middle-sized businesses. Specific criteria are assessed by answers to the following questions:

- Management and participation
    - Do the key roles in a successful worksite health promotion involve company owners or senior managers, who are directly liable to the owners of a small- or middle-sized business?

- Do the leading employees integrate the health factors at a workplace in their daily routine?
- Do all employees participate in planning and decision-making procedures, especially in the issues of organization of work, time schedule, working conditions, and smoothness of work processes?
- Does exemplary management behavior (appreciation of good results, the acceptance of critique from workers, and proper behavior in conflict situations) guarantee a good work atmosphere?
- Are there any suggested improvements, especially regarding organization of work, and monitoring of their implementation?

- Company procedures
    - Well-organized company procedures are based on three elements:
        1. Are all the necessary requirements for safe work, health at work, and protection of the environment well kept?
        2. Are there other measures to promote the health and lifestyle of employees besides the declared requirements?
        3. Does the company behave responsibly to its employees and to the community where it operates?
- Results
    - Managerial practice, based on the described criteria, ensures properly driven company procedures and contributes to the following results:
        - Is the satisfaction of employees with their work conditions monitored?
        - Is customer satisfaction monitored?
        - Is the health state of employees monitored, regarding health promotion (measured by basic indicators, work injuries, or the rate of work absence)?
        - Does the company compare financial results with the costs of health promotion for employees?

## Existing Research

Currently, there is no systematic research in the Czech Republic on the field of WHP. The research teams primarily focus on the relationship between physical activity and health and quality of lifestyle (Frömel et al., 2006; Frömel, Mitáš, & Kerr, 2009; Mitáš & Frömel, 2007; Pelclová, et al., 2009; Sigmund et al., 2009). Physical activity is linked to specific factors. The general topic of lifestyle is divided into more specific fields, such as environment and physical activity, demographic factors, cultural differences, and genetic, ethical, and political factors. WHP is only a marginal matter in this research. Research in the field of occupational health is primarily conducted by the Occupational Safety Research Institute of the Czech Republic. A number of research projects focusing on WHP are currently in progress, including the following:

- Stress in the workplace and the possibility of prevention
- The influence of changes in the working world on quality of life
- Real working conditions and working environment as indicators of health impairment and the shortening of time of professional abilities for specific professions
- Corporate culture and its structure, relationships, and influences

## Conclusion

The current worksite health promotion in the Czech Republic is characterized by:

- Low awareness of citizens and companies about WHP programs and medical and economic results of their implementation
- Lack of tradition and a preference for well-known, common medical preventive programs for health promotion (preventive checkups, vaccinations, etc.)
- Cheap labor and a high unemployment rate, which result in low care for employees
- Lack of legal regulation; therefore, companies regard it as optional and not economical
- Insufficiently incentivized in the legislative-based stimulus for health and sickness insurance (discounts, tax deductions, bonuses, etc.)

The opportunity to improve the current situation can be achieved by public education measures that aim to improve the awareness of WHP programs. The WHP movement should provide strong social, medical, and economic arguments in both the business sphere and the public sphere, including publishing research findings from particular EU countries. WHP in developing countries lacks a legislative framework, and therefore, receives less (or no) attention and support in times of economic crisis (government deficits, risky company finance, etc.).

## Summary

The Czech Republic is a central European country, formerly belonging to the Soviet Bloc. It is characterized by its lower socioeconomic status compared to more developed countries. Further, relatively few people have a university education (14.3% in 2008). The number of work hours per week is generally high. Present health issues, risk behaviors, and their trends are similar to those in other developed European countries. Public health insurance is obligatory and plays an essential role in financing health service. It guarantees the right for a free (standard) healthcare service. However, care for one's own health and changes in lifestyle can be viewed mainly as problems, depending on each individual's attitude. Workplace health promotion is currently an emerging trend whose importance is more realized by professionals and researchers in the field of health promotion than by employers. Government documents, the National Institute of Public Health, and some health insurance companies promote and declare support for complex WHP programs; whereas currently implemented programs in firms and companies usually consist of advanced preventive medical care (preventive check-ups, vaccination, spa therapy, etc.). At the company level, there are only a few complex programs that offer not only preventive medical care and healthcare consulting, but also include practical implementation at the workplace or in direct connection to the workplace.

## Review Questions

1. What are the primary causes of mortality and morbidity in the Czech Republic?
2. Describe the scope and responsibilities of the Czech Republic's Ministry of Health.
3. How are the roles of firms/companies, insurance companies, and state/regional authorities different? Similar?
4. List three examples of workplace health promotion best practices in the Czech Republic.
5. What are the legislative requirements for health promotion at a workplace in the Czech Republic?
6. Describe four research projects that focus on workplace health promotion in the Czech Republic.

## References

Český statistický úřad. (2009a).*Česká republika: hlavní makroekonomické ukazatele.* Retrieved July 21, 2009, from http://www.czso.cz/csu/redakce.nsf/i/cr:_makroekonomicke_udaje/$File/HLMAKRO.xls

Český statistický úřad. (2009b). *Základní informace o oČR, krajích, okresech a obcích; tab. č.3.* Retrieved July 27, 2009, from http://www.czso.cz/sldb/sldb2001.nsf/tabx/CZ0000

Český statistický úřad. (2005). *Vnitřní stěhování v ČR 1991 až 2004.* Retrieved July 23, 2009, from http://www.czso.cz/csu/2005edicniplan.nsf/t/5A003110D9/$File/402905a1.pdf

Eurostat. (2008). Retrieved July 30, 2009, from http://www.businessinfo.cz/cz/clanek/aktuality-z-eu-leden-2010/eurostat-cr-nejnizsi-riziko-chodoby-eu/1001863/56072/

Frömel, K., Bauman, A., Bláha, L., Feltlová, D., Fojtík, I., Hájek, J., … (2006). Intenzita a objem pohybové aktivity 15-69leté populace Český republiky. *Česká Kinantropologie, 10*(1), 13–27.

Frömel, K., Bláha, L., Dvořáková, H., Feltlová, D., Gajda, V., Hájek, J., … (2003). Physical activity of men and women 18 to 55 years old in the Czech Republic. In F. Vaverka (Ed.), *Movement and Health* (pp. 169–173). Olomouc, Czech Republic: Univerzita Palackého.

Frömel, K., Mitáš, J., & Kerr, J. (2009). The associations between active lifestyle, the size of a community, and SES of the adult population in the Czech Republic. *Health & Place, 15*(2), 447–454.

Hanuš, R., Šlachta, R., & Hrabalík, E. (2002). *Outdoor trénink a jeho využití v procesu firemního vzdělávání—Metodický materiál.* Olomouc, Czech Republic: Univerzita Palackého.

Institute of Health Information and Statistics of the Czech Republic. (2007). *Czech Health Statistics Yearbook 2007.* Retrieved July 10, 2009, from http://www.uzis.cz/info.php?article=8&mnu_id=5200&mnu_action=select

Komárek, L., Bencko, V., Mika, J., Rettich, F., Veselá, J., & Volf, J. (2005). *Kritéria kvality podpory zdraví na pracovišti.* Praha, Czech Republic: Státní zdravotní ústav v Praze.

Kožená, L. (2008). *Soutěž Podnik podporující zdraví.* Retrieved July 25, 2009, from National Institute of Public Health at http://www.szu.cz/tema/pracovni-prostredi/soutez-podnik-podporujici-zdravi-1

Ministry of Education, Youth, and Sports. (2002). *Zdraví 21—Dlouhodobý program zlepšování zdravotního stavu obyvatelstva ČR.* Retrieved July 21, 2009, from http://www.msmt.cz/vzdelavani/zdravi-21-dlouhodoby-program-zlepsovani-zdravotniho-stavu-obyvatelstva-cr-zdravi-pro-vsechny-v-21-stoleti-projednan-vladou-ceske-republiky-dne-30-rijna-2002-usneseni-vlady-c-1046?lred=1

Mitáš, J., & Frömel, K. (2007). Vliv faktorů socioekonomického statutu na životní styl obyvatel České Republiky. *Tělesná Kultura, 30*(1), 66–83.

Pelclová, J., Vašíčková, J., Frömel, K., Bláha, L., Feltlová, D., Mitáš, J., … (2009). Vliv vybraných faktorů na pohybovou aktivitu a sezení u zaměstnaných a osob v důchodu ve věku 55–69 let. *Eská Kinantropologie, 12*(4), 49–59.

Sigmund, E., Mitáš, J., Vašíčková, J., Sigmundová, D., Chmelík, F., Frömel, K., … (2009). Biosociální proměnné pohybové aktivity dospělých obyvatel vybraných metropolí České republiky. *Česká Kinantropologie, 12*(4), 9–20.

Škoda Auto a.s. (2008). Report about sustainable development in 2007/2008. Retrieved July 30, 2009, from Škoda auto a.s. at www.skoda-auto.cz/company/CZE/.../SustainabilityReport_2008_CZ.pdf

Sovinová, H. (2008). *Prevalence kuřáctví v dospělé populaci ČR*. Retrieved July 25, 2009, from National Institute of Public Health at http://www.szu.cz/tema/podpora-zdravi/prevalence-kuractvi-v-dospele-populaci-cr

Vavřinová, J. (2007). *Ocenění Podnik podporující zdraví v roce 2007 již potřetí*. Retrieved July 25, 2009, from National Institute of Public Health at http://www.szu.cz/tema/pracovni-prostredi/soutez-podnik-podporujici-zdravi-1

Chapter 7

# Denmark

Thomas Skovgaard and Finn Berggren

After reading this chapter you should be able to:

- Identify core strategies that are the focus of workplace health promotion efforts in Denmark
- Describe the historical evolution of Denmark's workplace health promotion efforts
- Explain the different approaches employed by corporate health promotion throughout Denmark
- Review the central disease states and health issues driving workplace health promotion in Denmark
- Name the components of, and the associated funding sources for, the Danish healthcare system
- Discuss the impact of culture on the health status and health promotion efforts within Denmark

| Table 7-1 **Select Key Demographic and Economic Indicators** | |
|---|---|
| Nationality | Noun: Dane(s)<br>Adjective: Danish |
| Ethnic groups | Scandinavian, Inuit, Faroese, German, Turkish, Iranian, Somali |
| Religion | Evangelical Lutheran 95%, other Christian (includes Protestant and Roman Catholic) 3%, Muslim 2% |
| Language | Danish, Faroese, Greenlandic (an Inuit dialect), German (small minority)<br>*Note:* English is the predominant second language |
| Literacy | Definition: age 15 and over can read and write<br>Total population: 99%<br>Male: 99%<br>Female: 99% (2003 est.) |
| Education expenditure | 8.3% of GDP (2005)<br>Country comparison to the world: 12 |

*continued*

| Table 7-1 Select Key Demographic and Economic Indicators, *continued* | |
|---|---|
| Government type | Constitutional monarchy |
| Environment | Air pollution, principally from vehicle and power plant emissions; nitrogen and phosphorus pollution of the North Sea; drinking and surface water becoming polluted from animal wastes and pesticides |
| Country mass | Total: 43,094 sq km<br>Country comparison to the world: 133<br>Land: 42,434 sq km<br>Water: 660 sq km<br>*Note:* includes the island of Bornholm in the Baltic Sea and the rest of metropolitan Denmark (the Jutland Peninsula, and the major islands of Sjaelland and Fyn), but excludes the Faroe Islands and Greenland |
| Population | 5,500,510 (July 2010 est.)<br>Country comparison to the world: 109 |
| Age structure | 0–14 years: 18.1% (male 511,882/female 485,782)<br>15–64 years: 65.8% (male 1,817,800/female 1,798,964)<br>65 years and over: 16.1% (male 387,142/female 498,940) (2010 est.) |
| Median age | Total: 40.7 years<br>Male: 39.8 years<br>Female: 41.6 years (2010 est.) |
| Population growth rate | 0.28% (2010 est.)<br>Country comparison to the world: 175 |
| Birth rate | 10.54 births/1,000 population (2010 est.)<br>Country comparison to the world: 184 |
| Death rate | 10.22 deaths/1,000 population (July 2010 est.)<br>Country comparison to the world: 57 |
| Net migration rate | 2.48 migrant(s)/1,000 population (2010 est.)<br>Country comparison to the world: 32 |
| Urbanization | Urban population: 87% of total population (2008)<br>Rate of urbanization: 0.5% annual rate of change (2005–2010 est.) |
| Gender ratio | At birth: 1.055 male(s)/female<br>Under 15 years: 1.05 male(s)/female<br>15–64 years: 1.01 male(s)/female<br>65 years and over: 0.78 male(s)/female<br>Total population: 0.98 male(s)/female (2010 est.) |

*continued*

Table 7-1 **Select Key Demographic and Economic Indicators,** *continued*

| | |
|---|---|
| Infant mortality rate | Total: 4.34 deaths/1,000 live births<br>Country comparison to the world: 203<br>Male: 4.39 deaths/1,000 live births<br>Female: 4.29 deaths/1,000 live births (2010 est.) |
| Life expectancy | Total population: 78.3 years<br>Country comparison to the world: 45<br>Male: 75.96 years<br>Female: 80.78 years (2010 est.) |
| Total fertility rate | 1.74 children born/woman (2010 est.)<br>Country comparison to the world: 166 |
| GDP—purchasing power parity | $197.8 billion (2009 est.)<br>Country comparison to the world: 52 |
| GDP—per capita | $36,000 (2009 est.)<br>Country comparison to the world: 31 |
| GDP—composition by sector | Agriculture: 1.2%<br>Industry: 23.8%<br>Services: 74.9% (2009 est.) |
| Agriculture—products | Barley, wheat, potatoes, sugar beets, pork, dairy products, fish |
| Industries | Iron, steel, nonferrous metals, chemicals, food processing, machinery and transportation equipment, textiles and clothing, electronics, construction, furniture and other wood products, shipbuilding and refurbishment, windmills, pharmaceuticals, medical equipment |
| Labor force participation | 2.84 million (2009 est.)<br>Country comparison to the world: 106 |
| Unemployment rate | 4.3% (2009 est.)<br>Country comparison to the world: 38 |
| Industrial production growth rate | -12 % (2009 est.)<br>Country comparison to the world: 151 |
| Distribution of family income (GINI index) | 29 (2007)<br>Country comparison to the world: 118 |
| Investment (gross fixed) | 18.8 % of GDP (2009 est.)<br>Country comparison to the world: 107 |
| Public debt | 41.6% of GDP (2009 est.)<br>Country comparison to the world: 63 |
| Market value of publicly traded shares | $203.2 billion (December 31, 2008)<br>Country comparison to the world: 31 |
| Current account balance | $9.103 billion (2009 est.)<br>Country comparison to the world: 22 |

*continued*

| Table 7-1 Select Key Demographic and Economic Indicators, *continued* | |
|---|---|
| Debt (external) | $607.4 billion (June 30, 2009)<br>Country comparison to the world: 16 |
| Debt as a % of GDP | ——— |
| Exports | $91.49 billion (2009 est.)<br>Country comparison to the world: 35 |
| Exports—commodities | Machinery and instruments, meat and meat products, dairy products, fish, pharmaceuticals, furniture, windmills |
| Exports—partners | Germany 17.53%, Sweden 12.68%, United Kingdom 8.49%, United States 6.05%, Norway 6.01%, Netherlands 4.84%, France 4.57% (2009) |
| Imports | $84.74 billion (2009 est.)<br>Country comparison to the world: 31 |
| Imports—commodities | Machinery and equipment, raw materials and semimanufactures for industry, chemicals, grain and foodstuffs, consumer goods |
| Imports—partners | Germany 21.07%, Sweden 13.18%, Norway 7%, Netherlands 6.97%, China 6.22%, United Kingdom 5.53% (2009) |
| Stock of direct foreign investment at | |
| Home | $145.7 billion (December 31, 2009 est.)<br>Country comparison to the world: 26 |
| Abroad | $185.3 billion (December 31, 2009 est.)<br>Country comparison to the world: 20 |

Source: CIA. (2010). *The world factbook*. Retrieved December 16, 2010, from https://www.cia.gov/library/publications/the-world-factbook/

# Introduction

## From Olsen to Mahler

"When one is in good health, one sleeps well, eats well, plays well, and works well" (Alfred B. Olsen, 1912, original quote translated by the authors of this article). The quote is from a book published about a century ago by the Danish doctor Alfred B. Olsen.

For its time, Olsen's work was a nuanced attempt at health promotion and education to be used, as it states, "in all sorts of homes." The book carries the title *Health for All*, which is interesting because many people associate the *health for all* slogan with more recent times. By the end of the 1970s, the World Health Organization (WHO) started to promote an extended view on what determines human health and well-being. Today there is a broad consensus that a wide range of determinants (also designated by names such as *factors* or *correlates*) impact our health.

Interestingly enough, there is notable common ground between Olsen's work of 1912 and the doings of one of his more contemporary countrymen. Thus, one of the main architects of the modern version of *Health for All* was also a Dane and a doctor: Halfdan Mahler, director-general of WHO from 1973 to 1988.

In spite the many years between them, Olsen and Mahler share a common dynamic perspective on health. Health, well-being, and quality of life are lost and gained in a constant flux—until the end. The individual feat, and the major challenge for people working professionally with health-related issues, is to strive for health as a resource in everyday life.

Such are some of the prime reasons why we persistently subscribe to general (public) health objectives such as increasing life expectancy free of disability or illness for everyone at all ages. Workplace health promotion most certainly has a role to play in this endeavor, especially in a country like Denmark where about 8 out of 10 men and women between 16 and 66 years are active in the labor market (Statistics Denmark, 2009).

## Prevailing Health Issues and Risk Behaviors

In the beginning of 2008, the Danish government appointed a broad-based committee to analyze the present and possible future challenges and opportunities as regards public health and efficient ways to prevent sickness and promote health. The commission published its final report 1 year later, in April 2009 (Forebyggelseskommissionen, 2009). Building on this, a new national plan for prevention and health promotion was launched in October 2009, containing 30 action points in total. Some of these specifically highlight the workplace as one of the everyday settings for promoting health (Government of Denmark, 2009).

The work of the Prevention Committee has in many ways taken place during promising times with regard to the status and trends in health and health behavior in Denmark. Thus, the proportion of daily smokers is dropping, the number of physically active people is on the increase, and the share of the population that consumes a sensible diet is growing. However, Danes, in general, have high levels of alcohol consumption and a small but growing number of adults report that they often feel a great deal of stress. Age groups in active employment feel especially stressed. Furthermore, the overall picture of major lifestyle areas indicates that inequalities in health behavior are related to social and economical variables. In other words, poor health and poor health behaviors clearly cluster in lower social classes. A descriptive analysis of the available data on proximal determinants of health leads to the following observations with regard to smoking, diet, alcohol, and exercise.

## Smoking on the Decline

The proportion of daily smokers has steadily decreased over the last 30 years. Today, less than 30% of the population light up every day. However, among those who smoke, the prevalence of heavy smokers (more than 15 cigarettes a day) is on the rise. Furthermore, it has proven to be a challenge to keep young people from taking up smoking. The number of smokers is highest in the group with the least education and lowest among the group with formal education of considerable length. Smoking is the lifestyle factor that costs the most human lives and has the greatest negative impact on health. For instance, smoking causes 3 out of 10 cases of heart disease and about 90% of all lung cancers (Kjøller & Falk, 2007). The most cost-effective prevention measures to reduce both active and passive smoking are major and noticeable increases in the price of (in particular) cigarettes and legislation making it difficult and/or illegal to smoke in certain settings. Various counseling schemes—for instance, based at or facilitated by the workplace—to quit smoking are also recommended (Kjøller & Falk, 2007).

## Health-Enhancing Physical Activity

Data from national surveys show that the share of adults (16+ years) who engage in strenuous physical activities 4 hours or more a week has been increasing over the years and is now at about 25–30%. In addition, the number of people achieving no fewer than 4 hours of low-intensity to moderate activity a week—like walking and biking at a leisurely pace or doing light gardening—has since the mid-1990s been stable at approximately 5–6 out of 10 (Jensen & Nielsen, 2002; Kjøller, 2007; National Institute of Public Health, 2009).

Despite such positive trends, it remains true that a major part of the Danish adult population is not physically active to the degree of the primary public recommendation of a minimum 30 minutes of moderate-intensity physical activity per day (National Institute of Public Health, 2007b).

## Diet

Current dietary recommendations emphasize eating more foods of plant origin and limiting the intake of red and processed meat. Among other things, higher consumption of plant foods most probably protects against a number of common chronic diseases (World Cancer Research Fund/American Institute for Cancer Research, 2007).

The developments in dietary habits are generally positive. The average intake of vegetables and fruit has increased and the amounts of fatty foods people eat are decreasing. However, only 2 out of 10 adults meet the recommendations for dietary fat and a disappointing 12% consume the recommended 600 or more grams of vegetables and fruits a day. Also, there is a strong social gradient in dietary habits; low socioeconomic status is associated with poor performance in relation to meeting official recommendations in this health behavior area.

An unhealthy diet, together with sedentary living, increases the risk of overweight and thereby the risk of complications such as noninsulin-dependent diabetes and cardiovascular diseases (Groth & Fagt, 2007).

## Alcohol

In Denmark, the main alcoholic drinks are beer, cider, wine, spirits, and liquor. Danes drink quite a lot. For the last 40 years the annual consumption has, on average, been about 11–12 liters of pure alcohol per adult per year. A growing number of Danes are unfortunately exceeding the maximum of standard drinks recommended by the Danish National Board of Health. Young people in Denmark are, compared to just about any other place in the world, very heavy drinkers at an early age (Grønhaek, 2007). Evidently there is reason to work hard on lowering the number of heavy consumers of alcohol among the young, middle-aged, and senior citizens alike. The collective framework for reducing drinking should be discussed and agreed upon at the national and municipal levels, at workplaces, in schools, in sports clubs, and elsewhere. One obvious first move is developing policies on alcohol consumption in everyday settings such as the workplace. At the societal level it must be ensured that alcohol-related health promotion is included in the training of relevant frontline personnel (Government of Denmark, 2002).

# Healthcare System

Denmark has what is usually called a tax-financed, universal health system. Basically this means that anyone who is a permanent resident in Denmark has access to the bulk of health-related examinations, services, and treatments free of charge. Thus, the Danish system is for all intents and purposes managed and developed by public authorities at the national, regional, and local levels. Administratively, the overall guiding principle is that responsibility for the provision of a given service lies with the lowest possible level, most times the regional or municipal councils (Vallgaarda, 2007).

As in most developed countries, health spending in Denmark is rising faster than income. Such increases are, among other things, due to demographics, technologic and pharmaceutical developments, and higher public expectations of the health system (DREAM, 2009).

In many ways, the increased investment is paying off. For instance, after poor developmental trends in the 1970s and 1980s, the growth in average life expectancy for Danish men and women is now at a reasonable level. However, with a life expectancy of 78.1 years at birth, Danes are still underperforming compared to what is sometimes called *EU-15*, an acronym for 15 Western European countries (WHO Europe, 2009).

There is an optional private healthcare sector in Denmark. The importance of this has been growing over the last decade, as the number of people who supplement their public insurance coverage with a private scheme has markedly increased. This is, in part, due to a growing number of employer-provided health insurances. Premiums for private health insurance are not included as a part of salary and therefore are not taxed. Thus, the insurance plans constitute a form of indirect public financing of health services. The number of private hospitals has also been on the rise. Compared to the situation 10–20 years ago, it is now much better business to provide private healthcare services. Still, the private sector continues to play a minor part compared to the vastly larger public health system. The best "guesstimate" for the future is that private insurance plans, covering fees for medicine, dental care, necessities like eyeglasses, health promotion interventions, and hospital treatments, will continue to gain momentum and volume within the Danish healthcare system. Some concerns have been expressed that this will entail growing inequalities with regard to access to and visibility of, first and foremost, health promotion initiatives and hospital treatment. One element in this potential development is the division between those who have insurance plans paid by their employer and those who do not (Vallgaarde & Krasnik, 2007).

A recent major health initiative in 2005 and the succeeding extensive structure reform in Denmark obligated municipality authorities to be the driving force in prevention and health promotion matters. In the required coordinated local and regional health plans, municipalities often mention the workplace as an obvious setting through which to reach the adult population in order to promote health and well-being. Hopefully, public authorities, as major employers themselves and supervisors for workplaces in general, can facilitate a situation where the workplace setting is a potent component in the overall ambition to support health for all and make free choice and self-determination in relation to health a real possibility.

## Influence of Culture and Mentality

It would be fair to describe Denmark as a social-liberal society. This is very much reflected in societal discussions on fundamental questions like: How far should collective responsibility for the individual extend? What should be the responsibility of the individual? Generic questions such as these also form the cornerstone in public debates regarding health-related issues.

However, until very recently, workplace health promotion has not played any major role in the running debate of targets and strategies for public health in Denmark. Apart from the most basic occupational health issues like work safety and primary prevention of hazards, the workplace traditionally has not been the starting point for broader lifestyle and wellness initiatives. Thus, the majority of Danish workplaces have hitherto failed to consider health promotion as a task in which they play any major role. With the stronger political messages of the last 10–20 years concerning the workplace as an important setting for health promotion and disease prevention, it has been possible to see much movement and shift of perspective among the many important decision makers in this nexus. This positive development has been supported by the fact that Danes increasingly expect strong partners like public authorities and workplaces to take responsibility and action in order to secure reasonable opportunities for health and health-enhancing lifestyles. Danes firmly accept and appreciate the personal responsibility of choice in health behaviors. At the same time, they demand that a setting like the workplace is structured in ways that make the healthy choice obvious and possible (Mandag Morgen, 2008).

Unfortunately a number of barriers consistently work against the further development of workplace health promotion. These have a lot to do with practical ostacles like the varying work hours many Danish employees have (more or less by choice); so-called limitless work wherein the boundary between work and private life is becoming more and more blurred for more and more employees; no possibility of interrupting a work function due to piece-work rates; and an increasing amount of the workforce spending a lot of time commuting. Based on a solid Danish tradition of voluntary participation and respect for individuals, issues like the ones mentioned must be taken into consideration in order to strengthen workplace health promotion and link the many separate initiatives to general efforts made by public authorities to improve workplace health and safety (The Danish National Board of Health, 2009).

## Drivers of Workplace Health Promotion

The single most important driver for workplace health promotion programs has been legislation on work-related safety and health. In Denmark, the focus has largely been confined to the prevention of physical accidents at work. Employers are legally bound to provide for the safety of their employees but not equally required to provide further health services in relation to lifestyle issues, etc. Thus, the employers' incentive to support workplace health promotion is not very pronounced.

This does not, however, mean that workplace health promotion is not happening in Denmark. In fact, 9 out of 10 workplaces are engaged in at least 1 major health-enhancing initiative, with programs on tobacco and alcohol being the most common. Possibly the most distinctive feature in relation to workplace health promotion in Denmark is that it, only to a limited degree, is a product of strong and forward-looking strategic planning. The latest overview, published by the National Board of Health in 2007 and covering about 1,900 public and private businesses, shows that even though 1 out of 3 employers state that they have a written health policy, more than two thirds include this policy as but one among many components in the general personnel strategy. In total, only 7% of Danish workplaces have an independent, high-profile health policy. Twenty percent of workplaces with a health policy have implemented it strategically in day-to-day operations, and very few have formulated measurable impact goals for their health policy. About half of the workplaces (47%) set aside financial means for health promotion activities and programs. A mere 7% have at their disposal an employee with time dedicated to realize and assess the company health policy. The described state of affairs contrasts the fact that most employers feel a high level of responsibility as regards creating an optimal working environment, including employees' possibilities to cope with (negative) stressors and in relation to behavior areas like diet, physical activity, smoking, and alcohol (The Danish National Board of Health, 2008b).

## Who Is Most Active and Who Has a Major Interest in the Field of Workplace Health Promotion?

Nationwide campaigns, organizations, and networks, such as the Danish National Board of Health and WHO/Healthy Cities Network, have highlighted ways in which the workplace can serve as a potent setting for health promotion and prevention initiatives.

Major patient associations, such as the Danish Cancer Society, the Danish Heart Foundation, and the Danish Diabetes Association, have also initiated health promotion programs in a number of workplaces. For-profit companies are increasingly moving into the workplace health promotion market. Wellness and health-oriented initiatives are increasingly becoming a standard perk and a feature used by companies to attract and hold on to their most crucial assets—qualified, high-performing employees. Supplying health promotion services and products is thus becoming a real and profitable business in Denmark, as it has been for a number of years in many other countries.

Looking at the nonprofit sector, the sports associations have especially engaged in the development of workplace-related health promotion. During the last 15 years, the Danish company Sports Federation has, for instance, become a strong player in the area.

## What Role Do Government Authorities Play?

The Danish National Board of Health has for a number of years been supportive as regards workplace health promotion. This has resulted in a variety of educational and setting-based initiatives dealing with the promotion of health and well-being. Also, in the last ten years, the government has produced and published a number of guidelines on the implementation of health promotion at workplaces (e.g., The Danish National Board of Health, 1997a, 1997b). At the end of 2009, the National Board launched a new comprehensive program, Health and Well-being at the Workplace—Inspiration to Systematic and Strategic Implementation of Health Promotion (The Danish National Board of Health, 2009). It will be interesting to follow what kind of impact this latest initiative will have on the area of workplace health promotion in Denmark. When it comes to funding, it has many times proven to be difficult for central authorities to allocate the resources needed to really demonstrate what works in relation to workplace health promotion, and from this, (1) design and produce solid guidelines for efficient implementation and (2) single out interventions that seem more cost-effective than other feasible alternatives.

# Programs and Good Practices

Marked interest in workplace health promotion first emerged in the mid-1980s, around the time when the Danish government presented the first comprehensive Government Preventive Program, influenced by WHO's strategy Health for All—Year 2000 (Ministry of Health, 1989).

In the years around 1990, some of the main reasons for implementing measures to promote good health at work were connected to expected outcomes like reduced absenteeism and increases in work efficiency. Today, frequently cited aims include promoting social relations between employees; strengthening the social profile and brand of the company; attracting and retaining employees; and contributing to the overall work environment (Skovgaard & Berggren, 2006; The Danish Working Environmental Council, 2009).

Thus it seems fair to state that Danish employers are interested in using health activities as a means of promoting their employees' well-being.

As already mentioned, the Danish National Board of Health has conducted a number of surveys on the prevalence and focus of workplace health promotion programs in Denmark. The latest figures from 2007 and 2009 show that just about all workplaces have campaigns and programs in relation to tobacco and alcohol. One out of two workplaces has schemes focusing on diet; physical activity; easy, employer-subsidized access to services such as physiotherapy, chiropractor or massage; and/or the promotion of mental well-being at work which, among other things, means handling work-related stress. Of course, it varies quite a lot as to how many resources and how much energy and focus workplaces put into their health promotion programs. Some support a very limited number of activities via the investment of little means while others display a comprehensive strategy covering a wide number of health and health behavior dimensions. Perhaps not surprisingly, the size of the workplace appears to have an effect on the extent to which health promotion opportunities are provided. Thus, companies with more than 100 employees are highly more likely to have broad-based arrangements (The Danish National Board of Health, 2008a; The Danish Working Environment Council, 2009).

In a time in which evidence-based, or at the very least data-driven, practice is heavily in vogue, it is interesting that only a minority of Danish workplaces can be said to conduct a systematic, regular assessment of their health promotion schemes and activities. This is not, however, a distinctively Danish phenomenon, but rather an indication of a general trend whereby the majority of health promotion programs are not subject to evaluation. Useful evaluation demands adequate resources, including the availability of time, money, and regular staff or consultants skilled in carrying out evaluation activities. Company budgets rarely allow room for such ideal provisions. However, an enlightened development of workplace health promotion in Denmark must include the use of relevant indicators to make solid performance measurements possible.

## Novo Nordisk: A Global Strategy

Novo Nordisk is a global healthcare company with more than 29,000 employees, of whom about half are located in Denmark. The company is a world leader in diabetes care.

In early 2008, Novo introduced a joint company health program building on four global standards. This program has been implemented with respect for the cultural differences that characterize Novo's various branches and offices.

The standards ensure that all employees have:

- Access to a smoke-free work environment and smoking cessation programs
- Access to healthy foods and beverages at the workplace
- Access to physical activities
- The possibility of a personal health check and individual lifestyle counseling every 2nd year

By upholding these four global standards, Novo strives to make the healthy choice easy and obvious. The standards and the company's other health and safety initiatives are systematically promoted via various social marketing techniques and channels. Information and communication technology plays an important role in this connection, for instance through use of NovoTube (inspired, of course, by YouTube).

The entire health strategy—which also contains specific goals on work/life balance, job security and employability, etc.—is managed by a global human resources board and figures explicitly in the annual reporting system. The goal-attainment rates of the various strategic initiatives are evaluated using performance data. Novo is committed to moving forward and expanding its efforts as regards workplace health promotion (The Danish National Board of Health, 2009; Nova Nordisk, 2010).

## Outcomes and Indicators

Ideally, solid indicators and scientifically based evaluation methods should be systematically applied in order to make valid assessments concerning the effectiveness of workplace health initiatives and how the initiatives work. Like all other core parts of a given enterprise (be it private, public, or something in between), health promotion should be integrated into the company's quality assurance system, wherein key functions and results are monitored and reported to relevant decision makers.

In the real world, however, the majority of Danish workplaces put limited effort into evaluating the process and impact of health promotion initiatives. This is problematic; remember the dictum, "What gets measured gets done." Put in a different way, if we want to strive for excellence and solid improvement of workplace health promotion, we must evaluate the quality (in relation to a number of dimensions agreed upon by all parties involved) of our present efforts in order to decide on the best way to move forward. Not many would disagree with this last idea. But the numbers show that Danish workplaces, as a rule, do not follow up on their health promotion initiatives—not even when these constitute visible strategic ventures.

A recent report, published by the national working environment authorities, shows that only a minority of workplaces have written objectives for health promotion activities. The written objectives are primarily attached to the following health-related issues: smoking, alcohol, psychosocial work environment, and absenteeism. Forty to fifty percent of workplaces have written objectives in these areas. In relation to, for instance, diet and physical activity, only 1 out 10 employers states that it written objectives. Many of the workplaces that have formulated objectives do not assess to what degree these have been attained (The Danish Working Environment Council, 2009). Thus, in many instances, Danish workplaces do not seem to be very attentive to exactly what the outputs and final outcomes are of health promotion initiatives. Some of the reasons for this unfortunate situation have been mentioned earlier (see "Programs and Good Practices"). Let it suffice to state that probably the best and maybe the only way to increase workplaces' evaluation of health promotion programs is not to ask for *state of the art* assessments. Instead, through mutual support and inspiration supplemented with fair but firm formal demands and regulations, workplaces should be inspired and empowered to produce and put forward the best possible evaluations on both the effects of health promotion efforts and information about organization and implementation of such efforts (see "Conclusion" for further remarks on the issue of assess-ment/evaluation).

## Existing Research

The field of workplace health promotion in Denmark is in a state of change. New knowledge is being generated, and best practices are being developed. The research-based evidence that already exists on effective interventions is communicated better today than even a few years ago. This is a positive development that must be supported by continuing the work in gathering evidence on effective methods and initiatives.

There are, however, still many areas in which we have scarce knowledge regarding key questions like how best to reach targeted populations; how to develop organizational support to deliver specific workplace interventions; and how to ensure that the selected interventions are delivered as prescribed in order to be effective in expected ways (The Danish National Board of Health, 2008a). Thus, at a time when business administrators, policy makers, practitioners, planners, and researchers frequently stress workplace health promotion as an important action zone for the coming years, we know quite a lot about the determinants of health and well-being. Unfortunately, we are still lacking solid evidence on the relative effectiveness of various health promotion and preventive interventions and to what extent promising programs are transferable across subgroups of, for instance, settings and target populations (The Danish National Board of Health, 2008a).

In a recent review of both national and international literature on workplace health promotion, the Danish Institute for Health Services Research concludes that (1) there exist relatively few solid publications on the effectiveness of workplace health promotion, and (2) only a few intervention models have been thoroughly tested and evaluated in more than one study. These overall conclusions were reached after compiling and summarizing the available evidence on workplace interventions in relation to diet, alcohol, smoking, physical activity, stress, and integrated programs dealing with more than one health-behavior area. On top of randomized, controlled trials, the review also includes quasiexperimental studies using, for instance, matched controls or cluster randomization designs. Well-ordered and carefully reported before-and-after measurements are also reviewed (Højgaard, 2008).

Before we become too downhearted by our apparent poor ability to generate solid evidence on both the results and process of workplace health promotion programs, it must be remembered that the demand is not for studies that establish causality under ideal conditions. The need is for real-world investigations to establish results under typical conditions. In technical terms, the call is for assessments of both the internal and external validity of specified workplace health interventions. Such appraisals are indeed requested within research, policy, and practice. They are, however, not always that easy to produce. This is due to gaps in the empirical knowledge and a lack of agreement on what makes up a theoretical and methodological toolbox suitable for addressing the complex challenges with which most workplace health promotion issues present us (Leeuw & Slovgaard, 2005; The Danish National Board of Health, 2008a).

Still, recognizing that there are many unanswered questions in relation to what works best for whom when using the workplace as an arena for health promotion, a publication released by the Danish National Board of Health in 2009 put forward the following five central messages in relation to workplace health promotion.

1. Working systematically within health promotion at and through the workplace pays off. There is, so to speak, good return on investment.
2. The gains and positive effects increase if workplace health promotion plays an active role in forward-looking strategies on, for instance, organizational performance.
3. Health promotion is about lifestyle, work–life balance, and corporate social responsibility.
4. Public and private workplaces of any size and in various lines of business can all make a real difference in relation to the health and well-being of their employees, even though the conditions vary.
5. Workplace health promotion programs must have positive and widespread effect in order to be tailored to the company in question (The Danish National Board of Health, 2009).

This last issue touches on how a given intervention and its effects can be maintained over time—a matter of crucial importance. Where the individual employee is concerned, the maintenance issue could zoom in on the ability to keep up changes in health-related habits and routines brought about by a given intervention. At the workplace level, the maintenance issue could circle around the feasibility of making interventions part of day-to-day operations.

In general, making health promotion an integrated part of the work environment appears to have at least a short-term positive effect on the maintenance issue. However, the biggest challenge of a workplace health promotion program is to sustain long-term interest and enthusiasm. This conclusion goes for both the individual and organizational level. Workplaces wanting to support long-term efforts must be prepared to invest many types of resources (e.g., human, financial, and organizational). Another challenge is engaging the more sedentary part of the workforce. Participation rates in workplace health promotion programs are not always that impressive, and many times those who do take part tend to be the employees whose general health and health behavior profile are better than average. Thus, in order to strengthen our knowledge and understanding of what works and why in relation to workplace health promotion, we must improve the quality and quantity of reports on both specific, short-term interventions and multicomponent programs running for longer periods of time. Using common and explicit standards on how to produce and communicate the design, implementation, and effectiveness of real-world health promotion and preventive measures constitutes a solid step forward. A major barrier for making this happen is that, as already stated, few employers make provisions for systematic evaluation of their health promotion programs through user surveys, measurement of results, etc.

## Conclusion

This chapter makes the case that, on the whole, workplace health promotion in Denmark has been gaining ground, especially since the late 1990s. Thus, there seems to be support for the conclusion that employers are interested in using health activities as a means of promoting their employees' well-being. If this is correct, future effort should, among other things, ensure that volunteers and paid professionals engaged in health promotion at workplaces receive better training and education in health-related issues. With a view to encourage the development of educational programs for individuals who wish to engage in careers in WHP, national guidelines should be considered in order to increase the learning standard. A future objective could be to implement a common reference system in the European Union and maybe even beyond. One possible starting point is the general quality criteria for workplace health promotion developed by the European Network for Workplace Health Promotion.

Furthermore, we need to build a more solid and reliable evidence base as regards best practices in workplace health promotion. The aim should be to generate practice-based knowledge, building on empirical findings from interventions implemented in everyday settings. To this end, a strong commitment must be made to put together monitoring and evaluation systems that provide information on the character and performance of particular workplace health promotion programs and wider policies. Ideally, such assessment systems should not only focus on the short time frame of instrumental utility. An effort should also be made to contribute to the growth of a more general, contextually oriented body of knowledge in the broad topic of workplace health promotion. This type of knowledge is crucial in the move further towards evidence-informed health promotion that combines the question of what interventions work with queries like *how and why do health interventions and programs work, at what cost, and in what kind of settings?* (Harrison, 2003).

Public authorities, private companies, and research institutions must work together on this matter. To do so they have to be convinced that there is something in it for them. There is a need to identify workable and sustainable ways to link these many and varying interests.

The field of workplace health promotion is indeed in a state of change and motion in Denmark. These are exciting and challenging times. Great challenges are well known to be inspired by, and themselves inspire, great words. So, let us end with Halfdan Mahler's reading of the core of the matter that eventually ended up as a prime statement in what has been called the cornerstone of new public health: The Ottawa Charter adopted in 1986.

> Health is created and lived by people within the settings of their everyday life; where they learn, work, play and love. Health is created by caring for oneself and others, by being able to make decisions and have control over one's life circumstances, and by ensuring that the society one lives in creates conditions that allow the attainment of health by all its members. (Mahler, 1986)

## Summary

Increased political and general social interest has, since the late 1990s, led to a significant strengthening of the workplace as a setting for health promotion and prevention in Denmark. Some of the most frequently cited reasons for employers to engage in health promotion activities are to promote social relations between employees; to strengthen the social profile and brand of the company; to attract and retain employees; and to contribute to the overall work environment. One of the distinctive features in workplace health promotion in Denmark is that it, to only a limited degree, is a product of strong and forward-looking strategic planning. Thus, only 7% of Danish workplaces have an independent, high-profiled health policy, and only very few of these contain measurable impact goals.

In many ways, we are still lacking solid evidence on the relative effectiveness of various workplace health promotion and preventive interventions and to what degree promising programs are transferable across subgroups of, for instance, settings and target groups. However, new knowledge is being generated and best practices are being developed. The research-based insight that exists on effective interventions is conveyed better today than just a few years ago. This is a positive development that must be supported by continuing the work of generating evidence on effective initiatives as regards workplace health promotion.

## Review Questions

1. What did Alfred Olsen mean by "Health for All" in his 1912 tome?
2. What did the government of Denmark determine were the prevailing health issues in their 2009 commission report?
3. What are the components of Denmark's healthcare system, and how are they funded? Regulated? Managed?

4. What was the major Danish health law passed in 2005, and what are its implications?
5. What is the driving force behind Denmark's workplace health promotion programs?
6. Identify and describe two of the national campaigns Denmark has used to promote workplace health promotion.
7. Describe the role of the Danish government in workplace health promotion activities in Denmark.
8. Are Danish workplace health promotion programs effective at producing useful analytics of their programs? Explain.
9. List the five central messages in relation to workplace health promotion that the Danish National Board put forward in 2009.

# References

The Danish National Board of Health. (1997a). *På vej mod en sundere arbejdsplads.* Copenhagen, Denmark: Author.

The Danish National Board of Health. (1997b). *På vej mod en sundere arbejdsplads—Fokus på Motion.* Copenhagen, Denmark: Author.

The Danish National Board of Health. (2008a). *Evidence in health promotion and disease prevention.* Copenhagen, Denmark: Author.

The Danish National Board of Health. (2008b). *Sundhedsfremme på arbejdspladsen—2007.* Copenhagen, Denmark: Author.

The Danish National Board of Health. (2009). *Sundhed og trivsel på arbejdspladsen.* Copenhagen, Denmark: Author.

The Danish Working Environment Council. (2009). *Sundhedsfremmeaktiviteter på arbejdspladsen.* Copenhagen, Denmark: Rambøll Management Consulting.

DREAM. (2009). *Langsigtet økonomisk fremskrivning 2009.* Copenhagen, Denmark: Author.

Forebyggelseskommissionen. (2009). *Vi kan leve længere og sundere.* Copenhagen, Denmark: Schultz.

Government of Denmark. (2002). *Healthy throughout life.* Retrieved February 4, 2010, from http://www.folkesundhed.dk/ref.aspx?id=190

Government of Denmark. (2009). *Sundhedspakke 2009. Godt på vej mod et sundere Danmark.* Copenhagen, Denmark: Author.

Grønbaek, M. (2007). *Alkohol.* In M. Kjøller, K. Juel, & F. Kamper-Jørgensen (Eds.), *Folkesundhedsrapporten*, Danmark 2007. Copenhagen, Denmark: National Institute of Public Health, 209–220.

Groth, M.V., & Fagt, S. (2007). *Kost*. In M. Kjøller, K. Juel, & F. Kamper-Jørgensen (Eds.), *Folkesundhedsrapporten, Danmark 2007*. Copenhagen, Denmark: National Institute of Public Health, 247–260.

Harrison, T. (2003). Evidence-based multidisciplinary public health. In J. Orme, J. Powell, T. Taylor, T. Harrisson, & M. Grey. (Eds.). *Public health for the 21st century*. Berkshire, England: Open University Press.

Højgaard, B. (2008). *Effekten af sundhedsfremme på arbejdspladsen— hvor meget dokumentation er der?* Copenhagen, Denmark: DSI.

Jensen, J. N., & Nielsen, N.S. (2002). *Fysisk Aktivitet*. In M. Kjøller & N. K. Rasmussen (Eds.), *Sundhed og sygelighed i Danmark 2000 & udviklingen siden 1987*. Copenhagen, Denmark: National Institute of Public Health, 338–349.

Kjøller, M., & Falk, J. (2007). *Rygning*. In M. Kjøller, K. Juel, & F. Kamper-Jørgensen (Eds.), *Folkesundhedsrapporten, Danmark 2007*. Copenhagen, Denmark: National Institute of Public Health, 221–234.

Kjøller, M., & Rasmussen, N.K. (2002). *Danish Health and Morbidity survey 2000 & trends since 1987*. Copenhagen, Denmark: National Institute of Public Health.

Kjøller, M. (2007). *Fysisk Aktivitet*. In M. Kjøller, K. Juel, & F. Kamper-Jørgensen (Eds.), *Folkesundhedsrapporten, Danmark 2007*. Copenhagen, Denmark: National Institute of Public Health, 235–246.

Leeuw, E. De, & Skovgaard T. (2005). *Utility-driven evidence for Healthy Cities: Problems with evidence generation and application. Social Science & Medicine*, 61(6): 1331–1341.

Mahler, H. (1986). Towards a new public gealth. *Health Promotion International, 1*, 409–411.

Mandag Morgen. (2008). *Fremtidens Forebyggelse— ifølge danskerne*. Copenhagen, Denmark: Author.

Ministry of Health. (1989). *The health promotion programme of the government of Denmark*. Copenhagen, Denmark: Author.

National Institute of Public Health. (2007a). *Public health report, Denmark 2007*. Copenhagen, Denmark: Author.

National Institute of Public Health. (2007b). *Sundheds—og sygelighedsundersøgelsen 2005: Interviewskema med svarfordeling*. Copenhagen, Denmark: Author

National Institute of Public Health. (2009). *KRAM-undersøgelsen i tal og billeder*. Copenhagen, Denmark: Author.

Novo Nordisk. (2011). Homepage. Retrieved August 4, 2010, from http://www.novonordisk.com

Olsen, A. B. (1912). *Sundhed for alle*. Copenhagen, Denmark: Author.

Skovgaard, T., & Berggren, F. (2006, fall). The prevalence and focus of workplace fitness programs in Denmark: Results of a national survey. *The Sports Journal, (9)*, 4.

Statistics Denmark. (2009). *Denmark in figures.* Copenhagen, Denmark: Author.

Vallgaarda, S. (2007). *The Danish Health System.* In S. Vallgaarda & A. Krasnik (Eds.), *Health Services and Health Policy*. Copenhagen, Denmark: Gyldendals Akademisk, 133–198.

Vallgaarda, S., & Krasnik, A. (2007). *Health services and health policy.* Copenhagen, Denmark: Gyldendals Akademisk.

WHO Europe. (2009). *The European health report 2009: Health and health systems.* Copenhagen, Denmark: WHO.

World Cancer Research Fund/American Institute for Cancer Research. (2007). *Food, nutrition, physical activity, and the prevention of cancer: A global perspective.* Washington, DC: Author.

Chapter 8

# Finland

Antero Heloma

After reading this chapter you should be able to:

- Identify core strategies that are the focus of workplace health promotion efforts in Finland
- Describe the historical evolution of Finland's workplace health promotion efforts
- Explain the different approaches employed by corporate health promotion throughout Finland
- Review the central disease states and health issues driving workplace health promotion in Finland
- Name the components of, and the associated funding sources for, Finland's healthcare system
- Discuss the impact of culture on the health status and health promotion efforts within Finland

Table 8-1 **Select Key Demographic and Economic Indicators**

| | |
|---|---|
| Nationality | Doun: Finn(s)<br>Adjective: Finnish |
| Ethnic groups | Finn 93.4%, Swede 5.6%, Russian 0.5%,<br>Estonian 0.3%, Roma (Gypsy) 0.1%, Sami 0.1% (2006) |
| Religion | Lutheran Church of Finland 82.5%, Orthodox Church 1.1%,<br>other Christian 1.1%, other 0.1%, none 15.1% (2006) |
| Language | Finnish 91.2% (official), Swedish 5.5% (official), other 3.3%<br>(small Sami- and Russian-speaking minorities) (2007) |
| Literacy | Definition: age 15 and over can read and write<br>Total population: 100%<br>Male: 100%<br>Female: 100% (2000 est.) |
| Education expenditure | 6.4% of GDP (2005)<br>Country comparison to the world: 33 |

*continued*

Table 8-1 **Select Key Demographic and Economic Indicators,** *continued*

| | |
|---|---|
| Government type | Republic |
| Environment | Air pollution from manufacturing and power plants contributing to acid rain; water pollution from industrial wastes, agricultural chemicals; habitat loss threatens wildlife populations |
| Country mass | Total: 338,145 sq km<br>Country comparison to the world: 64<br>Land: 303,815 sq km<br>Water: 34,330 sq km |
| Population | 5,250,275 (July 2010 est.)<br>Country comparison to the world: 112 |
| Age structure | 0–14 years: 16.4% (male 438,425/female 422,777)<br>15–64 years: 66.8% (male 1,773,495/female 1,732,792)<br>65 years and over: 16.8% (male 357,811/female 524,975)<br>(2010 est.) |
| Median age | Total: 42.1 years<br>Male: 40.5 years<br>Female: 43.7 years (2009 est.) |
| Population growth rate | 0.098% (2010 est.)<br>Country comparison to the world: 191 |
| Birth rate | 10.38 births/1,000 population (2010 est.)<br>Country comparison to the world: 187 |
| Death rate | 10.07 deaths/1,000 population (July 2010 est.)<br>Country comparison to the world: 61 |
| Net migration rate | 0.68 migrant(s)/1,000 population (2010 est.)<br>Country comparison to the world: 60 |
| Urbanization | Urban population: 63% of total population (2008)<br>Rate of urbanization: 0.8% annual rate of change (2005–2010 est.) |
| Gender ratio | At birth: 1.04 male(s)/female<br>Under 15 years: 1.04 male(s)/female<br>15–64 years: 1.02 male(s)/female<br>65 years and over: 0.68 male(s)/female<br>Total population: 0.96 male(s)/female (2010 est.) |

*continued*

Table 8-1 **Select Key Demographic and Economic Indicators,** *continued*

| | |
|---|---|
| Infant mortality rate | Total: 3.47 deaths/1,000 live births<br>Country comparison to the world: 216<br>Male: 3.78 deaths/1,000 live births<br>Female: 3.15 deaths/1,000 live births (2010 est.) |
| Life expectancy | Total population: 78.97 years<br>Country comparison to the world: 37<br>Male: 75.48 years<br>Female: 82.61 years (2010 est.) |
| Total fertility rate | 1.73 children born/woman (2010 est.)<br>Country comparison to the world: 167 |
| GDP—purchasing power parity | $178.8 billion (2009 est.)<br>Parity country comparison to the world: 56 |
| GDP—per capita | $34,100 (2009 est.)<br>Country comparison to the world: 36 |
| GDP—composition by sector | Agriculture: 3.6%<br>Industry: 30.3%<br>Services: 66.1% (2009 est.) |
| Agriculture—products | Barley, wheat, sugar beets, potatoes, dairy cattle, fish |
| Industries | Metals and metal products, electronics, machinery and scientific instruments, shipbuilding, pulp and paper, foodstuffs, chemicals, textiles, clothing |
| Labor force participation | 2.68 million (2009 est.)<br>Country comparison to the world: 107 |
| Unemployment rate | 8.5% (2009 est.)<br>Country comparison to the world: 98 |
| Industrial production growth rate | -11.8% (2009 est.)<br>Growth rate country comparison to the world: 147 |
| Distribution of family income (GINI index) | 29.5 (2007)<br>Income (GINI index) country comparison to the world: 115 |
| Investment (gross fixed) | 20.6% of GDP (2009 est.)<br>Country comparison to the world: 83 |
| Public debt | 44% of GDP (2009 est.)<br>Country comparison to the world: 60 |
| Market value of publicly Traded shares | $NA (December 31, 2009)<br>Traded shares country comparison to the world: 28 |
| Current account balance | $2.916 billion (2009 est.)<br>Country comparison to the world: 33 |

*continued*

| Table 8-1 Select Key Demographic and Economic Indicators, *continued* | |
|---|---|
| Debt (external) | $364.9 billion (June 30, 2009 est.)<br>Country comparison to the world: 21 |
| Debt as a % of GDP | ——— |
| Exports | $62.93 billion (2009 est.)<br>Country comparison to the world: 39 |
| Exports—commodities | Electrical and optical equipment, machinery, transport equipment, paper and pulp, chemicals, basic metals, timber |
| Exports—partners | Germany 10.32%, Sweden 9.79%, Russia 9%, United States 7.85%, Netherlands 5.9%, United Kingdom 5.24%, China 4.1% (2009) |
| Imports | $58.98 billion (2009 est.)<br>Country comparison to the world: 41 |
| Imports—commodities | Foodstuffs, petroleum and petroleum products, chemicals, transport equipment, iron and steel, machinery, textile yarn and fabrics, grains |
| Imports—partners | Russia 16.28%, Germany 15.76%, Sweden 14.65%, Netherlands 6.99%, China 5.29%, France 4.22% (2009) |
| Stock of direct foreign investment at | |
| Home | $80.9 billion (December 31, 2009 est.)<br>Country comparison to the world: 39 |
| Abroad | $117.7 billion (December 31, 2009 est.)<br>Country comparison to the world: 23 |

Source: CIA. (2010). *The world factbook*. Retrieved December 16, 2010, from https://www.cia.gov/library/publications/the-world-factbook/

# Introduction

Finland is a Nordic country and democracy situated in the Fenno-Scandian region of northern Europe. It borders Sweden on the west, Russia on the east, and Norway on the north, while Estonia lies to its south across the Gulf of Finland (Figure 8-1). The capital city is Helsinki. Finland has been a member of the European Union since 1995.

## Total Area and Population

Finland is comprised of 338,000 square kilometers, of which 10% is water and 69% forest; there are 187,888 lakes, 5,100 rapids, and 179,584 islands. Finland, including the semi-autonomous province of Åland, has Europe's largest archipelago. Finland has a total population

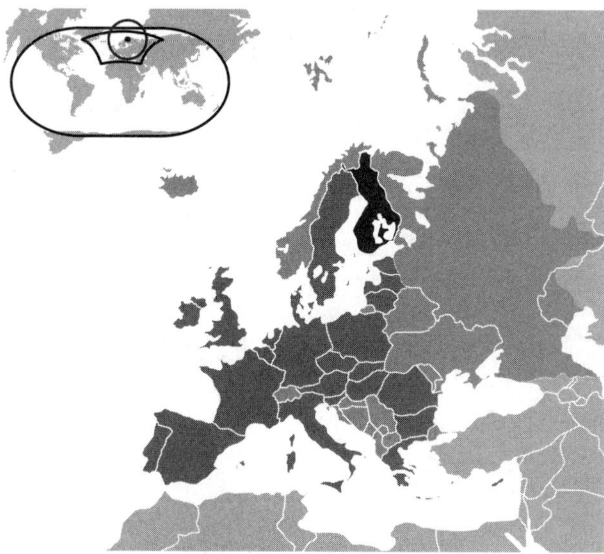

Figure 8-1 Finland on the map.
Source: Statistics Finland, www.stat.fi

of 5.3 million, with a density of 15.7 inhabitants per square kilometer. Seventy-one percent of the population lives in towns or urban areas and 29% in rural areas. The principal cities in Finland are Helsinki (564,000), Tampere (206,000), Turku (175,000), Oulu (130,000) and Lahti (100,000). About 1.25 million people live in the Helsinki metropolitan area (Official Statistics of Finland, 2009).

## Ethnic Breakdown of the Population

At the end of 2008, the number of Finnish citizens who were permanent residents in Finland was 5,183,058, of whom 90,516 had been born abroad as shown in Figure 8-2. Foreign citizens residing in Finland numbered 143,256 or formed 2.7% of the population. The number of foreign citizens grew by 10,548 persons during 2008. The largest groups of foreign citizens were from Russia (26,909 persons), Estonia (22,604 persons), Sweden (8,439 persons) and Somalia (4,919 persons). The total number of persons born abroad but residing in Finland was 218,626. (Official Statistics of Finland, 2009). The official languages of the country are Finnish and Swedish. The main religions are Lutheran (82%) and Orthodox (1.1%) (Official statistics of Finland, 2009).

## The Economy

In 2008, Finland's GDP per capita was approximately 34,800 Euros (Table 8-2). The unemployment rate in September 2009 was 7.3%, an increase from 5.9% in 2008, as shown in Table 8-3.

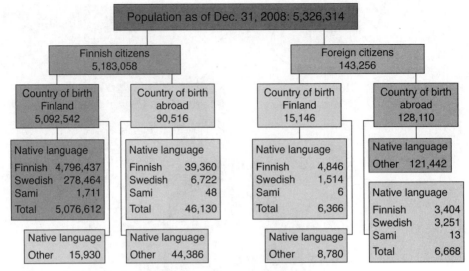


Figure 8-2 Ethnic breakdown of the population.

Source: Statistics Finland, www.stat.fi

**Table 8-2 Gross Domestic Product**

| | Billion € | € per person |
|---|---|---|
| 1998 | 117.1 | 22,716 |
| 1999 | 122.7 | 23,753 |
| 2000 | 132.2 | 25,541 |
| 2001 | 139.8 | 26,945 |
| 2002 | 143.8 | 27,650 |
| 2003 | 145.8 | 27,968 |
| 2004 | 152.2 | 29,107 |
| 2005 | 157.1 | 29,946 |
| 2006* | 167.0 | 31,713 |
| 2007* | 179.7 | 33,970 |
| 2008* | 184.7 | 34,769 |

* preliminary data

Source: Data from Official Statistics of Finland, 2009.

Table 8-3 **Changes in the Labor Force, September 2008–September 2009**

| | Month/year | | Change |
|---|---|---|---|
| | 09/2008 | 09/2009 | 09/2009 – 09/2008 |
| | Thousands of persons | | Percent (%) |
| Population aged 15–74 | 4,009 | 4,030 | 0.5 |
| Labor force, total | 2,670 | 2,628 | –1.5 |
| Employed, total | 2,511 | 2,436 | –3.0 |
| Employees | 2,179 | 2,094 | –3.9 |
| Self-employed persons and unpaid family workers | 332 | 342 | 3.0 |
| Unemployed persons | 158 | 192 | 21.5 |
| Total persons not in labor force | 1,339 | 1,401 | 4.7 |
| | Percent (%) | | Percent (%) |
| Employment rate (persons aged 15–64) | 70.0 | 67.6 | –3.4 |
| Unemployment rate, % | 5.9 | 7.3 | 23.7 |
| Labor force participation rate, % | 66.6 | 65.2 | –2.1 |

Unrounded figures are used in the Change column. The data comply with the ILO/EU definition.
Source: Data from Labor Market Statistics. Labor Force Survey, 2009.

## Population Projection 2007–2040

The current population of Finland with respect to age and gender is illustrated in Figure 8-3. Official Statistics of Finland (2009), has made the assumption that the population of Finland will keep growing until 2030. The population growth will be mainly sustained by immigration. Currently, the older age groups over 50 are large, and the annual number of deaths will exceed births by 2030.

By 2030, the proportion of persons in the population aged over 65 is estimated to rise from the present 16% to 26% and then remain almost unchanged for the next decade. Respectively, the proportion of persons aged 15 and under will diminish from the present 17% to 15.5% by 2040. By the same year, the working age population will be reduced from the present 67% to 58%. This will happen mainly because the postwar baby boom generation, born between 1945 and 1950, will reach retirement age after 2010. Consequently, the demographic dependency ratio, as shown in Figure 8-4, that is, the number of children and elderly people per 100 persons of working age, will rise from 50% to 75% between 2008 and 2040. This will cause a substantial increase in pension costs. The proportion of persons aged over 85 is forecast to rise from the present 1.8% to 6.1% by 2040. Thus, their numbers will increase from 94,000 to 349,000.

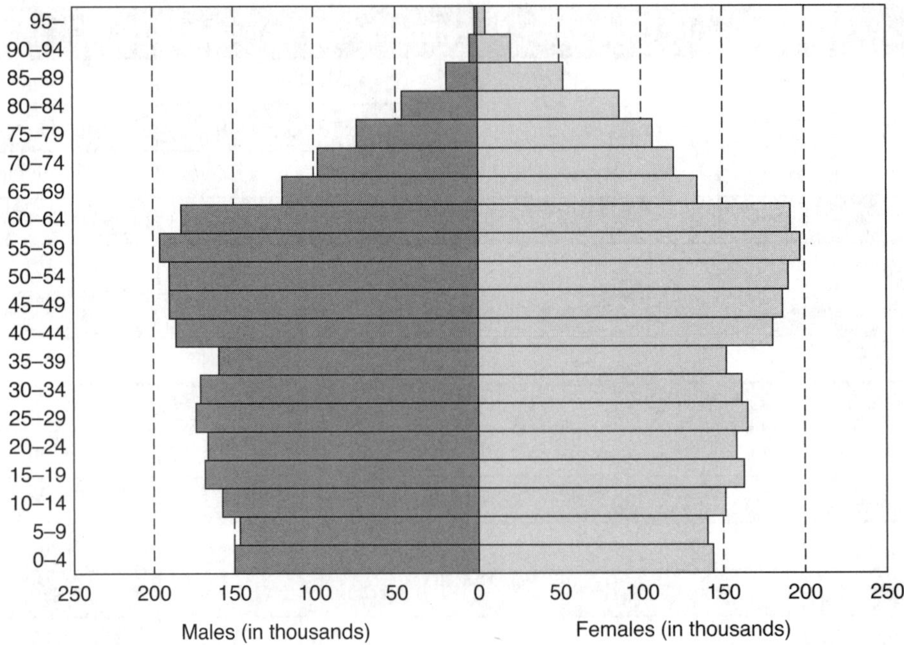


Figure 8-3 Population by age.

Source: Statistics Finland, www.stat.fi

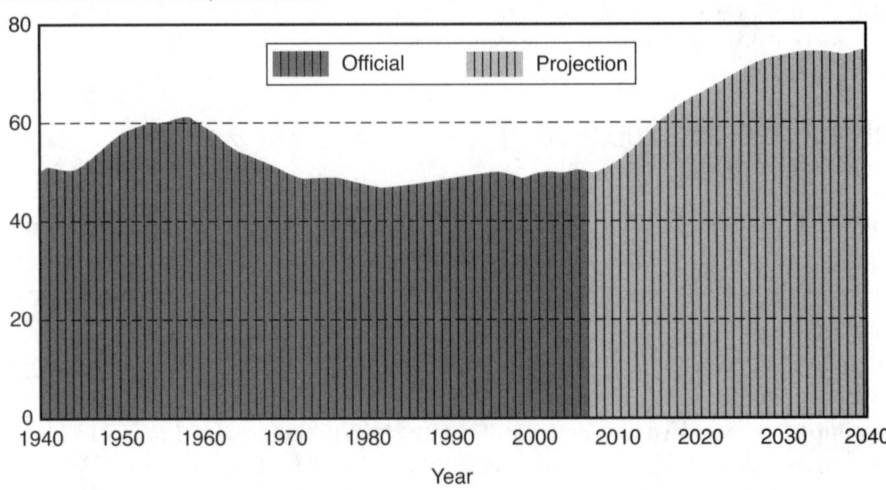


Figure 8-4 Demographic dependency ratio.

Source: Statistics Finland, www.stat.fi

Assuming that the present trend in internal migration continues, the population of sparsely populated rural areas will contract further when young people in particular move from these areas to so-called growth centers. These comprise regions around Helsinki, Tampere, Oulu, and a few other bigger cities. Their populations are estimated to grow by approximately 10% from the present to 2020 (Labour Market Statistics, 2009).

# Prevailing Health Issues and Risk Behaviors

## Life Expectancy and Mortality

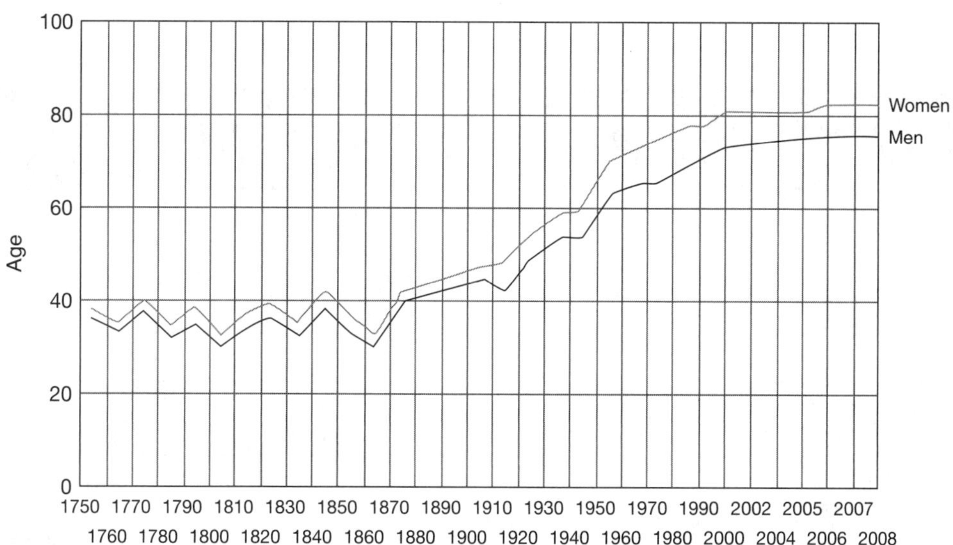


Figure 8-5 Life expectancy in Finland 1750–2008.

Source: Statistics Finland, www.stat.fi

Life expectancy in Finland (Figure 8-5) has increased considerably since the 1950s, mainly as a result of reduced cardiovascular mortality. However, there are still large mortality differences between population groups: those with a high education level (college and university) live longer than people who have only a basic education. Until the 1950s, life expectancy improved as a result of a lowered incidence of tuberculosis and other infectious diseases as well as a lowered child mortality rate. In the late 1950s, this improvement slowed down as mortality from circulatory diseases increased, especially among men.

Since 1970, life expectancy has rapidly increased, and Finland's international ranking has improved. In 2007, the life expectancy for men was 76 years and for women 83 years. The difference in this regard between Finland's population and the most long-lived populations in Europe has clearly narrowed compared with the situation in the 1950s.

Infant mortality (3/1,000) and the risk of death in children aged 1 to 15 (2/1,000) are now among the lowest in the world. Mortality in the middle-aged population has decreased by around 50% since the 1970s, mainly due to a decrease in cardiovascular diseases. Mortality has also declined considerably in the elderly population (Aromaa, Huttunen, Koskinen, & Teperi, 2005; Health Statistics, 2009).

## Future Outlook and Major Challenges

It is expected that the life expectancy of both men and women will continue to rise. However, unemployment and other factors causing social marginalization, increased obesity and alcohol use, and other changes with adverse health effects may slow down this process or even bring it to a halt. Table 8-4 presents 2007 data on the main causes of death for the working population, ages 15–64, per gender.

Table 8-4 **Main Causes of Death Among Working Age Population (15–64) by Gender in 2007**

| Rank | Men: Cause of death | No. of deaths | % | Rank | Women: Cause of death | No. of deaths | % |
|---|---|---|---|---|---|---|---|
| 1. | Alcohol causes | 1,425 | 18.7 | 1. | Alcohol causes | 371 | 11.5 |
| 2. | Coronary heart disease | 1,213 | 15.9 | 2. | Cancer of breast | 332 | 10.3 |
| 3. | Accidents (all) | 948 | 12.4 | 3. | Accidents (all) | 241 | 7.5 |
| | - traffic | 194 | 2.5 | | - traffic | 74 | 2.3 |
| | - falls | 206 | 2.7 | | - falls | 39 | 1.2 |
| | - occupational | 40 | .5 | | - occupational | 5 | .2 |
| 4. | Suicides | 618 | 8.1 | 4. | Coronary heart disease | 206 | 6.4 |
| 5. | Lung cancer | 400 | 5.2 | 5. | Suicides | 199 | 6.2 |
| 6. | Stroke | 315 | 4.1 | 6. | Lung cancer | 189 | 5.9 |
| 7. | Other causes | 2710 | 35.5 | 7. | Other causes | 1,681 | 52.2 |
| | All deaths in working age | 7,629 | 100.0 | | All deaths in working age | 3,219 | 100.0 |

Source: Data from Health Statistics, 2009.

Gender differences in smoking and alcohol use have decreased, which will contract the mortality difference between men and women. Mortality differences between socioeconomic groups will continue to increase unless there is an effective intervention into their causes. This is because smoking and unhealthy eating habits, as well as alcohol use, for example, are much more common in low-education and low-income groups than in those population groups who are better off. Also, long-term unemployment and social marginalization among the most underprivileged groups may serve to increase mortality differences (Aromaa et al., 2005; Health Statistics, 2009).

## Health Behavior

An annual postal survey entitled, "Health Behavior and Health Among the Finnish Adult Population" has been carried out since 1978. The primary purpose of this monitoring is to obtain information on the current health behavior of the working-age population and on its long- and short-term changes. The survey examines key aspects of health behavior such as smoking, food habits, alcohol consumption, and physical activity.

In 2008, 24% of men and 18% of women smoked daily. In the long term, food habits have moved in the direction of dietary recommendations. In 2008, 49% of men and 55% of women reported engaging in a minimum of 30 minutes of leisure-time physical activity at least three times a week. Regional differences with respect to daily smoking and healthy food habits have diminished. The differences in alcohol consumption, however, remain clear; alcohol consumption was the highest among those living in the southernmost region of Uusimaa. On the other hand, in Uusimaa, healthy food habits were the most common and overweight the most uncommon. Leisure-time physical activity has increased in all regions (Helakorpi, Paavola, Prättälä, & Uutela, 2009).

# Healthcare System

## Health Care

Health care is primarily based on public funding. Primary care is given in municipal health centers. The health centers are based in areas having a population of, at minimum, 20,000 people. Specialist care is provided by hospital districts.

Particularly in large cities, there are many private clinics. These clinics mainly provide outpatient health services. There are few private hospitals, but they are increasing in number.

In the two-tier Finnish healthcare system, private health care is also partly financed by public funds. Those who use private clinics can get a part of the fees refunded by the national health insurance.

In the public healthcare system, there is a waiting list limitation for nonurgent care: the maximum time for a patient on a hospital waiting list is 6 months. Emergencies and serious illnesses (e.g., cancer cases) are treated immediately.

## Healthcare Financing

### Healthcare Expenditure

Finland is one of only two EU member states (along with Estonia) in which total expenditures on health have declined as a proportion of GDP, falling from 7.6% in 1996 to 7.5% in 2005. Public spending as a proportion of total health expenditures has risen slightly from 75.8% in 1996 to 77.8% in 2005. Out-of-pocket payments fell (as a proportion of total spending) from approximately 20% in 1996 to approximately 18% in 2005 (Aromaa et al., 2005; Health Statistics, 2009; Nordin, Chen, Nieminen, & Heloma, 2008).

### Coverage and Benefits

The publicly financed health system covers all residents for a comprehensive range of benefits. Cost sharing is applied to most health services, but in 2000, an annual maximum out-of-pocket amount was introduced, and children under the age of 18 are exempt from primary care charges. Supplementary private health insurance mainly covers children and plays a very small role.

### Collection of Funds

The health system is mainly financed through central and local taxes. In 2004, the 416 municipalities financed approximately 40% of public spending on health care, the central government approximately 20%, and national health insurance approximately 17%. Owing to the economic recession of the early 1990s, there has been a shift toward increased financing by municipalities and the national health insurance. National health insurance is financed by employers and employees.

### Pooling

The size of the health budget is determined nationally and locally. The national budget is allocated to the municipalities based on risk-adjusted capitation, but municipal variation in per capita health expenditure remains an issue. National health insurance revenue is pooled separately and is mainly used to reimburse outpatient health care provided by private physicians and dentists and outpatient pharmaceutical expenditure.

### Purchasing Health Services

As municipalities own most hospitals and primary care centers, there is no real purchaser–provider split for tax-financed services. Hospital districts comprising several municipalities organize specialist care. The national health insurance reimburses part of the costs of privately provided outpatient physician, dental care, and pharmaceuticals. Patients have a limited choice of health centers and free choice of private doctors. Referral is required for public sector specialist care.

### *Provider Payment*

Primary care centers are allocated prospective budgets. Hospital districts increasingly use diagnosis-related groups to pay hospitals. Hospital and most municipal doctors are salaried employees (with some additional fee-for-service payments) and some hospital doctors also practice privately. Health centers that operate a personal doctor system pay doctors a mixture of salary, capitation, and fee-for-service payments. Private providers are reimbursed on a fee-for-service basis (Aromaa et al., 2005).

## Influence of Culture and Mentality

Finland, one might say, is a place where east and west meet. People in eastern Finland have in their culture many more traditions from the East and Russia than do people in western Finland and the south coast, including the Greek-Orthodox religion, which is rare in the western parts. The coastal regions in the west and south have the largest proportion of Swedish-speaking people. Nevertheless, the country's people throughout history have been much more homogenous than those of most European countries. This homogeneity was not challenged very much before the 1980s, when immigration from other countries began on a larger scale. Still, today Finland has far fewer immigrants than do her Scandinavian neighbors (Sweden, Norway, and Denmark). Due to a rapidly aging workforce, Finland is in need of more immigrants to fill the posts of those retiring.

According to a common belief—which is very much true—Finns are considered somewhat reserved people who do not talk very much. It is not very easy to start a conversation with a Finn, and even harder for a Finn to start one. However, as the ethnic structure of the population is getting more diversified, this mentality is gradually changing and people socialize more easily. Today, young people live in a much different society from that of their parents, who were born as products of the postwar baby boom generation.

In the 1960s–1970s, middle-aged Finnish men, particularly in eastern Finland, had one of the highest coronary heart disease rates in Europe. As a result, the North Karelia project was started (Puska, Vartiainen, Laatikainen, Jousilahti, & Paavola, 2009). The project tackled unhealthy eating habits, smoking, and inadequate physical activity, and promoted healthy lifestyles. Coronary deaths before age 65 have decreased considerably since then, and part of the credit for this success belongs to the North Karelia project. People with a low education level still have the poorest health status and the most unhealthy lifestyles.

# Drivers of Workplace Health Promotion

Workplace health promotion in Finland is based on the Workplace Health Care Act. It is the responsibility of the employer to organize preventive occupational health care for employees. Provisions for other kinds of health care, such as treatment of health problems and illnesses not related to work, are not mandatory. However, most firms of more than 20 employees voluntarily purchase healthcare services for their employees. By their doing so, the national health insurance will reimburse them 50–60% of costs incurred (Occupational Health Care Act, 1978; Occupational Health Care Act, 2001).

## Arrangement of Workplace Health Promotion in Finland

Employers have four different ways of organizing the occupational health care of their employees.

1. Establish their own occupational healthcare units (largest workplaces)
2. Set up an occupational healthcare unit organized and financed by several employers together (large and medium-sized workplaces)
3. Purchase occupational health care from a private clinic (small workplaces)
4. Purchase occupational health care from a municipal health center (small workplaces)

Finland's total workforce comprises 2.5 million employees. Preventive workplace health promotion covers around 90% of them, although ideally it should cover 100%. The coverage gap stems primarily from small workplaces of fewer than 10 employees. Around 80% of employees are also covered for sickness by a special outpatient occupational healthcare system paid by employers and the national health insurance together. Because of the Finnish two-tier system, people are also covered for primary health care by the municipal health centers. Specialized hospital care is covered for all Finnish people (whether working or not) by hospital districts and is seldom paid by employers.

The aim of workplace health promotion is that the employer, the employee, and occupational healthcare professionals together should:

- prevent work-related illnesses and accidents
- promote workplace health and the safety of the work environment
- promote the health of workers and employees and their working ability throughout their careers

The employer, together with workplace health professionals, has an obligation to:

- create a workplace health and safety plan
- arrange health check-ups for employees
- investigate employees' physical, functional, and psychological working abilities and arrange rehabilitation when needed

- give information, advice, and guidance regarding workplace safety and health
- provide first aid
- audit workplaces for quality and effectiveness of workplace health promotion

Problems related to work that are reflected most in occupational health care include:

- musculoskeletal diseases
- mental health disturbances, physical and psychological stress, burnout
- problems with learning new things and new work methods, often linked with aging
- problems in work atmosphere
- poor work organization
- employees' insecurity about maintaining their present jobs
- administrational changes

(Government Resolution Occupational Health 2015, 2004)

## The Main Strategic Elements in Workplace Health Promotion Until 2015

### *Improving the Quality of Working Life*

A safe and healthy working environment, together with a modern work organization, are essential for increasing employment and improving productivity and social cohesion.

The European Commission has released a communication entitled *Employment and Social Policies: A Framework for Investing in Quality*. In this communication, the commission has identified 10 dimensions of quality of work. These include job qualification requirements, access of workers to the labor market, career development and subjective job satisfaction of employees, the working environment and health and safety at work, and gender equality and nondiscrimination.

Finland complies with this EU strategy and represents a large consensus of all three parties (employers, employees, and the state) in order to ensure a healthy work environment, good work organization, and reconcilement of work and family life in a way that supports the health and work ability of employees.

## Promoting Health in the Workplace and Maintaining Work Ability

The main purposes of workplace health promotion and occupational health care are to prevent occupational accidents and diseases and to promote health and work ability. First, the work must be carried out without putting the workers' health at risk, and second, a safe and well-managed work environment must be guaranteed for all. These things will help to maintain work ability throughout the employees' entire careers and to prevent early retirements due to illnesses.

Enhancement of measures requires constant evaluation, monitoring, and development of the healthiness and safety of the work environment and working conditions. Workplaces, workplace communities, and each employee, entrepreneur, and self-employed person should have the opportunity to influence and participate in decisions that affect their health and working ability.

New working environment problems and other problems related to workplace health and work ability require workplace health promotion to develop new procedures and methods. Significant public health problems are being prevented, and public health promoted, in accordance with the government program *Health 2015*.

### Providing Comprehensive Occupational Health Services to All Employees

Occupational healthcare services should be available to every workplace, employee, entrepreneur, and other self-employed person. In providing occupational healthcare services, the major challenges are atypical working conditions, small workplaces, and entrepreneurs and other self-employed persons.

What are needed are networking of health center services, the creation of regional service structures, and cooperation among companies in producing occupational healthcare services. Structural changes in working life and changes in the content and procedures of working, together with the demographic shift in the working population, require development of new service structures and new methods of occupational health care—including revision and amendment of legislation if necessary—in order to keep pace with new needs.

Apart from preventive occupational healthcare services, the voluntary medical care and other healthcare services provided by the employer are important for ensuring the health, working ability, and well-being at work of employees throughout their careers.

## Programs and Good Practices

### Veto Program

The Veto program was implemented in 2003–2007. The aims of this action program were to ensure citizens' full participation in working life; affect the extension of working life; improve the reconciliation of work, family life, and free time; improve equality; and increase the attractiveness of work as an option in different situations. The program consisted of four sectors that had the following themes:

- high quality of working life and good safety culture
- efficient occupational health services and rehabilitation
- diversity and equality in working life
- minimum income guarantee and working life incentives

The program was led by the Ministry of Social Affairs and Health together with a steering group and was carried out in cooperation with other ministries, labor market organizations, and entrepreneurial organizations, research institutes, insurance and pension funds, and rehabilitation organizations.

In the Veto program, the strategic policies of the Ministry of Social Affairs and Health were implemented, and the projects of the already finished National Programme on Aging Workers and National Well-Being at Work Program, which ended in 2003, were continued. In addition, the program functioned in synergy with other ongoing national development and action programs.

In the Veto program, specific quantitative indicators were created to evaluate the results of the program. These indicators, presented in the "Outcomes and Indicators" later in this chapter, can also be used in other workplace health promotion programs.

Different parameters of actions, feedback, evaluation surveys, and evaluation discussions have been utilized in compiling the qualitative evaluation. The key results of the evaluation of the Veto program are as follows:

1. The central objectives of the program, namely postponing the retirement age and improving the employment rate, were achieved. However, the significance of the program's role in positive development is difficult to distinguish from other factors. There have also been advances in developing workplace health promotion and occupational health services and making the minimum income guarantee and pension schemes more encouraging.
2. The results of other objectives of the program, such as reducing absenteeism and occupational accidents, as well as reducing the use of alcohol and tobacco and increasing physical activity, were not scientifically measured by the quantitative indicators. Nevertheless, it seemed that the results were not achieved in the desired extent. The reasons for the lack of greater success in these areas lie partly in factors that are independent from the program, such as reduced alcohol prices.
3. The program has had an impact on aged people's attitudes toward work. According to the feedback received, media campaigns affecting attitudes and regional seminars focusing on well-being at work were considered successful.
4. Looking for, supporting, and distributing good practices are useful ways to implement the program. To distribute good practices, the communications and training related to them have to be planned carefully. Good, distributable practices must not be strictly defined, and they need to enable modifications, as no workplace is capable of adopting the experiences of another workplace without amendment.

5. The Veto program contributed to the creation of a more comprehensive approach to developing the factors that affect the attractiveness of working life. The Veto program created an umbrella that supported communication and interaction, under which issues related to the quality of work, working conditions, and working life could be developed further. In the management of the Ministry of Social Affairs and Health's administrative sector, the Veto program and its objectives could be seen as a theme steering the activities of agencies and institutes in the administrative sector.
6. The program gathered together several researchers, authorities, organizations, and experts working with the same subjects. The cooperation among the programs coordinated by different ministries, and the wider network created from them, were particularly beneficial.
7. The strategic objectives of the program were clear, and the keeping of a record of the objectives with the help of the developed and gathered indicators made the discussion on available means more vigorous.

## Well-Being at Work Program

In Finland, the mean retirement age is 59 years, which is too young and thus presents a burden for retirement funds and the national economy. The government's aim is to enhance well-being at work in order to encourage workers and employees to work longer in life (Forum for Well-Being at Work, 2009).

The success of an organization is based on people and their health and well-being. Therefore, the health of employees must be a paramount concern, and their working skills must be appreciated, because the success of the organization depends on a healthy and motivated workforce. Good management skills are a necessity in order to achieve well-being at work.

The aims of the program are the following:

- to increase willingness to stay at work after age 60 and to extend employees' working years
- to strive for a positive attitude change toward increasing well-being at work
- to strengthen the positive effect of a good working life on workers' health and welfare
- to reduce occupational accidents and diseases
- to decrease absenteeism
- to increase worker participation in issues concerning well-being at work
- to launch a European network of actors in the Well-Being at Work sector

## Druvan Model

The Druvan model was developed in the Swedish-speaking municipality of Dragsfjärd in southwestern Finland at the beginning of the 2000s. The word *druvan* means a grape in a bunch. In Dragsfjärd, absenteeism had risen dramatically between 1999 and 2001. In addition, workers were unwell and sought early retirements. The Druvan model was implemented as a workplace health promotion model to support employees' well-being at work and to increase productivity. The Druvan project lasted 3 years, until 2004.

In 2001, the municipality spent 20 euros per year per worker for occupational health care and workplace health promotion. After the initiation of the Druvan model, the sum was multiplied twentyfold.

Together with their foremen, employees began to plan how to improve their own workplaces. Their goal was better leadership, better well-being at work, and better productivity. The idea of the Druvan model is that these things correlate positively. The earlier invented metal age concept, discussed on pp. 178–179, was also integrated into the Druvan model, a practical program that stresses the participation of all employees and includes physical exercise for the purpose of improving work ability.

The Druvan project decreased absenteeism and pension costs, and improved workplace well-being. The model can be adopted by any kind of workplace. The documented effects of the Druvan model are based on good management, employee commitment, knowledge of difficulties, practical development projects, and a lifestyle change.

Studies of the Druvan model indicated that it improved the work ability and job satisfaction of employees. This consequently resulted in an increase in effective working hours and better productivity. Sick leave and pension costs decreased concomitantly. The project resulted in an annual profit of 46% to the capital that was invested in it (Näsman & Ahonen, 2008). Figure 8-6 illustrates the expected effects and their relations.

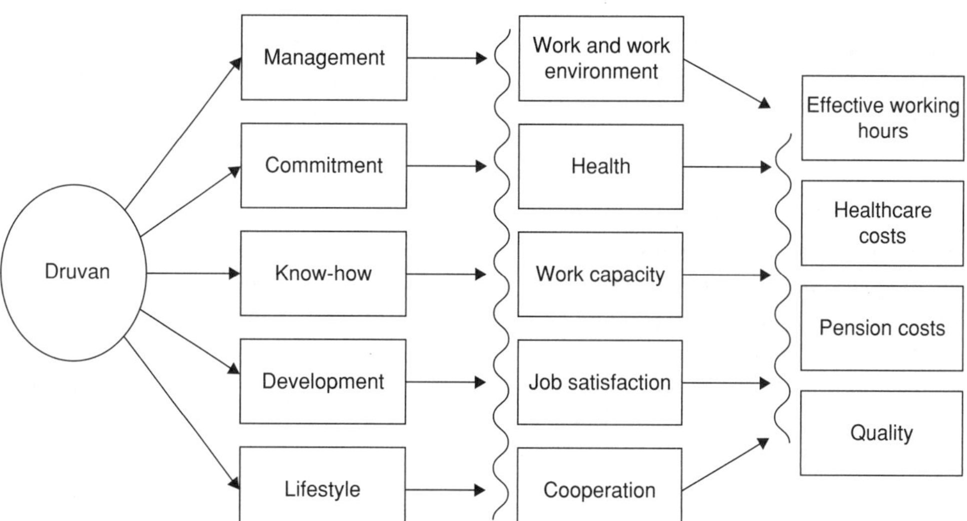


Figure 8-6 Expected effects and their relations in the Druvan model.

Source: Centre for Occupational Safety, Finlamd

The main focus of the Druvan model is the prevention of different factors that induce ill health and poor work ability. Secondary to this, when problems have already arisen, are remedies such as rehabilitation.

In the Druvan model, occupational health care acts as an engine by implementing workplace development projects and providing the organization and management with professional help (Rissa, 2007). Examples of practices that have been included in the Druvan model include lifestyle change and motion and improved management.

Lifestyle change and motion:

- "Should we talk?" A short intervention for alcohol and substance abuse.
- Smoking cessation and provision of nicotine replacement therapy.
- Exercise breaks for office workers.
- Water exercise/swimming/gym.
- Option to use the gymnasium for indoor ball games twice a week.
- Metal age concept for workplace health promotion.

Improved management:

- Continuous training of managers at all levels.
- Thematic training days for managers twice a year.
- Development discussions with the staff.

## Metal Age

Within the framework of the National Programme on Aging Workers, Fundia Wire Ltd., a manufacturer of long steel products, developed metal age. Metal age is a tool for participatory planning of workplace health promotion, aimed at improving working conditions and maintaining the work ability of aging workers. Although its original target group was aging workers in the metal industry, the program proved applicable to the promotion of a healthy workplace for employees of all ages in all sectors. It has now been used successfully in the steel industry as well as in hospitals, schools, and cleaning companies. Overall, the response has been positive. Metallgruppen, the Swedish organization of metal industry employers, also adopted metal age and incorporated it into its training program.

Fundia Wire Ltd. set up a working group of five staff, comprising three representatives from occupational health care and two from human resources. They designed an action program aimed at raising the average retirement age in the company while, at the same time, curbing the overall rise in the average age of employees (European Foundation for the Improvement of Living and Working Conditions, 2004).

The action program was divided into the following areas:

- *Maintaining the work input of aging workers.* In cooperation with the Finnish Institute of Occupational Health and the Ilmarinen Mutual Pension Insurance Institution, key employees were trained in how to promote a healthy workplace. Site-specific instructions for promoting a healthy workplace were reviewed and amended or replaced. According to new rules set by thc company, 25 years of service would be rewarded with an extra 2 weeks of holiday time, and 35 years of service with an extra 4 weeks.

- *Adapting working methods, work content, and the working environment.* In accordance with employees' individual needs, and particularly with regard to aging, the company reduced the number of workers taking early retirement by offering all employees of the appropriate age the option of part-time pensions, provided their work could be suitably arranged.
- *Developing professional skills.* Training that focused on new technology (particularly information technology) and language skills was provided to aging workers.
- *Human resources planning and recruitment.* Trained young people were recruited in advance to replace retiring workers.

# Outcomes and Indicators

## Main Indicators of Success in Workplace Health Promotion and the Outcomes

The Veto program and the Ministry of Social Affairs and Health, together with the National Institute for Health and Welfare, have defined indicators that can be used for measuring the impact of workplace health promotion programs (Helakorpi et al., 2009; Myhrman, Gröhn, Parvikko, & Säntti, 2006).

The aim of the Veto program was to increase the participation rate of the labor force in different age groups and to extend working life by 2–3 years from its current level. The goal was to achieve this by improving both well-being at work and the economic incentives to encourage working. Figures 8-7, 8-8, 8-9, and 8-10 describe specific Veto program indicators. Figures 8-11, 8-12, 8-13, and 8-14 describe general indicators created by the National Institute for Health and Welfare.

The Veto program indicators have been, as a rule, constructed so that the base year of the program is 2002. The success of the program is evaluated in terms of two possible alternatives. Alternative 1 represents a path in accordance with the government's employment target, and alternative 2 a path in which employment rates remain at the level of those in 2002.

The indicators in Figures 8-11, 8-12, 8-13, and 8-14 are nonspecific indicators that show the national trends from 1978 to 2008. The effect of the Veto program on these indicators has not been studied, although the Veto program included measures to reduce smoking and alcohol use and to encourage physical exercise among employees.

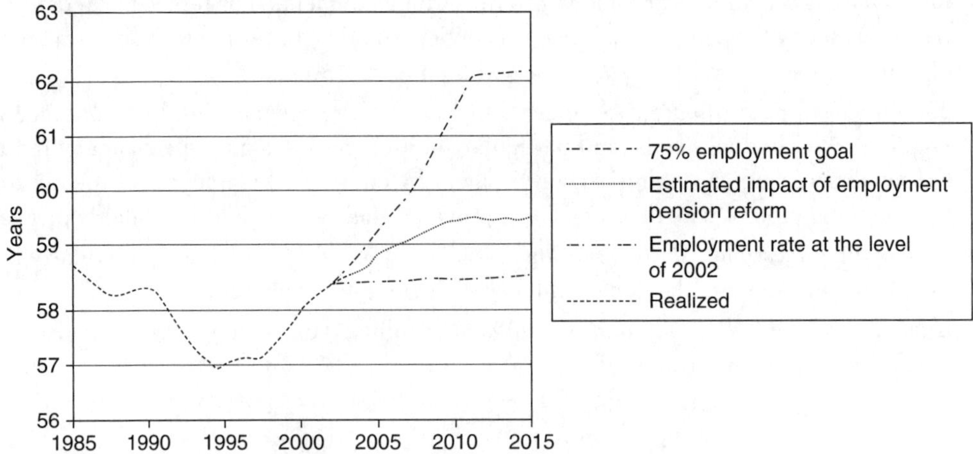


Figure 8-7 Expected retirement age by factor, 1985–2018.

Source: National Institute for Health and Welfare

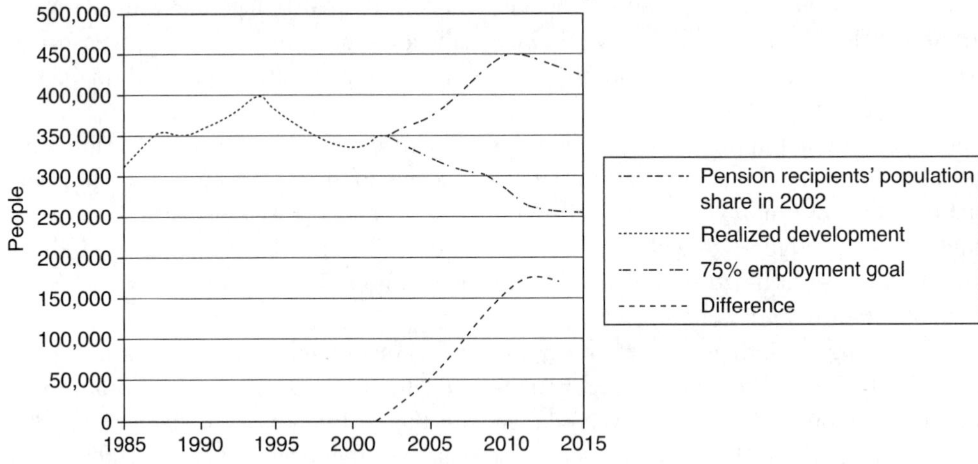


Figure 8-8 Expected number of pension recipients under 65.

Source: National Institute for Health and Welfare

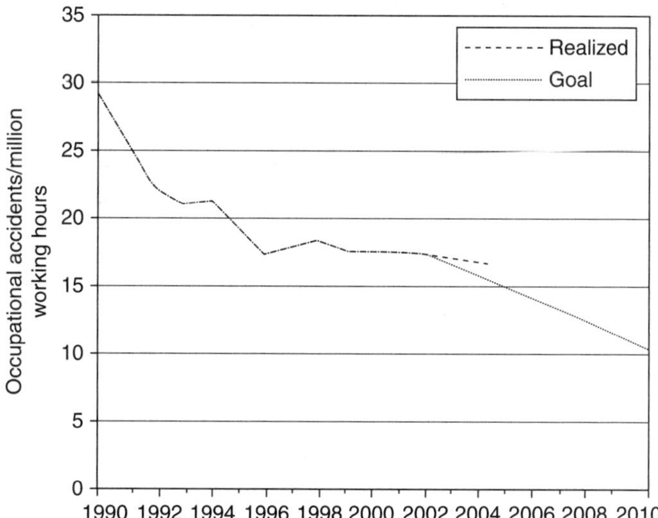


Figure 8-9 Wage earners' occupational accidents per 1,000 wage earners 1990–2003 and goal for 2003–2010.

Source: National Institute for Health and Welfare

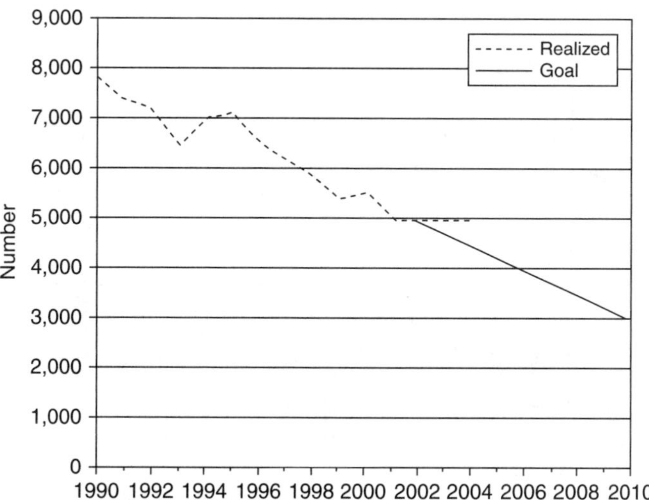


Figure 8-10 Employees' occupational diseases and suspected cases of occupational diseases 1993–2002 and goal for 2003–2010.

Source: National Institute for Health and Welfare

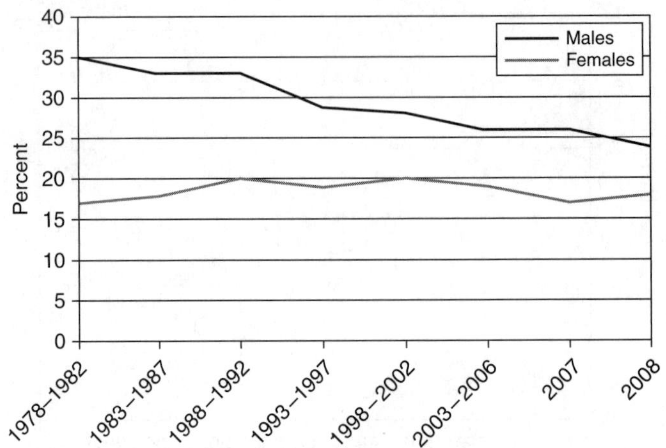


Figure 8-11 Proportion of daily smokers in population by sex (%).

Source: National Institute for Health and Welfare

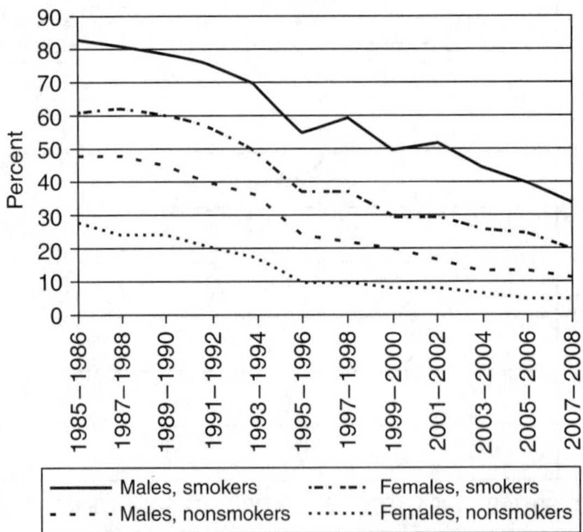


Figure 8-12 Proportion of persons exposed to secondhand smoke at work by sex and smoking status (%).

Source: National Institute for Health and Welfare

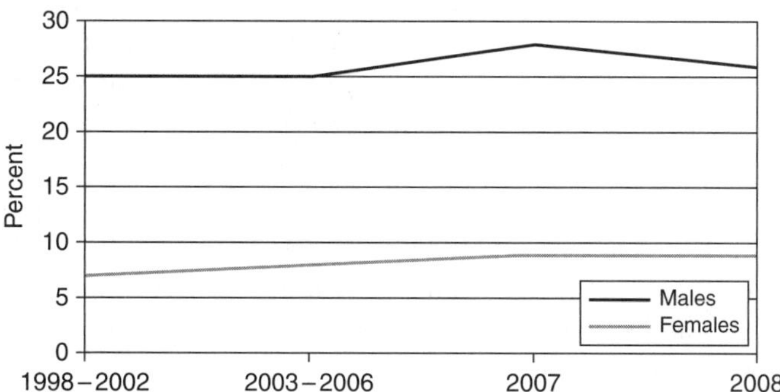


Figure 8-13 Proportion of respondents who consume six or more portions of alchohol on one occasion at least once a week (%).

Source: National Institute for Health and Welfare

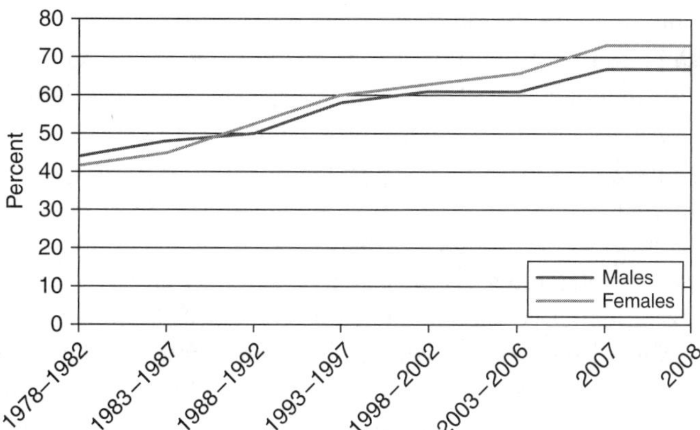


Figure 8-14 Proportion of persons who practice physical exercise on their leasure time at least 2 times a week by sex (%).

Source: National Institute for Health and Welfare

## Existing Research

In the 1990s and early 2000s, a great deal of prominent and important occupational health research was performed in Finland with a focus on work ability and well-being at work. For example, this research includes cutting-edge data on the impact of work-related psychosocial factors on coronary heart disease.

Some of the research articles listed in the references deal with the most important issues in Finnish workplace health promotion and the occupational health policies of today. Well-being at work is essential for better productivity and work ability. The research results also show that employee well-being is the best way to encourage workers to stay longer in working life, which is beneficial to the national economy.

## Conclusion

Working life today presents many challenges. In Finland, these include a rapidly aging working age population, increasing pension costs, and the changing requirements of the work itself. Workplace health promotion plays a key role in finding solutions to meet these challenges. Good management and work environment, employee commitment, and promotion of healthy lifestyles are important ways to reduce absenteeism due to physical and psychological ill health, to increase productivity, and to prevent too-early retirement.

Workplace health promotion in Finland is based on the Occupational Health Care Act, first enacted in 1978 and amended in 2001. The legislation includes mandatory preventive measures that concern all workplaces and employees. Outpatient occupational medical care has been voluntarily adopted by a great majority of employers. Employers are reimbursed by the national health insurance up to 60% of occupational health costs.

In the 2000s, a number of development programs were implemented to increase the attraction of working life and to encourage employees to stay longer at work. Some of these programs and projects have also created new models for workplace health promotion. Important goals of the projects have included better well-being at work and increased productivity. A forum for well-being at work was launched in 2008 as a component of the government's policy program for employment, entrepreneurship, and working life. Its objective is to boost network cooperation and partnerships in workplace health and safety promotion by joining forces to achieve common goals.

Two projects that have been implemented at the local level and are described in the chapter are the Druvan model and metal age. These projects have started from specific local needs and lacked the large structures of national programs. The results of the projects have been encouraging, and they have been adopted by other firms even outside Finland.

## Summary

Finland is a country in northern Europe with 5.3 million inhabitants. It is highly industrialized, and 71% of the population live in urban areas. The GDP per inhabitant is 34,800 (2008), and the unemployment rate is 7.3% (2009). Life expectancy has risen rapidly from the 1970s, and as of 2007 was 83 years for women and 76 years for men.

The main problems in health behavior are increased alcohol use and obesity, while smoking and suicides have decreased. Finland has a rapidly increasing older population, a fact that may lead to a lack of an experienced workforce and a steep rise in the demographic dependency ratio in the near future. However, increasing immigration of skilled workers from other countries may ameliorate the problem and its stress on the economy.

The occupational healthcare system covers workplace health promotion for all employees and outpatient occupational health care for a majority of employees. All people's primary and hospital care is covered, whether they are working or not, and is funded mostly by state and municipal taxes.

In workplace health promotion, larger firms have implemented projects to improve company management and to create a healthy working environment. Their goal has been to prevent too-early retirement and increase the attractiveness of working life. Among these projects are the Druvan model and metal age.

The government has carried out programs that aim for healthier lifestyles of employees and increased work ability among people of older working age. These include Health 2015, Occupational Health 2015, the Veto program, and the Well-Being at Work program.

## Review Questions

1. Describe the population projection for Finns over the next 2 decades. How may it impact health programs?
2. What are the main causes of death among working persons in Finland?
3. Explain the two-tier Finnish healthcare system.
4. How is health care financed in Finland?
5. How can employers organize the occupational health care of employees?
6. Describe the Veto program. How is it different from or the same as the Druvan model?
7. How did the Occupational Health Care Act impact workplace health promotion in Finland?

# References


Ahonen, G., Hussi, T., & Schuder-Tatzber, S. (2007). Work-related well being: A precondition for intellectual capital. In C. Chaminade & B. Catasús (Eds.), *Intellectual capital revisited.* Cheltenham, UK: Edward Elgar Publishing, Ltd.

Aromaa, A., Huttunen, J., Koskinen, S., & Teperi, J. (Eds.). (2005). *Health in Finland.* Helsinki, Finland: Duodecim.

European Foundation for the Improvement of Living and Working Conditions. (2004). *Managing the challenge of an ageing workforce—Case example of the Finnish national strategy on ageing.* Retrieved from http://www.eurofound.europa.eu/emcc/publications/2004/ef0479en_2.pdf

Forum for Well-Being at Work. (2009). *Making well-being at work a strength—Activities and opportunities for participation.* Retrieved from http://www.stm.fi/c/document_library/get_file?folderId=39503&name=DLFE-6307.pdf

*Government Resolution Occupational Health 2015.* (2004). Publications of the Ministry of Social Affairs and Health 2004:5. Helsinki, Finland: Ministry of Social Affairs and Health. Retrieved from http://www.stm.fi/c/document_library/get_file?folderId=28707&name=DLFE-3947.pdf&title=Government_Resolution__Occupational_Health_2015_en.pdf

*Government resolution on the Health 2015 public health programme.* Retrieved from http://www.terveys2015.fi/english.html

*Health statistics.* (2009). Helsinki, Finland: Statistics Finland. Retrieved from http://www.tilastokeskus.fi/til/ter_en.html

Helakorpi, S., Paavola, M., Prättälä, R., & Uutela, A. (2009, February). *Health behaviour and health among the Finnish adult population, spring, 2008.* Helsinki, Finland: National Institute of Health and Welfare.

Ilmarinen, J. E. (2001). Aging workers. *Occupational and Environmental Medicine, 58,* 546.

Kivimäki, M., Elovainio, M., Vahtera, J., & Ferrie, J. E. (2003). Organisational justice and health of employees: Prospective cohort study. *Occupational and Environmental Medicine, 60,* 27–34.

Kivimäki, M., Head, J., Ferrie, J. E., Hemingway, H., Shipley, M. J., Vahtera, J., & Marmot, M. G. (2005). Working while ill as a risk factor for serious coronary events: The Whitehall II Study. *American Journal of Public Health, 95,* 98–102.

Labour market statistics. (2009). Helsinki, Finland: Statistics Finland. Retrieved from http://www.tilastokeskus.fi/til/tym_en.html

Myhrman, R., Gröhn, K., Parvikko, O., & Säntti, R. (2006). Longer careers? The Veto Programme indicators. *Reports of the Ministry of Social Affairs and Health 2006.* Helsinki, Finland: Ministry of Social Affairs and Health.

Näsman, O., & Ahonen, G. (2008). Druvan-projekti [The Druvan project] [in Finnish]. *Työterveyslääkäri 26,* 58–65.

Nordin, P., Chen, S., Nieminen, J., & Heloma, A. (2008, February). Present and future challenges for health care employment: European and Finnish experiences. *Publications of the State Provincial Office of Southern Finland, Health and Social Affairs Department.* Helsinki, Finland: State Provincial Office of Southern Finland. Retrieved from http://www.poliisi.fi/lh/biblio.nsf/0A96237133D1BC18C22574350028F422/$file/sto_0208.pdf

Occupational Health Care Act 743/1978. (1978). Helsinki, Finland: Finnish law. Retrieved from http://www.finlex.fi

Occupational Health Care Act (Revision) 1383/2001. (2001). Helsinki, Finland: Finnish law. Retrieved from http://www.finlex.fi

Official statistics of Finland. (2009). Helsinki, Finland: Statistics Finland.

Puska, P., Vartiainen, E., Laatikainen, T., Jousilahti, P., & Paavola, M. (Eds.). (2009). *The North Karelia project: From North Karelia to national action.* Helsinki, Finland: National Institute for Health and Welfare.

Rissa, K. (2007). *The druvan model: Well-being creates productivity.* Helsinki, Finland: The Centre for Occupational Safety.

Vahtera, J., Kivimäki, M., Pentti, J., Linna, A., Virtanen, M., Virtanen, P., & Ferrie, J. E. (2004). Organisational downsizing, sickness absence, and mortality: 10-town prospective cohort study. *British Medical Journal, 328,* 555.

## Acknowledgments

Mr. Jarkko Honkonen, BSocSc, and Ms. Arja Mikkelinen are gratefully acknowledged for their help in the collection of graphic data and drawing of figures.

Chapter 9

# Germany

Kerstin Baumgarten and Gerhard Huber

After reading this chapter you should be able to:

- Identify core strategies that are the focus of workplace health promotion efforts focus in Germany
- Describe the historical evolution of Germany's workplace health promotion efforts
- Explain the different approaches employed by corporate health promotion throughout Germany
- Review the central disease states and health issues driving workplace health promotion in Germany
- Name the components of, and the associated funding sources for, the German healthcare system
- Discuss the impact of culture on the health status and health promotion efforts within Germany

**Table 9-1 Select Key Demographic and Economic Indicators**

| | |
|---|---|
| Nationality | Noun: German(s)<br>Adjective: German |
| Ethnic groups | German 91.5%, Turkish 2.4%, other 6.1% (made up largely of Greek, Italian, Polish, Russian, Serbo-Croatian, Spanish) |
| Religion | Protestant 34%, Roman Catholic 34%, Muslim 3.7%, unaffiliated or other 28.3% |
| Language | German |
| Literacy | Definition: age 15 and over can read and write<br>Total population: 99%<br>Male: 99%<br>Female: 99% (2003 est.) |
| Education expenditure | 4.6% of GDP (2004)<br>Country comparison to the world: 82 |
| Government type | Federal republic |

*continued*

| Table 9-1 Select Key Demographic and Economic Indicators, *continued* | |
|---|---|
| Environment | Emissions from coal-burning utilities and industries contribute to air pollution; acid rain, resulting from sulfur dioxide emissions, is damaging forests; pollution in the Baltic Sea from raw sewage and industrial effluents from rivers in eastern Germany; hazardous waste disposal; government established a mechanism for ending the use of nuclear power over the next 15 years; government working to meet EU commitment to identify nature preservation areas in line with the European Union's Flora, Fauna, and Habitat directive |
| Country mass | Total: 357,022 sq km<br>Country comparison to the world: 62<br>Land: 348,672 sq km<br>Water: 8,350 sq km |
| Population | 82,329,758 (July 2010 est.)<br>Country comparison to the world: 15 |
| Age structure | 0–14 years: 13.7% (male 5,768,366/female 5,470,516)<br>15–64 years: 66.1% (male 27,707,761/female 26,676,759)<br>65 years and over: 20.3% (male 7,004,805/female 9,701,551)<br>(2010 est.) |
| Median age | Total: 44.3 years<br>Male: 43 years<br>Female: 45.6 years (2010 est.) |
| Population growth rate | -0.053% (2010 est.)<br>Country comparison to the world: 210 |
| Birth rate | 8.18 births/1,000 population (2010 est.)<br>Country comparison to the world: 220 |
| Death rate | 10.9 deaths/1,000 population (July 2010 est.)<br>Country comparison to the world: 44 |
| Net migration rate | 2.19 migrant(s)/1,000 population (2010 est.)<br>Country comparison to the world: 39 |
| Urbanization | Urban population: 74% of total population (2008)<br>Rate of urbanization: 0.1% annual rate of change (2005–2010 est.) |
| Gender ratio | At birth: 1.06 male(s)/female<br>Under 15 years: 1.05 male(s)/female<br>15–64 years: 1.04 male(s)/female<br>65 years and over: 0.72 male(s)/female<br>Total population: 0.97 male(s)/female (2010 est.) |
| Infant mortality rate | Total: 3.99 deaths/1,000 live births<br>Country comparison to the world: 210<br>Male: 4.41 deaths/1,000 live births<br>Female: 3.55 deaths/1,000 live births (2010 est.) |

*continued*

| Table 9-1 **Select Key Demographic and Economic Indicators,** *continued* | |
|---|---|
| Life expectancy | Total population: 79.26 years<br>Country comparison to the world: 32<br>Male: 76.26 years<br>Female: 82.42 years (2010 est.) |
| Total fertility rate | 1.42 children born/woman (2010 est.)<br>Country comparison to the world: 196 |
| GDP—purchasing power parity | $2.812 trillion (2009 est.)<br>Country comparison to the world: 6 |
| GDP—per capita | $34,100 (2009 est.)<br>Country comparison to the world: 37 |
| GDP—composition by sector | Agriculture: 0.9%<br>Industry: 26.8%<br>Services: 72% (2009 est.) |
| Agriculture—products | Potatoes, wheat, barley, sugar beets, fruit, cabbages, cattle, pigs, poultry |
| Industries | Among the world's largest and most technologically advanced producers of iron, steel, coal, cement, chemicals, machinery, vehicles, machine tools, electronics, food and beverages, shipbuilding, textiles |
| Labor force participation | 43.51 million (2009 est.)<br>Country comparison to the world: 14 |
| Unemployment rate | 7.5% (2009 est.)<br>Country comparison to the world: 71 |
| Industrial production growth rate | -11% (2009 est.)<br>Country comparison to the world: 145 |
| Distribution of family income (GINI index) | 27 (2006)<br>Country comparison to the world: 125 |
| Investment (gross fixed) | 17.9% of GDP (2009 est.)<br>Country comparison to the world: 115 |
| Public debt | 72.1% of GDP (2009 est.)<br>Country comparison to the world: 19 |
| Market value of publicly traded shares | NA (December 31, 2008)<br>Country comparison to the world: 9 |
| Current account balance | $135.1 billion (2009 est.)<br>Country comparison to the world: 3 |
| Debt (external) | $5.208 trillion (December 30, 2009 est.)<br>Country comparison to the world: 3 |

*continued*

| Table 9-1 Select Key Demographic and Economic Indicators, *continued* | |
|---|---|
| Debt as a % of GDP | ——— |
| Exports | $1.159 trillion (2009 est.)<br>Country comparison to the world: 3 |
| Exports—commodities | Machinery, vehicles, chemicals, metals and manufactures, foodstuffs, textiles |
| Exports—partners | France 10.2%, United States 6.7%, Netherlands 6.7%, United Kingdom 6.6%, Italy 6.3%, Austria 6%, China 4.5%, Switzerland 4.4% (2009) |
| Imports | $966.9 billion (2009 est.)<br>Country comparison to the world: 3 |
| Imports—commodities | Machinery, vehicles, chemicals, foodstuffs, textiles, metals |
| Imports—partners | Netherlands 12.71%, France 8.3%, Belgium 7.19%, China 6.89%, Italy 5.88%, United Kingdom 4.76%, Austria 4.55%, United States 4.25%, Switzerland 4.07% (2009) |
| Stock of direct foreign investment at | |
| Home | $1.008 trillion (December 31, 2009 est.)<br>Country comparison to the world: 4 |
| Abroad | $1.454 trillion (December 31, 2009 est.)<br>Country comparison to the world: 4 |

Source: CIA. (2010). *The world factbook.* Retrieved December 16, 2010, from https://www.cia.gov/library/publications/the-world-factbook/

# Introduction

The Federal Republic of Germany, consisting of 16 states (*Länder*), is located in central Europe. Germany has 82.5 million inhabitants and is densely populated with around 230 inhabitants living per square kilometer (the European average is 116 inhabitants per square kilometer) (Statistisches Bundesamt, 2009a). Just over 7 million inhabitants (8.8%) do not hold German citizenship. Over the few past years, the most important demographic feature of the country has been the continuous increase of the proportion of older adults within the population. The share of the population below 15 years of age decreased from 25% in 1970 to 15% in 2008, while the share of inhabitants who are over 64 years old remained at around 15% until 1993 and has since increased to 19%. The percentage of the age group above 80 years has remained stable over the last 10 years, at around 3.8%, and is predicted to rise further in the coming years (Busse & Riesberg, 2004).

The rapid change in Germany's population structure was caused by a combination of a decrease in birth rates between 1950 (2.16 children per woman) and 2008 (1.35 children per woman) and an increase in life expectancy at birth. According to statistics published by the World Health Organization (WHO), the female life expectancy is at an average of 82.44 years, while the male life expectancy is at an average of 77.16 years (WHO, 2006).

In 2008 the gross domestic product (GDP) amounted to a total of €2,489 billion (Statistisches Bundesamt, 2009b). The unemployment rate in Germany ranked above the Organisation for Economic Co-operation and Development (OECD) average, with about 3.1 million people unemployed in 2008. This is a rate of 7.2% of the workforce (Bundesagentur für Arbeit: Der Arbeits- und Ausbildungsmarkt in Deutschland, 2009). Table 9-2 shows a general overview of facts concerning the German labor market.

Table 9-2 **Basic Facts of the Labor Market in Germany, 2008**

| Indicator | Share |
|---|---|
| Unemployment rate | 7.2% |
| Employed inhabitants | 43.41 million |
| Self-employed | 4.47 million |
| Employees | 35.89 million |
| Employees in the agriculture sector | 0.86 million |
| Employees in the manufacturing industry | 10.22 million |
| Employees in the services sector | 29.27 million |

Source: Data from www.destatis.de

As Table 9-2 shows, the service sector is by far the most important sector of the labor market in Germany, followed by the manufacturing industry.

## Prevailing Health Issues and Risk Behaviors

In the context of health-related risk factors, issues of particular importance include the spectrum of diseases, the main causes of death, and employee absenteeism in connection to various types of diseases.

Just as in other industrialized western countries, risk factors like smoking, obesity, physical inactivity, hypertension, and impaired fat metabolism foster the burden of disease of German residents. These risk factors are mainly caused by the personal behaviors and lifestyle of the individuals in western civilization. Currently there are approximately 4 million people in

Germany living with diabetes as a result of this lifestyle, and this number is increasing continuously (Robert Koch Institute [RKI], 2005a). The following section reviews the prevalence of the most important risk factors in Germany.

## Smoking

Every third adult person in Germany smokes (RKI, 2006). About 25% of the German population smoke regularly and 4% belong to the category of occasional smokers. With regard to these numbers, gender-specific differences need to be taken into consideration. Currently, 35% of the male and 22% of the female population are smokers (Deutsche Krebsgesellschaft, 2008). While surveys show that the smoking habits of men in general have been decreasing; unfortunately, such surveys have also shown an increase among teenagers above 15 years of age (RKI, 2006).

## Alcohol Consumption

Alcohol consumption within the German population has been declining slowly over the last decades. Using international statistics, Germany is in fifth place (RKI 2008a). With 10.2 litres of pure alcohol consumption per person in 2003, German alcohol consumption is above the EU average of 9.2 litres of pure alcohol per year (Busse & Riesberg, 2004).

## Overweight and Obesity

For several decades, the percentage of the German population suffering from overweight and obesity has been rising. This trend affects children and teenagers as well as adults. About half of all German adults are overweight (RKI, 2005c). Fifty-five percent of men and 49% of woman have a body mass index of 25.0–29.9. About one fifth of the German population is obese. Nineteen percent of men and 20% of women have a BMI of 30 or more (WHO, 2006). The share of obese children in Germany is 7% (RKI, 2005c). This fact shows that the problem of being overweight begins during childhood.

## Physical Inactivity

Looking at physical activity of the German population, different results can be seen due to different study designs. According to the results of the Bundes-Gesundheits survey carried out in 1998, only about 13% of the German adults reach the recommended minimum level of physical activity (Mensink, 2003). This means that 78% of the German population do not follow the recommendation to engage in physical activity at least 3 days a week. Furthermore, a national survey of people between 18 and 79 years discovered that one third of the German population has no involvement in sports (RKI, 2005b). In this age group, 73% of men and 57% of women report 2 hours of physical activity per week. Nevertheless, it needs to be stated that physical activity diminishes enormously with increasing age of the male and female population (RKI, 2005b).

## Disease Profile and Main Causes of Death

The disease profile in Germany is dominated by cardiovascular diseases and cancer. In both males and females, the largest mortality rate in Germany is due to cardiovascular diseases (WHO, 2006). Among cardiovascular diseases, ischemic heart disease is the biggest issue in Germany; it caused 21% of all deaths in 2002 (Table 9-3).

Cancer is the second most frequent cause of death after cardiovascular diseases in the male and female population. Each year more than 400,000 people are diagnosed with cancer; the same number of people die as a result of cardiovascular diseases (RKI, 2006). Cancer accounted for about 27% of deaths in Germany in 2002 (WHO, 2006). Lung cancer is the most common cancer, with tobacco being the most important risk factor.

Concerning the prevalence of cancer, gender-specific differences need to be taken into account. In the male population, prostate cancer, colon cancer, and lung cancer are the most common types of cancer. The most frequent types in the female population are breast cancer, colon cancer, and lung cancer (RKI, 2008b).

Table 9-3 reflects the burden of disease of the German population.

**Table 9-3 Top Ten Causes of Death for All Ages, 2002**

| Causes | Estimated number of deaths (in thousands) | Estimated percentage (%) of deaths |
|---|---|---|
| All causes | 815 | 100 |
| Ischemic heart disease | 173 | 21 |
| Cerebrovascular disease | 79 | 10 |
| Trachea, bronchus, lung cancer | 42 | 5 |
| Colon and rectum cancers | 32 | 4 |
| Chronic obstructive pulmonary disease | 22 | 3 |
| Diabetes mellitus | 21 | 3 |
| Lower respiratory infections | 21 | 3 |
| Breast cancer | 20 | 3 |
| Hypertensive heart disease | 18 | 2 |
| Cirrhosis of the liver | 18 | 2 |

*Note:* Total Population in 2002: 82,414
Source: Data from WHO, 2004.

## Work-Related Health Issues

With regard to key work-related health issues, it is necessary to analyze absenteeism data. Most German health insurance companies focus on work-related health data in their annual health reports. Table 9-4 illustrates the 10 diseases most frequently responsible for the absenteeism of insured people from the health insurance company Deutsche Angestellten Krankenkasse. The data show that 53% of absenteeism days in 2007 are related to 3 disease groups:

- Musculoskeletal disorders
- Respiratory tract diseases, and
- Injuries (DAK, 2008)

Musculoskeletal disorders comprise the most frequent and most expensive group of symptoms in Germany and have advanced to the top of Deutsche Angestellten Krankenkasse's sickness figures (accounting for 21.9% of days absent). Musculoskeletal disorders have the second highest incidence rate. Within this disease group, back pain is the most important diagnosis.

Table 9-4 **Employee Absenteeism in 2007 by Type of Disease**

| Illness | Percent of total days absent | Percent of disability cases caused by each disease category |
|---|---|---|
| Musculoskeletal disorders | 21.9% | 14.4% |
| Respiratory tract diseases | 16.8% | 29.1% |
| Injuries | 14.3% | 9.2% |
| Mental disorders | 10.2% | 4.1% |
| Disorders of the digestive system | 7.4% | 13.7% |
| Cardiovascular diseases | 4.7% | 2.8% |
| Symptoms | 4.6% | 5.7% |
| Infections | 4.5% | 8.8% |
| Nervous system, eyes, ears | 4.1% | 4.5% |
| Malignant neoplasm | 3.8% | 1.2% |
| Other | 7.7% | 6.5% |

Source: Data from DAK, 2008.

Absenteeism statistics from the health insurance company Allgemeine Ortskrankenkasse indicate that during the last ten years mental disorders have risen steadily. This is consistent with the data from many health insurance companies. The number of cases of absenteeism due to mental disorders has been increasing enormously, with an increase of 58% between 1996 and 2007 (Badura, Schröder, & Vetter, 2008).

Mental diseases such as depressive disorders and panic disorders have been gaining major significance and play an important role in early retirement. Fifteen percent of German men and 8% of German women suffer from a period of depression during their life (RKI, 2006).

## Healthcare System

Germany is recognized as the first country to have introduced a national social security system. The development of the specific framework of the German healthcare system dates back to 1883 when the parliament made nationwide health insurance compulsory. In the following decades, the principles of statutory social insurance, called the Bismarck system, were extended to include the following areas:

- Alleviation of risks of work-related accidents and invalidity (1884)
- Old age and disability (1889)
- Unemployment (1927)
- The need for long-term nursing care (1994)

The prominence and structural continuity of social insurance remains one of the key features of the historical development of Germany's healthcare system until the present day.

Health insurance contributions, as well as representation in the governing boards, are shared equally between employees and employers. Insurance for work-related accidents and invalidity is entirely financed by employers.

In 2003, about 87% of the population was covered by statutory health insurance. Ten percent of the population took out private health insurance, 2% were covered by governmental schemes, and 0.2% were not covered at all (WHO, 2006). Since 1996, almost every person has had the right to choose a health insurance company freely and companies are obligated to accept any applicant. The government partially reimburses the cost for low-wage earners, whose premiums are capped at a predetermined value. Higher wage workers covered by statutory health insurance pay a premium based on their salary. They may also opt for private insurance, which is generally more expensive. The cost of private insurance varies for each individual and is based on the individual's health status.

The 292 health insurance companies collect contributions and purchase proactively or pay retroactively for health and long-term care services for members (WHO, 2006). Health promotion was made mandatory for health insurance companies in 1989. It was then eliminated in 1996 and reintroduced again in a modified form in 2000.

Furthermore, it must be noted that healthcare costs in Germany have been expanding continuously for decades. Total health expenditure accounted to 10.4% of GDP in Germany in 2007 (OECD, 2008). This corresponds to an amount of €2,970 per citizen per year. The share of GDP that is spent on health care in Germany is 1.5 percentage points higher than the Organization for Economic Co-Operation and Development (OECD) average of 8.9% in the OECD countries (OECD, 2008). Only the United States and Switzerland allocated more of their GDP to health than Germany.

# Influence of Culture and Mentality

Issues like health awareness, eating patterns, and physical activity have to be taken into account in the context of the German culture and mentality.

## Awareness of Health Issues

In a study carried out in 2006 (WHO, 2006), most Germans stated that they were satisfied with their health. Of the German population, 80.8% reported their health to be good or very good (WHO, 2006).

The awareness of the importance of health issues among the German population has been growing enormously during the last few years. Currently, the maintenance of health is of high value to German residents. The results of a survey from Berger in 2007 (MED-Magazin, 2007) show that 70% of the German population rate health as more important than love, partnership, or friendship. In addition to their health insurance costs, Germans spend approximately €900 per year to support and improve their health. This significant amount is primarily spent on medical check-ups, complementary and alternative medicine, wellness, sports, and healthy nutrition (MED-Magazin, 2007). However, people from lower income groups spend relatively less than people from higher income groups.

## Eating Patterns

Germans' caloric intake is about the same as that of their European Union neighbors; however, they eat fewer fruits and vegetables (Busse & Riesberg, 2004).

A representative survey on nutrition in Germany (Nationale Verzehrstudie) shows the following results concerning nutrition habits of the German population (Bundesforschungsinstitut für Ernährung und Lebensmittel, 2008):

- High consumption of meat (men, 103 grams daily; women, 53 grams daily)
- Low consumption of fish
- Sixty percent of Germans do not eat enough fruits and vegetables (based on five a day recommendation)

Organic products have become very popular in Germany, making the associated bioindustry a growth sector.

The main meal in Germany is lunch. Accordingly, company catering is a main part of the catering sector in Germany. Roughly 1.4 billion customers spent about €4 billion on catering in 2003 (Deutsche Gesellschaft für Ernährung e.V., 2008). In view of the facts stated above, healthy catering in cafeterias is an appropriate starting point for WHP interventions.

## Infrastructure for Physical Activity

German structures for physical activity are well developed and varied. Sports clubs are a major characteristic of the German sports infrastructure. In 2008, 27 million inhabitants (29% of the German population) were members in 86,000 sports clubs (DOSB, 2009). Specifically, company sports clubs offer opportunities for physical activity at the workplace. Additionally, 7 million Germans (8.75% of the population) are members of commercial fitness centers (Fuchs, 2007).

The well-developed system of public transportation in Germany helps individuals keep physically active. People who use public transportation walk more than people who ride by car on a daily basis. Furthermore, there is a good infrastructure of bicycle paths available. This makes cycling a very common sport in Germany, and many people use bikes in everyday life. Through health promotion campaigns that promote biking to work, health insurance companies support the use of bikes in order to increase the amount of daily physical activity.

## Challenges

The above facts demonstrate that the cultural conditions, health-related values, eating habits, and available structures for physical activity in Germany offer a significant basis for work-related health promotion strategies. On the other hand, a challenge to WHP is the high sensitivity to data privacy. Employees typically perceive health as a personal issue not in the realm of company activities. Therefore, skepticism arises when the occupational health department or the human resources department asks employees for health-related data, even if collected anonymously.

# Drivers of Workplace Health Promotion

Health insurance companies are the main providers as well as financing agencies for WHP in Germany. In fact, Germany is one of the few countries worldwide in which workplace health promotion has a legal foundation. Workplace health promotion in Germany is mainly based on Article 20 of the general social insurance law (SGB V). Based on this law, health insurance companies have been developing and implementing projects in the field of workplace health promotion since 1989. Article 20 was amended with the health reform law in 2001 and recognizes the recommendations for modern, comprehensive health promotion based on the Ottawa Charter. In addition, since 2004, Article 84 of SGB IX requires employers to offer disability management and return-to-work programs (independent of company size, in order to protect the health of employees and retain work ability (AOK, 2007).

WHP interventions financed by health insurance companies aim to improve the health status and health resources of insured employees. Table 9-5 highlights the main areas of activity and principles of intervention within workplace health promotion projects based on Article 20.

Table 9-5 **Main Areas of Activity and Principles of Workplace Health Promotion Based on Article 20**

| Areas of activity | Principles of intervention |
|---|---|
| Work-related physical strain | • Prevention and reduction of work-related strain of the musculoskeletal system |
| Company catering | • Healthy catering at the workplace |
| Psychological stress | • Promotion of individual competencies to cope with stress at the workplace<br>• Leadership that supports health |
| Addictive drug consumption | • Smoke-free enterprise<br>• Zero blood alcohol level at the workplace |

Source: Data from Arbeitsgemeinschaft der Spitzenverbände der Krankenkassen, 2008.

German health insurance companies have been increasing the number of interventions in the field of WHP over the last several years. In 2003, there were 2,164 documented WHP intervention cases. The cost of these interventions was €32.2 million in 2007 (Drupp, 2009).

WHP interventions must follow quality management guidelines prepared by the German WHP network in 2001. The network is the first and only network for WHP in Germany to address all aspects of working life, and it is open to all stakeholders in the field of WHP for the national exchange of experience and information. The network's secretariat is funded by the BKK Federal Association and the German Federation of Institutions for Statutory Accident Insurance and Prevention. There are quality guidelines concerning the qualification of the providers of interventions in the four main areas of activity (see Table 9-5).

Health insurance companies either run health promotion interventions at the workplaces themselves, in collaboration with employers' liability insurance associations, or they employ private companies. The AOK (largest health insurer in Germany) in Lower Saxony has been running an innovative bonus project with considerable success. For example, AOK grants a discount for the government's social security health insurance (in both employee and employer payments) to companies that implement health promotion programs according to criteria based on the European Foundation of Quality Management. A study on the impact of the program showed that 14 participating companies realized a reduction of 28% in absenteeism compared to an industry average of 20%, as well as lower accident rates and improved employee satisfaction (AOK, 2004).

An additional reward system for the support of WHP interventions was implemented in the field of income tax law in January 2009. Based on Article 3 No. 34 of the income tax law, employers have the opportunity to claim an amount of €500 per employee per year for WHP interventions (based on Article 20 SGB V) as tax deductions. This development provides a new incentive, even if small, for employers to implement health promotion interventions at the workplace.

## Programs

Working conditions have undergone significant changes since 1990. The advancements and pervasiveness of new technology are pertinent to this change, and new technology has simultaneously created growth in the service sector. An important consideration here is the increasing age of the workforce, which is leading to a shortage of skilled employees. At the same time, employees are required to cope with heightened mental and psychological stress, a major change from the previous demands of hard physical labor (Anderson, Serxner, & Gold, 2001). In light of these massive changes, workplace health promotion programs offer a good possibility to reduce the negative consequences for both employee and employer. With that said, it is clear that both sides can enjoy the benefits. An integral requirement of this is that there is variation and tailoring of programs.

Germany has a long tradition of organizational approaches with regard to employee health through organizational development, optimization of the work process, leadership, improvement of company communication structures, and career development. This approach is widely viewed as an effective strategy to address work-related stress and mental disease—in particular as a necessary extension of individualistic approaches—and therefore has enjoyed greater popularity recently. One commonly used organizational intervention strategy is the health circle concept, which was developed in the 1980s in Germany. Health circles are discussion groups that are tasked with the development of change options for the improvement of potentially harmful working conditions, especially with regard to psychosocial health risks (Westermayer & Bähr, 1994). Health circles typically involve representatives from various disciplines dealing with workplace health and safety. Another proven approach is the integration of health-related issues, such as how to reduce musculoskeletal disorders, with existing continual improvement processes.

The workplace also offers an opportunity to address prevalent chronic disease and lifestyle-related behaviors, as it presents a captive audience including some people who are normally difficult to reach. There is a large variety of program modalities:

- During working hours
- Before or after working hours
- Within the company
- Outside the company
- With relationship to the specific conditions of the workplace
- Without relationship to the specific conditions of the workplace

WHP programs in Germany vary in many respects and are typically based on data that is gathered by the company-specific health reports. Activities range from health days or fairs to completely integrated programs with tailored activities (including rehabilitation programs). Very often, the programs are oriented to the interests of the employees in order to reach a large amount of consensus. A survey conducted by the University of Heidelberg in 2008 in the largest energy enterprise in Germany showed that the following activities were the most requested (MVV Gesundheitsbericht, 2008):

1. Ergonomic advice
2. Blood sugar screening
3. Sleep disorder programs
4. Sports (ball games)
5. Jogging groups
6. Work–life balance

It is important to develop more programs and resources for the many small and medium-sized enterprises. Occupational health statistics show that employees in small companies (fewer than 50 workers) have much worse health overall than employees in larger companies. This does not necessarily have to do with the fact that employees in larger companies work less or work more health consciously, but that in smaller companies there is inherently more dependence on each individual. In a three-person company, if one person has a sick day, then 33% of the workforce is not present. This would be the comparison of 330 people who are sick at the same time in a company with 1,000 employees. Due to this fact, it is even more necessary to encourage smaller companies to have WHP programs.

# Good Practice

A literature search of research studies has identified the following elements as good practice:

1. *Analysis of sick leave and disability data.* This data highlights basic health problems and their allocation to different employee groups, which provide evidence for the need to design WHP programs. It is also essential for the cost-benefit analysis. For example, the automobile company Daimler demonstrated a positive cost-benefit effect of a strength training program by reducing sick days related to back pain (Huber & Stroheker, 2005).
2. *Modular questionnaires.* Well-designed programs also use modular questionnaires that bring together aspects such as dissatisfaction at work, stress and work demands, and physical activity, as well as content, desired outcomes, and suggestions in order to create programs. The questionnaires can also uncover hints for creating motivation and tailoring programs to the employee population. A good example is the SF-36 questionnaire to measure health-related life quality (sf-36.org, n.d.).
3. *Workplace inspection with photographic documentation.* The focus on the individual employee and his or her specific work situation is a central requirement for workplace health programs. This evaluation can be completed during a work inspection while looking for already-existing solutions to compile and integrate into the program. Photos of workplaces are useful tools; e.g., for back pain programs.
4. *Interviews (exploration talks).* Carrying out interviews with individual employees can help clear up conflicts from an employee's point of view as well as deliver important information about program objectives and desired outcomes. Such talks serve as the basis for creating a positive social environment in the business. This is therefore an important building block of programs. These interviews are very useful in combination with questionnaires.
5. *Tracking presenteeism.* The recognition of presenteeism as a critical entity in workplace health promotion has not yet led to standard processes in data collection. In the United States of America, numerous instruments are used (for a review see Collins et al., 2005). The Stanford Presenteeism Scale has been translated into German and has been used in some preliminary studies (Koopman et al., 2002).

# Outcomes and Indicators

Health programs in the workplace are a perfect example of the so-called win-win situation. This means all participants profit from a provision. Research in Germany documents the following advantages from the side of the employee:

- Reduced work strains
- Reduced health complaints
- Increased well-being at work
- Increased satisfaction with work
- Better life quality
- Better social atmosphere at work

The employer may expect the following outcomes from workplace health programs:

- Decrease of the rate of sick days
- Decrease in turnover
- Increase in manufacturing quality and/or the service quality
- Increase in work satisfaction
- Improved corporate identity; supports a positive image of business, which at the same time is communicated from the inside and outside

An important development in Germany is the connection between workplace health promotion programs and the criteria of quality management in companies. Satisfied and healthy workers are the basis of making quality programs and ensuring that they remain at a high quality in all companies. If WHP programs would start to be understood as a part of each company's overall strategy, then the quality management part would need to be integrated.

Since quality management needs to be oriented around economic factors, these factors would also be applied. Companies are typically interested in the economic effects of health programs. Taking a look at the relationship of the costs and benefits is unavoidable. Many research methods from the United States cannot be used because of the different health systems; nonetheless, employers, particularly in the United States, believe that well-designed WHP programs that utilize appropriate measurements are very beneficial. Whereas close to 90% of U.S. employers offer WHP programs, the number is much smaller in Germany. Valid numbers are not available, but the percentage is clearly less than 25%. Due to this, there are few scientific investigations available about the effectiveness of WHP programs in Germany.

Nevertheless, the costs of these programs are known to be an important factor in the cost-benefit relationship (Pelletier, 2005), which has been transferred into the German context (Huber & Stroheker, 2005). The savings are created by reducing the following cost factors:

- Continuation of wages if the person becomes ill
- Apportionment to indirect costs for an ill worker (e.g., substitutes, materials)

- Direct and indirect sick costs to the corporation
- Costs to replace the ill person

According to the German Institute of Business (Langhoff, 2008), the costs run an average of 300 to 500 euros for every day that a person is unable to work. The costs per work hour are one of the most costly in the world at 25 euros an hour. However, WHP considerations should not be reduced to financial costs.

# Existing Research

As already mentioned, there are a lot of players and actors on the stage of workplace health promotion in Germany. There is no steering committee or coordinating mechanism, and generally accepted guidelines for workplace health promotion do not exist. Therefore, existing research is mainly driven by the interests of organizations, insurance companies, or vendors of programs and services. The published research is focused on two different areas—health reports and evaluation of programs.

## Health Reports

One of the main research areas with a history is the *Fehlzeiten Report* (Badura, Schröder, & Vetter, 2008), a report on sick days and different analyses of sick leave. It is published annually by a health insurance company and the University of Bielefeld and includes statistics on absenteeism of workers in all industries; the main reasons for absenteeism; and comparative data for different ages, professions, and job qualifications. In addition, it contains review papers from various authors dealing with specific topics that are representative of various research areas.

Since 2004, the following volumes have been published:

2009: Mental stress

2008: Corporate Health: Analyses of Costs and Benefits

2007: Work, Gender and Health

2006: Chronic Diseases

2005: Job Insecurity and Health

2004: Worksite Health Promotion in Hospitals

One of the services delivered by insurance companies for employers is specific health reports. These reports are very useful tools to adapt programs to the specific needs of a company and its employees and to employ science in creating useful information.

## Evaluation of Programs

The main reason for evaluation is the pressure to justify workplace health promotion programs. Evaluation methods are focused on the following outcome parameters:

- Quality of life
- Cost-benefit calculations

Outcome evaluation checks whether and to what extent the intended goals were reached. In order to measure quality of life in terms of health-related measures, the SF-36 questionnaire has proven to be very helpful in various studies (Bullinger, 1996; Bullinger & Kirchberger, 1998; Schüle & Huber, 2004). The SF-36 questionnaire shows a complete picture of the state of health, including health-related status as well as subjective quality of life data.

The cost-benefit calculation plays a crucial role in the justification and sustainable integration of WHP programs. A special form is the cost-benefit analysis (Schwartz, Wilhelm, Ulla, Bernt-Peter, & Schmidt, 1998). This analysis compares the costs of the interventions with the profitability of achieved effects. The effects are transferred into monetary units. These economic analyses are not easy to conduct but are often requested by the top-level management. The results of scientific studies including cost-benefit calculations are published very rarely, as they are often treated as a trade secret. The Initiative Gesundheit und Arbeit published a comprehensive review on the return on investment of WHP in 2007, and concluded that cost-benefit calculations were new in the German context and that most return on investment studies originated in the United States. The report also underlines the rising interest among employers and health insurance companies in cost-benefit calculation methods (Kramer & Bödeker, 2007).

The next focus of research in Germany will be presenteeism, which is viewed as having a much stronger impact on company productivity than absenteeism. So far, questionnaires on presenteeism have not found general acceptance in German workplaces; however, the Work Performance and Activity Impairment Questionnaire and the Stanford Presenteeism Scale have been used on occasion.

It is expected that a growing number of research studies will take on a European dimension (often driven by the European Union). Therefore, research methods that can be compared to other international methods should be expanded. Due to the great variety in culture, healthcare systems, and lifestyles, this international analysis will be a huge task for the future.

# Conclusion

In light of the described demographic trends, the common lifestyle-related risk factors (obesity, lack of physical activity, hypertension), growing work-related stress and mental disease, and increasing healthcare costs in Germany, workplace health promotion interventions that use the settings approach are important to improve the health status of the population.

Workplace health promotion has a legal foundation in Germany and is mainly based on Article 20 of the general social insurance law. On the basis of this law, health insurance companies have been implementing projects and activities in the field of workplace health promotion since 1989. Although there is an abundance of WHP activities currently being offered in Germany, there is a lack of tailored and systematic programs that have been evaluated and shown to be successful. In addition, a need is evident for more activities in small and medium-sized enterprises, where the majority of the working population is employed.

## Summary

Germany is facing similar challenges to many other developed nations with an aging workforce and rising chronic diseases. An alarming statistic is that 75% of men and 69% of women have a body mass index of 25 or above. In spite of significant unemployment (7.2% in 2008), a lack of skilled workers is already visible in a number of industries. To address these challenges, the retirement age was recently raised to 67 years, and for many years healthcare reform has been intensely debated.

Germany is one of the few countries with a legal foundation for workplace health promotion, as incorporated in Article 20 of the social security law (SGB V). Health insurance companies are required to offer health promotion programs at the workplace by identifying and improving health risks and potential health risks for employees. This has led to an abundance of workplace health promotion activities offered mostly by health insurance companies (statutory and private) since 1989. These efforts include both individual and organizational approaches to health and well-being. In addition, awareness of health issues is very high among Germans (e.g., organic foods are very popular). Germans spend approximately €900 per year on health-related services and products in addition to health insurance. Nevertheless, tailored and systematic WHP programs, which have been evaluated, are far and few between. Absence rates are still being used as the main outcome indicator although these have been low for many years, mainly due to economic pressures and job insecurity. Only recently has presenteeism been introduced as a possible health-related indicator. The main reasons for sick leave are musculoskeletal disorders and respiratory tract diseases (in that order), with mental disorders rising steadily.

In conclusion, the need for more tailored programs embedded in the business structure and evaluation of programs is evident, as is the need for enhanced resources and guidance for small- and medium-sized enterprises, where the majority of workers in Germany are employed.

## Review Questions

1. What are the most important health risk factors in Germany? Are they the same as the causes of absenteeism?
2. How is the German healthcare system funded, managed, and regulated?
3. In what way does the German culture affect population eating patterns and health behaviors?
4. What is the role of health insurance companies in regard to German workplace health promotion programs?
5. What are the factors that control savings in German workplace health promotion programs?
6. Identify two assessment tools that measure outcome for workplace health and wellness programs.

## References


Anderson, D. R., Serxner, S. A., & Gold, D. B. (2001, May–June). Conceptual framework, critical questions, and practical challenges in conducting research on the financial impact of worksite health promotion. *Am J Health Promot (United States): 15*(5), 281–288.

AOK. (2004). *Betriebliche Investionen in Gesundheit zahlen sich aus.* Retrieved February 11, 2009, from http://www.aok.de/nieders/tool/presse/index.php?cid=2&aid=94&search=&page=8

AOK. (2007). Betriebliches eingliederungsmanagement. *Praxis Handbuch.* Essen: CW Haarfeld.

Arbeitsgemeinschaft der Spitzenverbände der Krankenkassen. (2008). *Gemeinsame und einheitliche Handlungsfelder und Kriterien der Spitzenverbände der Krankenkassen zur Umsetzung von §§ 20 und 20a SGB V vom 21. Juni 2000 in der Fassung vom 2. Juni 2008.* Bergisch Gladbach, Germany: IKK Bunderverband.

Badura, B., Schröder, H., & Vetter, C. (2010). *Arbeit und Psyche: Belastungen Reduzieren—Wohlbefinden Fördern.* Berlin, Germany: Springer-Verlag.

Badura, B. S., Schröder, H., & Vetter, C. (2008). *Fehlzeiten—Report 2008. Betriebliches Gesundheitsmanagement. Kosten und Nutzen.* Heidelberg, Germany: Springer Medizin Verlag.

Breyer, F. Z. (1997). *Gesundheitsökonomie* (Bd. 2). Berlin, Germany: Springer.

Bullinger, M. (1996). Erfassung der Gesundheitsbezogenen Lebensqualität mit dem SF-36 Health Survey. *Die Rehabilitation, 1*(35), 17–30.

Bullinger, M., & Kirchberger I. (1998). SF-36 Fragebogen zum Gesundheitszustant—Handanweisung, Germany. Göttingen: Hogrefe.

Bundesagentur für Arbeit: Der Arbeits- und Ausbildungsmarkt in Deutschland. (2009). Nürnberg. Retrieved from www.pub.arbeitsamt.de

Bundesforschungsinstitut für Ernährung und Lebensmittel. (2008). Nationale Verzehrstudie. *Ernährung—Wissenschaft und Praxis, 2*(2), 77–81.

Busse, R., Riesberg, A. (2004). *Health care system in transition.* Copenhagen, Denmark: WHO Regional Office for Europe.

Collins, J., Baase, C. M., Sharda, C. E., Ozminkowski, R. J., Nicholson, S., Billotti, G. M., … Berger, M. L. (2005). The assessment of chronic health conditions on work performance, absence, and total economic impact for employers. *Journal of Occupational and Environmental Medicine 47*(6), 547–557.

Deutsche Angestellten Krankenkasse (DAK). (2008). *Gesundheitsreport 2008.* Hamburg, Germany: DAK Forschung.

Deutsche Gesellschaft für Ernährung e.V. (2008). *Ernährungsbericht 2008.* Bonn, Germany: DGE.

Deutsche Krebsgesellschaft. (2008). Abgerufen am February 2009 von Rauchen-Zahlen und Fakten. Retrieved from http://www.krebsgesellschaft.de/rauchen_datenzahlenfakten,1050.html

Deutscher Olympischer Sportbund (DOSB). (2009). *Bestandserhebung des Deutschen Olympischen Sportbundes 2008.* Frankfurt am Main, Germany: DOSB.

Drupp, M. (2009). Betriebliches Gesundheitsmanagement. Finanzierung, Bonussysteme und steuerliche Förderung. *Impulse* (63).

Fuchs, R. (2007). Bewegung, Gesundheit und Public Health. In Thomas von Lengerke (Hrsg.), *Public Health-Psychologie. Individuum und Bevölkerung zwischen Verhältnissen und Verhalten* (S. 77–91). Weinheim, Germany: Juventa.

Huber, G., & Stroheker, M. (2005, November). Betriebliches Gesundheitsmanagement, ein Ansatz der sich rechnet. *Journal of Public Health, 13,* 64.

Koopman, C., Pelletier, K. R., Murray, J. F., Sharda, C. E., Berger, M. L., Turpin, R. S. … Bendel, T. (2002). Stanford presenteeism scale: Health status and employee productivity. *Journal of Occupational and Environmental Medicine, 44*(1), 14–20. Retrieved from http://www.drpelletier.com/chip/pdf/CHIP-standford_presenteeism_scale.pdf

Kramer, I., & Bödeker, W. (2007). *IGA Report: Return on Investment im Kontext der betrieblichen Gesundheitsförderung und Prävention.* Essen, Germany: BKK Bundesverband.

Langhoff, T. (2008). Den demographischen Wandel erfolgreich gestalten. Heidelberg, New York, NY: Springer

MED-Magazin. (2007). *Studie zum zweiten Gesundheitsmarkt.* Retrieved February 16, 2009, from http://www.med-magazin.de/article4036.html

Mensink, G. (2003). *Bundesgesundheitssurvey: Körperliche Aktivität. Aktive Freizeitgestaltung in Deutschland.* Berlin, Germany: Robert Koch Institute.

MVV Gesundheitsbericht (2008). Unpublished Report University of Heidelberg.

Organization for Economic Co-Operation and Development (OECD). (2008). *OECD health data 2009: Statistics and indicators for 30 countries.* Retrieved February 4, 2009, from http://www.oecd.org/health/healthdata

Pelletier, K. R. (2005). A review and analysis of the clinical and cost-effectiveness studies of comprehensive health promotion and disease management programs at the worksite: Update IV 2000–2004. *Journal of Occupational and Environmental Medicine, 47*(10), 1051–1058.

Robert Koch Institute (RKI). (2005a). *Diabetes mellitus. Gesundheitsberichterstattung des Bundes. Heft 24.* Berlin, Germany: Robert Koch Institute.

Robert Koch Institute (RKI). (2005b). *Körperliche Aktivität. Gesundheitsberichterstattung des Bundes. Heft 26.* Berlin, Germany: Robert Koch Institute.

Robert Koch Institute (RKI). (2005c). *Übergewicht und Adipositas. Gesundheitsberichterstattung des Bundes. Heft 16.* Berlin, Germany: Robert Koch Institute.

Robert Koch Institute (RKI). (2006). *Gesundheit in Deutschland. Gesundheitsberichterstattung des Bundes.* Berlin, Germany: Robert Koch Institute.

Robert Koch Institute (RKI). (2008a). *Alkoholkonsum und alkoholbezogene Störungen. Gesundheitsberichterstattung des Bundes. Heft 40.* Berlin, Germany: Robert Koch Institute.

Robert Koch Institute (RKI). (2008b). *Krebs in Deutschland. Häufigkeiten und Trends 2003-2004. Gesundheitsberichterstattung in Deutschland.* Berlin, Germany: Robert Koch Institute.

Schüle, K. & Huber, G. (2004). *Grundlagen der Sporttherapie. Prävention, ambulante und stationäre Rehabilitation.* München, Germany: Urban & Fischer.

Schwartz, F., Wilhelm,W., Ulla, R., Bernt-Peter, & Schmidt, T. (1998). *Prävention.* In F. W. Schwartz, B. Badura, R. Leidl, H. Raspe, & J. Siegrist (Hrsg.). *Das Public Health Buch: Gesundheit und Gesundheitswesen* (pp. 151–170). München/Wien, Germany/Baltimore, MD: Urban & Schwarzenberg,

SF-36.org. (n.d.) *SF-36 health survey.* Available at http://www.sf-36.org

Statistisches Bundesamt. (2009a). *Die Bevölkerung in Deutschland. Wiesbaden.* Retrieved from www.destatis.de

Statistisches Bundesamt. (2009b). V*olkswirtschaftliche Gesamtberechnungen. Wiesbaden.* Rctrieved from www.destatis.de

Westermayer, G., & Bähr, B. (1994). *Betriebliche Gesundheitszirkel.* Göttingen, Germany: Verlag für Angewandte Psychologie.

World Health Organization (WHO). (2004). *Highlights on health in Germany.* Copenhagen, Denmark: WHO Regional Office for Europe. www.euro.who.int/__data/assets/pdf_file/0009/103221/E88527.pdf

World Health Organization (WHO). (2006). *Highlights on health in Germany.* Copenhagen, Denmark: WHO Regional Office for Europe.

Chapter 10

# Gulf Cooperation Council

Jalees K. Razavi and Wolf Kirsten

After reading this chapter you should be able to:

- Identify core strategies that are the focus of workplace health promotion efforts among the Gulf Cooperation Council (GCC) countries
- Describe the historical evolution of workplace health promotion within the GCC
- Explain the different approaches employed by corporate health promotion efforts throughout the GCC states
- Review the central disease states and health issues driving the GCC's health promotion needs
- Name the components of, and the associated funding sources for, healthcare systems within the GCC
- Discuss the impact of culture on the health status and health promotion efforts of GCC states

Table 10-1 **Gulf Corporation Council Demographic**

| | Bahrain | Qatar | Kuwait | Sultanate of Oman | United Arab Emirates | Kingdom of Saudi Arabia |
|---|---|---|---|---|---|---|
| Geography | | | | | | |
| Area (sq. km) | 741 | 11,586 | 17,818 | 309,500 | 83,600 | 2,149,690 |
| Terrain | Low desert | Barren desert | Desert | Desert/ mountains | Coastal plains/ desert | Desert |
| People | | | | | | |
| Population total | 728,709 | 833,285 | 2,692,526 | 3,418,085 | 4,798,491 | 28,686,633 |

*continued*

| Table 10-1 **Gulf Corporation Council Demographic,** *continued* | | | | | | |
|---|---|---|---|---|---|---|
| No. of Non-nationals | 235,108 | Not available | 1,291,354 | 577,293 | Not available | 5,576,076 |
| Age | | | | | | |
| 0–14 | 25.9% | 21.8% | 26.4% | 42.7% | 20.4% | 38.0% |
| 15–64 | 70.1% | 76.8% | 70.7% | 54.5% | 78.7% | 59.5% |
| 65 and over | 4.0% | 1.4% | 3.0% | 2.8% | 0.9% | 2.5% |
| Median | 30.4 | 30.8 | 26.2 | 23.9 | 30.1 | 21.6 |
| Life expectancy | 75.19 | 75.35 | 77.71 | 74.16 | 76.11 | 76.3 |
| Net migration rate | 0.2 | -3.58 | 16.01 | 0.24 | 22.98* | -7.6 |
| Government | Constitutional monarchy | Emirate | Constitutional emirate | Monarchy | Federation | Monarchy |
| Economy | | | | | | |
| GDP (billions) | 28.31 | 99.59 | 142.1 | 72.88 | 186.8 | 592.3 |
| GDP per capita | $38,800.00 | $119,500.00 | $52,800.00 | $25,000.00 | $38,900.00 | $20,600.00 |
| Labor force | 595,000 | 1.179 million | 2.04 million | 968,800 | 3,152,000† | 6,922,000 |
| Unemployment rate | 15% | 0.5% | 2.2% | 15% | 2.4% | 11.7% |
| Military expenditures (% of GDP) | 4.5% | 10% | 5.3% | 11.4%* | 3.1% | 10% |

* Number 1 in the world.

† Expatriates equal 85% of workforce.

## Introduction

This chapter will focus on the member states of the Gulf Cooperation Council (GCC). The GCC is an association of the Kingdom of Bahrain, Qatar, Kuwait, the Sultanate of Oman, the United Arab Emirates (UAE), and the Kingdom of Saudi Arabia. It was created in 1981 after the role model of the European Union to provide a common market for member states and support cross-country investment and services trade (Cooperation Council for the Arab States of the Gulf, 2010). This region has undergone tremendous development and economic growth since the 1980s, in large part due to the abundance of natural resources; i.e., oil and gas. Nomadic settlements have become modern cities with skyscrapers, world-class airports, and an influx of immigrants. The fascinating sociologic and economic changes play a key role with regard to the health of the people.

Alongside the recent, rapid economic development, the Arabian Gulf countries increasingly have been faced with chronic disease patterns in the population. The Arabian Gulf has adopted Western behaviors and lifestyles, which have contributed to an increase in major noncommunicable diseases, such as diabetes and hypertension. At the same time, communicable diseases, such as malaria, HIV, Ebola, yellow fever, polio, and others have not been eradicated. This double burden causes big challenges for the healthcare systems (Table 10-2).

Table 10-2 **Demographic Data for the GCC Region (Numbers per 1,000 Population)**

| Country | Population (× 1,000) | Mortality rate | % Unemployment | % GDP spent on health | Life Expectancy | Area (km²) |
|---|---|---|---|---|---|---|
| Bahrain | 1.05 | 3.1 | 6 | 3.8 | 74.9 | 736 |
| UAE | 4.106 | 1.5 | 3 | 2.6 | 75.9 | 83,600 |
| Qatar | 1.305 | 1.7 | 2.4 | 4.1 | 75.2 | 11,580 |
| Kuwait | 3.328 | 1.7 | 1 | 2.2 | 77.5 | 17,818 |
| Oman | 2.577 | 2.5 | - | 2.5 | 73.9 | 309,500 |
| Saudi Arabia | 24.242 | 3.9 | - | 3.4 | 74.1 | 2,000,000 |

Source: Data from WHO Data, 2006/2007; CIA. *The World Factbook*, 2009.

A striking characteristic of all GCC countries is the diversity of their populations. Different ethnic groups and nationalities can be found in all the nations. This ranges from over 80% of the population in the UAE being immigrants, to 65% in Kuwait, 70% in Qatar, 27% in Saudi Arabia, and 20% in Oman (Kapiszewski, 2006). Next to the native Arabian people, one will find largely Asian immigrants (such as Pakistanis, Indians, Filipinos, and Iranians), but also other Arabs from the Levant or North Africa. In addition, a considerable number of Western expatriates live and work in the GCC countries. The most common religion is Islam with the two major denominations, Sunni and Shi'a, making up on average 80–90% of the population. Prevalence of other religions, such as Hinduism and Christianity, is relatively low (10–20%). Arabic is the official language, while English is the second most important language in the GCC. Additional languages, such as Kurdish, Farsi, Hindi, and Urdu, are also spoken.

Education has been a major focus of development in recent years. Technical and vocational education in the Arab world has traditionally had little prestige and has attracted few resources. More recently, policies have emphasized the importance of specialized and professional knowledge. One can find high illiteracy rates in the GCC countries; in Bahrain, it is 13.5%; in the UAE, 22.1%; in Qatar, 11%; in Kuwait, 6.7%; in Oman, 18.6%; and in Saudi Arabia, 21.2% (UNDP, 2009). The lack of skilled workers still remains a challenge for the GCC countries, in particular within the national population.

The GCC governments have recognized the strong dependence on oil and have started to invest in nonoil sectors, such as finance, information technology, and tourism in order to contribute to the gross national product (GNP). Ways to develop more independence from oil differ across the GCC states. The UAE, especially Dubai, which does not have the same massive oil reserves as its neighbor Abu Dhabi, has managed to develop new economic sectors quite quickly and successfully (e.g., real estate, tourism, health care), even if it has been hit hard by the recent economic crisis. Other states have followed the diversification strategy and are looking to find their niche (e.g., education in Qatar and financial services in Bahrain).

This trend is leading to greater urbanization and more industrial working opportunities for the people. Historically, nomads and indigenous Arabs have not coped well with the new Western lifestyle. A genetic predisposition, as well as a reduced physiological ability to cope with a sedentary lifestyle and the digestion of processed foods—not unlike the Native Americans—has likely contributed to the alarming chronic disease rates. The common diet has changed from predominantly fresh fish to processed fast foods (served by both international and local outlets). In addition, physical activity has declined significantly due to increased automobile use and an infrastructure that is not conducive to activity. This lethal combination has led to growing rates of overweight and high diabetes. The suffering and associated costs are significant, and most GCC states have reacted to this by heavily investing in health care and curative medicine. The most notable example is Dubai's Health Care City, where state of the art medical care is available. Unfortunately, health promotion and prevention strategies and programs remain the exception. It seems that only the media has caught on to the importance of healthy lifestyles and the value of preventive measures. Some national governments have only recently recognized that without health promotion strategies, the chronic disease crisis cannot be turned around. For example, Qatar has established a health promotion board as an integral part of the Ministry of Health, and Bahrain has recently announced a national health promotion strategy.

## Prevailing Health Issues and Risk Behaviors

Health challenges differ across all GCC states, but heart disease remains the leading cause of death for all of them. Noncommunicable diseases dominate the mortality statistics. Communicable diseases have nearly disappeared in the rankings; only Oman and Saudi Arabia still have diarrheal diseases in position 10. Respiratory infections are the only remaining communicable diseases that are prevalent across the GCC region (World Health Organization, 2009). Noteworthy is the high ranking of accidents, mostly road traffic fatalities (see Table 10-3).

Table 10-3 **Mortality Scale—Top 10 Ranking**

| Diseases | Bahrain | UAE | Qatar | Kuwait | Oman | Saudi Arabia |
|---|---|---|---|---|---|---|
| **Heart** | 1 | 1 | 1 | 1 | 1 | 1 |
| **Cerebrovascular** | 5 | 3 | 5 | 7 | 4 | 7 |
| **Diabetes** | 3 | 7 | 3 | 6 | 3 | 6 |
| **Nephritis/ nephrosis** | 8 | 6 | 6 | 9 | 9 | 9 |
| **Lung diseases** | 7 TBLC | 5 RI | 9 TB | 8 RI | 5 RI | 4 RI |
| **Diarrheal diseases** | - | - | - | - | 10 | 10 |
| **Perinatal conditions** | - | - | 7 | 5 | 8 | 8 |
| **Accidents** | 4 | 2 | 2 | 3 | 6 | 5 |

(TBLC = Trachea, bronchus, lung cancer; RI = respiratory infection, TB = tuberculosis)

Source: Data from WHO Data, 2006/2007; CIA. *The World Factbook*, 2009.

It is important to note that disease trends and health status often differ considerably between nationals and foreigners (mostly from Asia) who are often employed as manual laborers in challenging conditions. Workers' rights, unsanitary living conditions, harsh working conditions (e.g., excessive heat) and poor safety practices have been the subject of media attention. Some countries have begun addressing these conditions; for example, the UAE banned work between the hours of 12:30 p.m. and 3:00 p.m. from July 1 through August 31 (see more under "Drivers of Workplace Health Promotion").

Cardiovascular and cerebrovascular diseases, as well as diabetes and nephritis, are on the rise. A study by the International Diabetes Federation in 2007 found that 5 out of 6 GCC states were on the list of the top 10 countries worldwide listed by prevalence of diabetes (Healthplus, 2009). The UAE alone has a prevalence of diabetes of 19.5%. The WHO expects the diabetes prevalence to be doubled by 2030 in the UAE, from its baseline in 2000, or even tripled in Kuwait and Oman. While women are less likely to smoke, smoking prevalence is especially high among Arab men, with a rate between 26% and 42% (World Health Organization, 2006). Because smoking has a long tradition in Arab countries, antismoking campaigns are facing some significant cultural barriers. The practice of smoking water pipes (*shisha*) or other forms of tobacco is widespread among Arabs and is often a part of daily social life. As in many countries, obesity is becoming a huge problem and is significantly contributing to the increase of chronic diseases. Arab women are on average more obese than men (see Table 10-4).

Table 10-4 **Overweight/Obesity and Smoking Prevalence (Female/Male)**

| Diseases | Bahrain | UAE | Qatar | Kuwait | Oman | Saudi Arabia |
|---|---|---|---|---|---|---|
| BMI >25 (%) | 67.4/61.0 | 69.7/66.9 | 64.1/57.9 | 79.0/69.5 | 47.8/43.4 | 63.8/63.1 |
| BMI >30 (%) | 35.2/21.2 | 39.4/24.5 | 29.3/17.4 | 52.9/29.6 | 14.8/7.7 | 33.8/23.0 |
| Smoking prevalence | 2.9/26.1 | 2.6/26.1 | 6.0/42.0 | 1.9/34.4 | 1.3/24.7 | 3.6/25.6 |

Source: Data from WHO, 2006.

The food consumption pattern has dramatically changed in some Arab countries as a result of the sudden increase in income from oil revenue. Research from Musaiger showed an increase in the calorie intake from 1971 to 1997 in the countries of the region, and a high percentage of these calories came from animal foods (Musaiger, 2002). Over the same period, the per capital daily fat intake increased, ranging from 13.6% in Sudan to 143% in Saudi Arabia (Musaiger, 2002). Musaiger and others from the Gulf States believe that government policies introduced in the 1960s and 1970s, such as the food subsidy policy, have adversely affected the food habits in the Gulf States by encouraging the intake of fat, sugar, rice, wheat flour, and meat. Other policies that targeted the urbanization of nomadic populations and the migration movement, particularly those carried out during the 1970s, had a great impact on the food practices in many Arab countries. Educating these populations about health was a much slower process than the successful urbanization efforts. Thus, serious yet preventable diseases such as iron deficiency anemias can still be found in the Arab world and GCC countries (Al-Assaf, 2007; Al-Quaiz, 2001). Mass media, especially televised food advertisements, also play an important role in modifying dietary habits.

About 81% of Saudi men age 19 or older are reported to be either completely inactive or only irregularly active. Physical activity is low for these individuals, mainly due to time constraints as a result of married life, working more than one shift, and/or having little time off from work during the week. In addition, physical inactivity is reported to be lower among individuals with less education or those working in the private sector. The 19% of Saudi men who are active on a regular basis report maintaining health and losing weight as the main drivers for engaging in physical activity (Rafaee, 2001).

Another crucial challenge to GCC governments is the high number of road traffic injuries (often resulting in death), especially among the young population. Accidents are among the top five death causes in most GCC states. According to figures compiled by the World Health Organization, the Arab world has only 2% of the world's motor vehicles, but records 6% of all traffic fatalities. The Eastern Mediterranean region has the highest rate of road traffic death among males (World Health Organization, 2004).

# Healthcare Systems

Healthcare expenditures in the GCC remain low by international standards; however, healthcare systems in the Arab world have undergone rapid changes. The progress is driven by a sharp increase in demand for health care due to changing attitudes toward lifestyle diseases and to increased life expectancies.

Although GCC countries have a much lower percentage of older people than Europe or North America, challenges have surfaced. On the one hand, the health system is not prepared for an increasing aging population; on the other hand, the growing population is overflowing the GCC states with young people and the economic market is not able to provide enough jobs. The high unemployment rates have negative effects on the economy as well as on the health system. This provides an additional hurdle for the field of health promotion, as the unemployed are typically unhealthier than their employed counterparts and harder to reach.

Access to health care in Saudi Arabia, Oman, and the UAE still does not reach 100% of the population. Especially in rural areas, the healthcare infrastructure is insufficient. An Arabian study reported that the Gulf region needs an extra 138,965 hospital beds, 140,334 physicians, and 227,079 nurses by 2050 to maintain current levels of care (Emirates Business 24/7, 2009). Major efforts, often by reputable international academic institutions such as Healthcare City in Dubai, are underway to train nationals in medicine, medical technology, and healthcare administration. However, this process takes time, and not enough young people are choosing this career path.

The governments are the main healthcare providers, shouldering three quarters of the total expenditure (NCB Capital, 2009). In principle, health care is free to everyone in the GCC states. The ministries cover up to 85% of total health expenditures; however, they struggle to provide standardized quality health services and to finance increasing costs. There is a gap between health care for the wealthy and health care for the economically disadvantaged, which often translates into nationals and migrant workers, respectively. Public health services are often overstretched and ill equipped to deal with chronic disease, leading many residents to turn to the private sector. A study found that more than 70% of UAE residents would seek medical treatment overseas if they fell seriously ill. Even Emiratis showed little faith in their healthcare system, with 57% saying they would seek treatment abroad (The National, 2009). The Ministry of Health of the UAE has traditionally paid for nationals to be treated abroad, including travel costs for the patient and accompanying individuals.

The gap regarding the quality of health care will grow, as currently all states are trying to support the private healthcare sector with incentives and new regulations. The UAE and Saudi Arabia have already implemented mandatory insurance systems for expatriates. Bahrain is in the process of introducing an insurance system, and Qatar and Oman are in the planning phase. All systems are conceptualized in such a way that they will cover nationals in the long term as well, which will most likely lead to a boom in the private health sector in the GCC states. The healthcare market in the GCC is expected to grow at about 9% annually, to reach between $47 billion and $55 billion by 2020 (Emirates Business 24/7, 2009).

To reach the goal of structured and coordinated health care, the GCC countries have to invest more money in public health, develop national strategies of health promotion, and start addressing the determinants of health. Bahrain is the only country so far that has developed a national strategy for health promotion. Oman has had some success through community health projects, such as the Nizwa Healthy Lifestyle Project (NHLP, 2007), but still invests insufficient money to achieve broad success. As documented in Table 10-5, health expenditures in GCC states are considerably lower than those in most industrialized countries.

Table 10-5 **Health Expenditures—GCC States**

| Country | % GDP for health | % of total gov. expenditures | % of health care gov. funded | % out of pocket |
|---|---|---|---|---|
| Bahrain | 3.8 | 10 | 66.5 | 69.2 |
| UAE | 2.6 | 8.6 | 71.6 | 77.9 |
| Qatar | 4.1 | 9.7 | 78.0 | 87.8 |
| Kuwait | 2.2 | 6.2 | 77.2 | 91.6 |
| Oman | 2.5 | 6.1 | 85.0 | 66.4 |
| Saudi Arabia | 3.4 | 8.7 | 76.2 | 16.5 |

Source: Data from WHO, 2005.

The GCC states had only slight increases in their health budget for the last few years, whereas the GDP has been rapidly growing. Therefore, the percentage of GDP invested in health is decreasing. The amount of investments in health is crucial, but so is how that money is spent. The focus should not be exclusively on providing curative care, as in the numerous new high-tech medical facilities, but also on promoting public health and offering prevention services to fight noncommunicable diseases. In addition, the social determinants of health, such as gender and social status, need to be tackled head-on, as recommended by the World Health Organization (WHO, 2008).

## Influence of Culture and Mentality

In the GCC, the majority of the population is of Muslim faith. In Islam, prevention of diseases is taught through a system of self-control, moderate eating habits, and activity (Qadri, 2006). Islamic foundations of health promotion can be found in the Quran and the Sunnah (authenticated scriptures provided by companions of Muhammed, the last Prophet of Islam). A paper by de Leeuw and Hussein (1999) analyzes to what extent the Ottawa Charter for Health Promotion is compatible with Islamic principles. For example, *Shuuura,* a process of mutual consultation between people and their leaders on the structure and development of society, including health care, can be linked to the Ottawa Charter principle reorienting health services. *Waqfs* represents the Islamic system of endowments toward social and health services and have played a key role in the establishment of libraries, hospitals, schools, and mosques. The Quran and Sunnah emphasize individual and community rituals, such as hygiene and the role of mosques as community units, which relate to the strengthening of community action and the personal skills highlighted in the Ottawa Charter (see Figure 10-1).

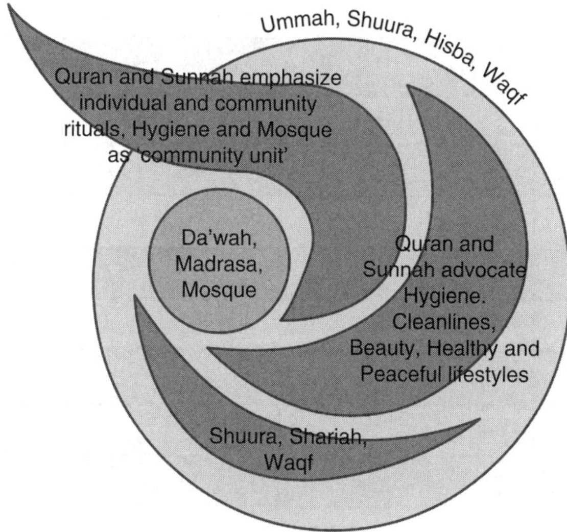


Figure 10-1 The Ottawa Charter.

Source: de Leeuw & Hussein (1999)

In particular, social organization, community life, and a sense of belonging—often lacking in modern Western societies—can be significant factors contributing to health enhancement.

The Quran has many verses that encourage primary and secondary prevention, such as, "O Children of Adam! Wear your beautiful apparel at every time and place of prayer: Eat and Drink: But waste not by excess, for Allah loveth not the wasters" (Jannah.org, 2009). One Hadith, a saying attributed to the Prophet Muhammed, says to keep a third of the stomach for food, another third for liquids, and the last third empty. The request for physical labor and activity is also mentioned. In one Hadith, Prophet Muhammed advises his followers to "teach your children swimming, archery and horse riding" (Jannah.org, 2009). The World Health Organization Regional Office for the Eastern Mediterranean developed a specific strategy for health promotion in Islam by issuing the Amman Declaration on Health Promotion (1989). The declaration states, "Islamic lifestyles embrace numerous positive patterns promoting health and rejecting any behavior which is contradictory to health."

Sociocultural factors such as gender discrimination, education, and women's employment have all impacted food consumption and obesity patterns in this region. Studies of gender inequality in some Arab countries can point to some preventable sources of ill health, such as inactivity among women, which leads to obesity. In many Islamic societies there is a division of gender roles. Traditionally, men are expected to work and earn money to feed their families, while women are expected to care for the children and the family's house. These defined roles have an impact on the physical activity level of women, as they spend a lot of time at home. The woman's role and position in society has changed in many countries, and literacy rates and education of women have also improved significantly. Employment numbers for women are gradually increasing but remain low compared to those of other developed countries (see Table 10-6).

Table 10-6 **Labor Force, Female**

| Country | 2000 | 2004 | 2007 |
|---|---|---|---|
| Bahrain | 35.5 | 35.3 | 25.2 |
| UAE | 35.4 | 39.5 | 40.8 |
| Qatar | 35.9 | 41.0 | 42.3 |
| Kuwait | 43.8 | 43.9 | 44.3 |
| Oman | 24.6 | 25.7 | 27.1 |
| Saudi Arabia | 17.4 | 19 | 20.0 |
| United States | - | - | 46 |

Source: World Bank, GenderStats, 2007; U.S. Department of Labor, 2007.

Family and privacy are highly valued in the Arab culture. Personal issues are rarely mentioned outside the family and physical activity in public places just recently began to become a normal sight. Today one can see numerous women (and men) briskly walking on the corniches of Bahrain and Kuwait, or along the creek in Dubai in the evening hours. Leisure-time offerings are limited in most Gulf countries, and people tend to spend most of their free time eating and shopping in malls. The hot weather restricts activities to the indoors for a large part of the year. The infrastructure also does not support physical activity (due to factors such as lack of sidewalks), as it is exclusively designed for automobile use. In addition, the comprehensive food offerings in the malls entice people to consume more calories than they expend. One might say that the odds are stacked against achieving a balance between calorie intake and expenditure, and with that, against living a healthy lifestyle.

The great hospitality of Arab people is famous and an important part of their lifestyle. Visitors to the Gulf region experience this part of Arab culture quickly. Unfortunately, a lot of the socializing is linked with eating and sitting, and to a degree smoking (especially *shisha*). People tend to eat more when dining with friends over a prolonged period of time.

The GCC boasts the largest expatriate working population in the world (as a percentage of overall population). The work environment in these countries is not different from that in most other countries, except for a few Islamic norms that must be followed in most of these countries. Most GCC nationals in responsible positions are foreign educated and are extremely friendly and professional in their work-related dealings. This attitude also stems from the warm culture that exists within the region and its similarity to the Turkish community with regard to hospitality.

Since the mid-1950s, the GCC governments have shown their appreciation of the importance of family and of social support for the expatriate workforce by making resident and visit visas easily obtainable. Many workers live in communities of their own nationality and are able to find stores and restaurants that sell their national products, whether from China, the Philippines, Pakistan, India, or continental Europe.

Large employers and their contractors often translate safety signs, posters, and literature into the languages of their workforce, including Urdu, Hindi, Tagalog, and Tamil. Some employers, such as Saudi Aramco, provide free Arabic language lessons for the European and North American workforce and their families.

Employers continue to struggle to find qualified and experienced nationals to fill positions in a growing economy. Most Gulf countries have embarked on national strategies, such as the UAE's "Emiratisation," to increase the percentage of nationals in the workforce and reduce dependence on foreigners.

## Drivers of Workplace Health Promotion

Since early 2000, there have been many positive changes in all of the GCC countries, especially Saudi Arabia, Bahrain, and the UAE, where rights for all workers (national or foreign) have become guaranteed through the development of workers committees to guard their interests and represent their issues and concerns to the employers or even to external judiciary bodies. The steps taken by the GCC countries to combat a small number of employers who may have exploited their workforce through delayed payments of salaries, uninsured health care, substandard living quarters, prolonged working hours, and lack of safety measures in the workplace were hailed by groups including the International Labour Organization as responsible steps in the right direction. Such actions were not new for the large regional corporations in these countries. But the GCC governments have recognized that workers in small and medium-sized companies with fewer than 100 employees often do not receive sufficient levels of specialized occupational health care, as there are no procedures for monitoring staff injuries and sickness. Large companies usually have effective occupational health policies in place to monitor the health and safety of their workers and sometimes even an in-house doctor. However, in some small and medium-sized businesses in the region, no such provisions exist. Workers who become sick or injured contribute significantly, in terms of lost productivity, compensation payments, and even higher insurance premiums, to the inevitable costs to companies that do not have such systems in place. Industries that employ a relatively low number of workers are being urged to develop strategies to tackle occupational health issues in accordance with guidelines from regional health and labor ministries, international trade and labor organizations, and the World Bank. Sickness and injury at work is estimated to cost businesses in the region millions of dollars every year due to absenteeism alone. While the cost of developing processes for monitoring and treatment may deter companies from addressing the occupational health needs of its workforce, the long-term financial benefits of preventing, treating, and managing work-related injuries and sickness outweigh the initial outlay.

As major employers are only gradually addressing chronic disease and the individual health risks of their employees, some governments, such as Qatar and Bahrain, are developing strategies and creating infrastructures to tackle this new challenge. Although the workplace has not been explicitly targeted as a setting in these initiatives, a spillover effect is anticipated.

## Programs and Good Practices

In the past few years, recognition in the Middle East of the value of preventive medicine has increased as a result of the efforts that healthcare providers and ministries of health in the region have made to treat advanced stages of chronic diseases and their complications. Healthcare providers are making great efforts to intervene during the initial stages of a disease, if possible, by preventing disease complications from developing.

Although health promotion and preventive medicine in the GCC states are still in a development phase, some enterprises have implemented workplace health promotion programs. These enterprises are pioneers in the region and should be recognized as role models for health promotion in companies in the GCC states. They all have in common the understanding that workplace health promotion is not just about occupational health and safety at work. They have assumed the responsibility for promoting healthy lifestyles and supporting their employees in becoming healthier individuals.

### Case Study: Saudi Aramco

The advantages of supporting prevention and incorporating it into medical practice are well recognized at Saudi Aramco, which has played a significant role in promoting the development and maintenance of the infrastructure of their vast areas of operations within the Kingdom of Saudi Arabia. As early as the mid-1930s, in the Arabian Peninsula, due consideration was paid in oil exploration to the essential needs of employees' and their dependents' health care. In the early 1940s and 1950s, Saudi Aramco began to look after its employees and their extended families through developing world-class community healthcare centers in Dhahran,

Ras Tanura, Abqaiq, and Al-Hassa. The company also invested in the infrastructure of these communities, developing highways and schools, and providing home loans (with restrictions based on peer-reviewed architectural engineering) to develop modern, healthy, and culturally sensitive communities. Saudi Aramco recognized the true value of citizenship and resolved to exert influence by leading by example. The company developed training programs to educate its contractors on safety, health, and the environment. These programs and adherence to their instructions were essential for Saudi Aramco in disseminating best practices and the universality of workers' rights. Teams from preventive medicine, environmental protection, and loss prevention conducted periodic, regular, and unannounced inspections of the contractors' labor camps, including the living quarters, the dining facilities, the quality of food, and the contractor clinics. The working environments were also monitored and the appropriateness of personal protective equipment were tested. These inspections and adherence to Saudi Aramco's standards form the basis for determining contract renewals.

Saudi Aramco developed close ties with the Saudi government in order to establish a preventive medicine program in the Eastern Province, which aimed to reduce the incidence of communicable diseases. Since then, Saudi Aramco has worked incessantly with the government to control the incidence and prevalence of communicable diseases in the Eastern and Central Provinces, in efforts including the Malaria Control Program, which led to complete eradication of malaria during the early 1960s in the Eastern Province.

The company provides health support through different sectors: Saudi Aramco Healthcare provides medical treatment in its own facilities, and the Preventive Medicine Services Division integrates the occupational medicine section. Aramco has an established surveillance system and conducts different health, safety, and environmental awareness programs in order to maintain health and encourage employees' healthy lifestyles, including individual counseling. Traditional occupational health and security programs, such as basic life support and first aid training, are also provided to employees. In recent times, there has been a serious shift of focus from communicable diseases and vaccination to early detection of diseases associated with chronic morbidity and mortality, such as diabetes mellitus, hypertension, and ischemic heart disease. Although immunization and screening tests remain an imperative, the most promising role for prevention in current medicine in Saudi Arabia is recognized in changing personal health behaviors. In 2004, Saudi Aramco conducted a landmark study on its firefighters (see "Existing Research") that led to comprehensive health and fitness programs for the firefighters, including small fitness centers at most Aramco fire stations throughout Saudi Arabia (Razavi, n.d.).

## Other Employers Leading in Health Promotion

The Emirates National Oil Company, a regional oil and gas group located in Dubai, UAE, has implemented a number of programs for the improvement of the health of its employees and has supported the Women's Initiative for Rheumatoid Arthritis, an awareness campaign on rheumatoid arthritis, and driver's education for female employees, to reduce accident rates. The Emirates National Oil Company also recently opened an in-house clinic in Dubai that offers staff members occupational health services, including health evaluations and awareness campaigns. The strategic health safety initiative is led by the Emirates National Oil Company's Environmental Health, Safety and Quality department (M. Newson-Smith, personal communication, June 15, 2009).

The Gulf Petrochemical Industries Company has been a long-standing leader in safety, health, and environment in the GCC Region. The Gulf Petrochemical Industries Company, located in Manama, Bahrain, is a producer of methanol, ammonia, and granulated urea. The Gulf Petrochemical Industries Company has achieved high international standards and has earned several awards in the area of traditional safety. The safety program was extended to behavior-based safety in 2008. In addition to regular worksite assessments and the qualification of first aiders, the company instituted an auditor system for safety issues in order to reach a broader range of employees. The program has since expanded to address pressing health issues, such as heat stress management (M. Latif, personal communication, June 15, 2009).

Dolphin Energy is a gas producer with branches in the United Arab Emirates and Qatar. The Quality, Health, Safety and Environment management system was implemented from the outset as a business objective. This included a health strategy with sectors on wellness and the prevention of occupational illness. Under these sectors, awareness campaigns promote healthy lifestyles and environments for the staff and their families. The system also offers seminars and workshops on different health-related topics, such as first aid instruction and information on health risks and diseases. Regular health assessments and an annual heat stress management program are conducted. Dolphin Energy's key to success is the commitment of senior management (H. Madhi, personal communication, June 15, 2009).

## Outcomes

Overall, a lack of evaluation and outcome data persists in the GCC. The larger, advanced employers (as previously mentioned) track absence rates, disability types and rates, vaccination rates, hospital admissions, days lost to injuries at work, and mortality cases. Health risk and productivity data are typically not tracked. This might be due to the fact that a countrywide minimum standard regarding working conditions and workplace safety has not yet been achieved. Many companies are still struggling to provide basic safety equipment or good working conditions and therefore have high rates of injury and sickness. For example, a study from Kuwait found that the number of violations against Kuwait labor law represented 17.7% of all private sector businesses (Arabianbusiness.com, 2008). The inspections found that nearly 84% of firms (3,170) had failed to provide the proper protections to prevent workplace accidents, and 32 companies did not provide basic workplace protection gear, including safety helmets. More than 155 employers did not provide suitable accommodations for their staff.

## Existing Research

In 2004, the Preventive Medicine Services Division of Saudi Aramco was tasked by the Saudi Aramco management with studying the issue of Saudi Aramco firefighters' fitness for work (Razavi & Kirsten, n.d.). The Preventive Medicine Services Division conducted a cross-sectional descriptive study of 275 firefighters who were tested for physical demand variables related to job-related fitness and general physical fitness. In job-related fitness, the capacity to perform operational firefighting without impacting the health and safety of the individual was identified as the most important variable. In general, physical fitness, aerobic capacity, muscular strength, and flexibility were identified as important variables. It was found that 89% of Saudi Aramco's firefighters were not fit enough to perform active firefighter duties, a statistic that included the younger firefighters (age groups 20–30 and 30–40). Therefore, emergency preparedness was not guaranteed and a major emergency could have dire consequences. These alarming findings led Saudi Aramco to launch a systematic fitness program embedded in a comprehensive health promotion approach. Soon after the results of the study were accepted by Saudi Aramco management, its fire protection department hired a dedicated physical fitness coordinator to oversee a physical fitness program for the Saudi Aramco firefighters. The program was rolled out and implemented throughout Saudi Aramco, and every fire station was provided with physical fitness equipment. Physical fitness became both an integral part of the performance appraisal program for all firefighters and an essential part of their job requirements. While 11% of firefighters met the standard during the SAFF 2005 study, now 45% have met the standard (Razavi & Kirsten, n.d.). Saudi Aramco has also introduced an annual firefighter fitness competition that brings teams from each division to compete against each other for a trophy.

Additional research studies on lifestyle issues have been referenced in the section entitled "Prevailing Health Issues and Risk Behaviors" (Musaiger, 2002; Al-Assaf, 2007; Al-Quaiz, 2001).

## Conclusion

The GCC countries are faced with tremendous challenges given the dire chronic disease trends, the lack of qualified professionals, and the multicultural workforce. However, the region has significant resources with which to deal with these challenges. Most GCC countries have amassed considerable wealth from the oil and gas boom and are gradually transitioning into more diversified economies.

Unfortunately, raising health awareness among people is proceeding much more slowly than are the successful urbanization efforts, which play a big role in promoting unhealthy lifestyles. It is time to move to more calculated growth, such as in the planning of cities, that takes environmental and health issues into serious consideration, and to address chronic disease suffering from a health promotion perspective. As investments in health care continue to rise and state-of-the-art facilities are built in the region, more focus needs to be directed to preventive and behavior-based approaches. Little expertise exists in the fields of public health and behavior change. Transforming this situation requires a shift in thinking, or a paradigm shift, from a purely biomedical model to a health promotion model. The workplace can serve as a favorable setting and employers can act as drivers, as some of the larger ones already are. While some companies are moving from focusing exclusively on how work affects the health of workers to how health affects work, there is still very little evidence on how workplace health promotion can make a difference in the GCC countries. This hinders the spreading of such programs. Therefore, baseline assessments and evaluations of health promotion programs are essential. It is envisioned that the national governments will play a key role in advancing health promotion in the future with strategies, policies, incentives, infrastructure, and overall guidance. Ideally, the GCC countries will continue to strengthen their cooperation and to learn from each other not only how to grow their economies, but also how to improve the health of their citizens.

## Summary

The Gulf Cooperation Council (GCC) includes the countries of Bahrain, Qatar, Kuwait, Oman, the United Arab Emirates, and Saudi Arabia. The GCC countries have undergone tremendous growth since 2000, in large part due to a thriving oil and gas business. This economic development has led to rapid urbanization and major lifestyle changes. While this has resulted in significant improvements in health care in all GCC countries, the resulting effects on population health have been negative, in the form of rising chronic diseases such as diabetes and heart disease, unhealthier diets, increased food consumption, and reduced physical activity. Investment in prevention and health promotion is minimal. The GCC's governments are gradually coming to terms with the challenge of chronic disease and the need to move beyond investing in health care and medical facilities.

Workplace health promotion is a very young field in the GCC. Only a small number of large employers have set up comprehensive occupational health and safety infrastructures such as the implementation of health awareness campaigns, individualized screenings, and health enhancement programs. Programs have not been evaluated, and evidence of the effectiveness of workplace health promotion in the GCC is lacking. The main drivers for implementing programs are first and foremost corporate social responsibility and corporate image, then absenteeism and worker productivity. Major challenges lie in the heterogeneity of the employee population, with the bulk of workers coming from abroad, mainly Asia, and in the region's lack of qualified health professionals.

## Review Questions

1. What is the corporate health promotion significance of membership in the Gulf Cooperation Council (GCC)?
2. What factors have led to growing rates of overweight and diabetes in the GCC?
3. Who is the main provider of health care in the GCC? How is it funded? How is quality control managed across states?
4. Explain the compatibility of health promotion efforts and the Muslim faith. Are there problems with incompatibility? Why or why not?
5. Is there a system in place for occupational health policies among GCC corporations? Explain your answer.
6. How are some corporations in the GCC promoting healthy lifestyles and/or supporting their employees in becoming healthier individuals?
7. Why is data tracking especially critical among GCC corporations?
8. Describe the future challenges to GCC corporations that want to implement workplace health promotion initiatives.

## References


Al-Assaf, A. (2007). Anemia and iron intake of adult Saudis in Riyadh City-Saudi Arabia. *Pakistani Journal of Nutrition, 6*(4), 255–258.

Al-Quaiz, J. (2001). Iron deficiency anemia: A study of risk factors. *Saudi Medical Journal, 6*(22), 490–496.

ArabianBusiness.com. (2008, May 26). Retrieved February 21, 2010, from Kuwait Health Initiative: http://kuwaithealth.wordpress.com/news/

Central Intelligence Agency (CIA). (2009). *The world factbook.* Retrieved February 16, 2010, from https://www.cia.gov/library/publications/the-world-factbook/

Cooperation Council for the Arab States of the Gulf. Secretariat General. (2010). *Member states.* Retrieved December 22, 2010, from http://www.gccsg.org/eng/index.php?action=GCC

de Leeuw, E., & Hussein, A. A. (1999). Islamic health promotion and interculturalization. *Health Promotion International, 14*(4).

Emirates Business 24/7. (2009, June 23). *Private sector needs to play key role in GCC healthcare system.* Retrieved September 15, 2009, from http://www.business24-7.ae/Articles/2009/6/Pages/22062009/06232009_3577792065ab4579a517bd24e88664f8.Aspx

Healthplus. (2009). *The diabetes heartland.* Berlin/Brandenburg, Germany: Health Capital.

International Labour Organization. (2002, April 18). *Boost of workers' rights in Saudi Arabia* [press release]. Geneva, Switzerland: ILO.

Jannah.org. (2009). Islam: The eternal path to peace. Retrieved November 15, 2009, from http://www.jannah.org/qurantrans/quran7. html

Kapiszewski, A. (2006). *Arab versus Asian migrant workers in the GCC countries.* Beirut, Lebanon: United Nations Secretariat.

Musaiger, A. (2002). Diet and prevention of coronary heart disease in the Arab Middle East countries. *Medical Principles and Practice: International Journal of the Kuwait University Health Sciences Centre, 11*(suppl. 2), 9–16.

The National. (2009, August 9). Most would go abroad for medical treatment. Retrieved September 15, 2009, from http://www.thenational.ae/apps/pbcs.dll/article?AID =/20090809/NATIONAL/708089856/0/FRONTPAGE

NCB Capital. (2009). *GCC economics. Healthcare in the GCC. Toward a brighter future.* Riyadh, Saudi Arabia: NCB Capital.

Nizwa Healthy Lifestyle Project (NHLP). (2007). The anti tobacco activities for the year 2007. Retrieved January 31, 2010, from http://www.emro.who.int/tfi/wntd2008/pdf/ Oman_Nizwah_Project_Report.pdf

Qadri, M. T. (2006). Islam on prevention of heart disease. Retrieved February 16, 2010, from http://www.therevival.co.uk/wp-site/155

Rafaee, S. a.-H. (2001). Physical activity profile of adult males in Riyadh City. *Saudi Medical Journal, 9*(22), 78–79.

Razavi, J. K. (n.d.) Evaluating fitness for duty among firefighters in Saudi Arabia: The Saudi Aramco experience. Manuscript submitted for publication.

Razavi, J. K., & Kirsten, W. (n.d.) Standardization of wellness and health programs for firefighters in Saudi Arabia: Setting realistic goals and achieving world class results: The Saudi Aramco experience. Manuscript submitted for publication.

United Nations Development Programme (UNDP). (2009). *Arab human development report 2009.* New York, NY: United Nations Publications.

United States Department of Labor. (2007). *Women in the labor force in 2007.* Retrieved February 6, 2009, from http://www.dol.gov/wb/factsheets/Qf-laborforce-07.htm

World Health Organization. (2004). *Road report on road traffic injury prevention.* Geneva, Switzerland: WHO Press.

World Health Organization. (2008). Closing the gap in a generation: Health equity through action on the social determinants of health. *Final report of the Commission on Social Determinants of Health.* Geneva, Switzerland: WHO Press.

World Health Organization. (2009). *World health statistics.* Geneva, Switzerland: WHO Press.

World Health Organization Regional Office for the Eastern Mediterranean. (1989). *Health promotion through Islamic lifestyles: The Amman declaration.* Retrieved November 12, 2009, from http://www.emro.who.int/publications/HealthEdReligion/AmmanDeclaration/index.htm

Chapter 11

# India

G. L. Khanna and Vishal Marwah

After reading this chapter you should be able to:

- Identify core strategies that are the focus of workplace health promotion efforts in India
- Describe the historical evolution of India's workplace health promotion efforts
- Explain the different approaches employed by corporate health promotion throughout India
- Review the central disease states and health issues driving workplace health promotion in India
- Name the components of, and the associated funding sources for, the Indian healthcare system
- Discuss the impact of culture on the health status and health promotion efforts within India

Table 11-1 **Select Key Demographic and Economic Indicators**

| | |
|---|---|
| Nationality | Noun: Indian(s)<br>Adjective: Indian |
| Ethnic groups | Indo-Aryan 72%, Dravidian 25%, Mongoloid and other 3% (2000) |
| Religion | Hindu 80.5%, Muslim 13.4%, Christian 2.3%, Sikh 1.9%, other 1.8%, unspecified 0.1% (2001 census) |
| Language | Hindi 41%, Bengali 8.1%, Telugu 7.2%, Marathi 7%, Tamil 5.9%, Urdu 5%, Gujarati 4.5%, Kannada 3.7%, Malayalam 3.2%, Oriya 3.2%, Punjabi 2.8%, Assamese 1.3%, Maithili 1.2%, other 5.9%<br>Note: English enjoys associate status but is the most important language for national, political, and commercial communication; Hindi is the most widely spoken language and primary tongue of 41% of the people; there are 14 other official languages: Bengali, Telugu, Marathi, Tamil, Urdu, Gujarati, Malayalam, Kannada, Oriya, Punjabi, Assamese, Kashmiri, Sindhi, and Sanskrit; Hindustani is a popular variant of Hindi/Urdu spoken widely throughout northern India but is not an official language (2001 census) |

*continued*

| Table 11-1 Select Key Demographic and Economic Indicators, *continued* | |
|---|---|
| Literacy | definition: age 15 and over can read and write<br>total population: 61%<br>male: 73.4%<br>female: 47.8% (2001 census) |
| Education expenditure | 3.2% of GDP (2005)<br>Country comparison to the world: 140 |
| Government type | Federal republic |
| Environment | Deforestation; soil erosion; overgrazing; desertification; air pollution from industrial effluents and vehicle emissions; water pollution from raw sewage and runoff of agricultural pesticides; tap water is not potable throughout the country; huge and growing population is overstraining natural resources |
| Country mass | Total: 3,287,263 sq km<br>Country comparison to the world: 7<br>Land: 2,973,193 sq km<br>Water: 314,070 sq km |
| Population | 1,156,897,766 (July 2010 est.)<br>country comparison to the world: 2 |
| Age structure | 0–14 years: 30.5% (male 187,197,389/female 165,285,592)<br>15–64 years: 64.3% (male 384,131,994/female 359,795,835)<br>65 years and over: 5.2% (male 28,816,115/female 31,670,841) (2010 est.) |
| Median age | Total: 25.9 years<br>Male: 25.4 years<br>Female: 26.6 years (2010 est.) |
| Population growth rate | 1.407% (2010 est.)<br>Country comparison to the world: 93 |
| Birth rate | 21.72 births/1,000 population (2010 est.)<br>Country comparison to the world: 90 |
| Death rate | 7.6 deaths/1,000 population (July 2010 est.)<br>Country comparison to the world: 115 |
| Net migration rate | -0.05 migrant(s)/1,000 population (2010 est.)<br>Country comparison to the world: 85 |
| Urbanization | Urban population: 29% of total population (2008)<br>Rate of urbanization: 2.4% annual rate of change (2005–2010 est.) |
| Gender ratio | At birth: 1.12 male(s)/female<br>Under 15 years: 1.1 male(s)/female<br>15–64 years: 1.07 male(s)/female<br>65 years and over: 0.91 male(s)/female<br>Total population: 1.08 male(s)/female (2010 est.) |

*continued*

| Table 11-1 **Select Key Demographic and Economic Indicators,** *continued* | |
|---|---|
| Infant mortality rate | Total: 50.78 deaths/1,000 live births<br>Country comparison to the world: 51<br>Male: 49.33 deaths/1,000 live births<br>Female: 52.4 deaths/1,000 live births (2010 est.) |
| Life expectancy | Total population: 66.09 years<br>Country comparison to the world: 161<br>Male: 65.13 years<br>Female: 67.17 years (2010 est.) |
| Total fertility rate | 2.65 children born/woman (2010 est.)<br>Country comparison to the world: 86 |
| GDP—purchasing power parity | $3.57 trillion (2009 est.)<br>Country comparison to the world: 5 |
| GDP—per capita | $3,100 (2009 est.)<br>Country comparison to the world: 163 |
| GDP—composition by sector | Agriculture: 17.5%<br>Industry: 28.2%<br>Services: 54.9% (2009 est.) |
| Agriculture—products | Rice, wheat, oilseed, cotton, jute, tea, sugarcane, lentils, potatoes, onions, dairy products, sheep, goats, poultry, fish |
| Industries | Textiles, chemicals, food processing, steel, transportation equipment, cement, mining, petroleum, machinery, software, pharmaceuticals |
| Labor force participation | 467 million (2009 est.)<br>Country comparison to the world: 2 |
| Unemployment rate | 10.7% (2009 est.) country comparison to the world: 120 |
| Industrial production growth rate | 8.2% (2009 est.)<br>Country comparison to the world: 9 |
| Distribution of family income (GINI index) | 36.8 (2004)<br>Country comparison to the world: 79 |
| Investment (gross fixed) | 32.3% of GDP (2009 est.)<br>Country comparison to the world: 17 |
| Public debt | 58% of GDP (2009 est.)<br>Country comparison to the world: 34 |
| Market value of publicly traded shares | $1.227 trillion (December 31, 2009)<br>Country comparison to the world: 14 |
| Current account balance | $-31.54 billion (2009 est.)<br>Country comparison to the world: 183 |

*continued*

| Table 11-1 **Select Key Demographic and Economic Indicators,** *continued* | |
|---|---|
| Debt (external) | $223.9 billion (December 31, 2009 est.)<br>Country comparison to the world: 25 |
| Debt as a % of GDP | ——— |
| Exports | $164.3 billion (2009 est.)<br>Country comparison to the world: 22 |
| Exports—commodities | Petroleum products, textile goods, gems and jewelry, engineering goods, chemicals, leather manufactures |
| Exports—partners | United Arab Emirates 12.87%, United States 12.59%, China 5.59%, (2009) |
| Imports | $268.4 billion (2009 est.)<br>Country comparison to the world: 14 |
| Imports—commodities | Crude oil, machinery, gems, fertilizer, chemicals |
| Imports—partners | China 10.94%, United States 7.16%, Saudi Arabia 5.36%, United Arab Emirates 5.18%, Australia 5.02%, Germany 4.86%, Singapore 4.02% (2009) |
| Stock of direct foreign investment at | |
| Home | $157.9 billion (December 31, 2009 est.)<br>Country comparison to the world: 24 |
| Abroad | $76.62 billion (December 31, 2009 est.)<br>Country comparison to the world: 26 |

Source: CIA. (2010). *The world factbook.* Retrieved December 16, 2010, from https://www.cia.gov/library/publications/the-world-factbook/

# Introduction

India is probably the most diverse country in the world. With 22 official languages, close to 200 spoken languages, and a thousand dialects, and each region having its distinct culture, tradition, and lifestyle, India may be seen as several countries within one. Sixty-two years after gaining independence from the British Colonial rule, India stands as the largest democratic nation in the world.

With a population of over 1 billion (World Bank, 2008), India is the second most populous country in the world. With an area slightly more than one third the size of the United States, India is the seventh largest country in the world and houses 17% of the world's population. Seventy-one percent of this population lives in villages. The population gender ratio, which is heavily skewed in favor of men (926 women per 1,000 men), has been a matter of concern (CIA, 2010). Ethnically, India is diverse, with Hinduism being the predominant religion (80%). Islam accounts for about 13%, Christianity for 2.3%, and Sikhism for 1.9%.

The preamble of the Constitution of India describes it as a sovereign, socialist, secular, democratic republic. The Indian republic consists of 28 states and 7 union territories with a parliamentary form of democracy. Though for several decades, postindependence India was drawn towards socialist ideology given its strong ties with the Soviet Union, an economic crisis in the early 1990s saw liberalization and market-based reforms in the Indian economy. Despite the fact that the communist left ideology has prevailed in a couple of states, namely Kerala and West Bengal, the country as a whole has transitioned towards globalization, and since 1990, India has seen an average economic growth rate of 5.8% per annum, and almost 8.4% in 2006–2007 (World Bank, 2008). With a GDP of 1.089 trillion dollars, India is the 12th largest economy in the world (4th largest considering purchasing power parity). Despite economic strides, India is facing problems of inequitable distribution of wealth across different regions and social strata. As of 2005, 28.3% of India's population lived below the poverty line (National Health Profile, 2007). While certain states have made significant socioeconomic progress, some have lagged behind. The states of Bihar, Madhya Pradesh, Rajasthan, and Uttar Pradesh have healthcare statistics significantly poorer than the national average (National Health Profile, 2007). One of India's strengths is its growing middle class, which is expected to be two thirds of the population by 2009–2010 (National Health Profile, 2007). As a greater percentage of the population moves into this bracket, it is expected that their healthcare needs and demands are likely to increase.

## Demographics of Workforce

Almost 92% of the workforce in India lies in the informal sector. While almost the entire farming sector can be considered to be informal, 80% of the nonfarming sector also lies in the informal category (Shakthivel & Joddar, 2006). India's workforce is predominantly young. As of 2009, India's total working age population (15–64 years) was about 765 million, which was about 17% of the world's working age population. Declining fertility rates have created this demographic dividend with a low dependency ratio (ratio of dependent population to the working age population). This working class is expected to be the engine of India's economic growth. The rapid economic expansion postglobalization has created ample opportunities in the service sectors. The educational sector, however, has struggled to keep up with the increasing demand for skilled labor, and a large section of the workforce remains unemployable as a result of lack of vocational training. The widening gap between demand and supply has made skilled labor a valuable commodity. There are also concerns about the health of the workforce, and the health needs of this working class are expected to increase. Unless India invests in the health of its human capital, she risks squandering the demographic advantage by loss of capital gains through expenditures in health care.

# Prevailing Health Issues and Risk Behaviors

## Vital Statistics

The life expectancy at birth is 67 years; 66 years for males and 68 years for females (CIA, 2010). This is a significant improvement given the fact that at the time of independence in 1947, the life expectancy was just over 33 years. The maternal mortality rate is 4.5 per 10,000 live births (CIA, 2010). Malnutrition among children is another problem, and reportedly 43.5% of children under 5 years are malnourished.

## Disease Burden

With respect to disease burden, India bears characteristics of both developing and developed countries. Infectious and parasitic diseases still remain a major problem and account for 33% of all deaths. With 17% of the global population, India accounts for 20% of the total global disease burden, 23% of child deaths, 20% of maternal deaths, 30% of tuberculosis cases, 68% of leprosy cases, and 14% of HIV infections (Ministry of Health and Family Welfare, n.d.). The HIV prevalence rate is around 0.3% (CIA, 2007), and although this is much lower than in African countries, it is still a matter of concern. Deaths due to infectious diseases have progressively declined over the years. Urban sedentary lifestyle, changes in dietary habits, and stress have all contributed to an increase in prevalence of chronic diseases such as coronary heart disease, obesity, stroke, and diabetes. Almost 31 million Indians are diabetics, and the number is expected to increase to 57 million by 2025 (PricewaterhouseCoopers, 2007a). The incidence of diabetes among urban adults was 2.1% in the 1970s, and now it is up to 12.1%, the incidence being much higher in southern states as compared to northern states (PricewaterhouseCoopers, 2007a).

The estimated prevalence of coronary heart disease is around 3–4% in rural areas and 8–10% in urban areas among adults older than 20 years, representing a twofold rise in rural areas and a sixfold rise in urban areas over the past 4 decades. About 29.8 million people were estimated to have coronary heart disease in India by 2003; 14.1 million in urban areas and 15.7 million in rural areas.

## Changing Disease Spectrum—A Shift Toward Noncommunicable Diseases

Noncommunicable chronic diseases are reaching epidemic proportions worldwide and are estimated to grow at an alarming rate in the decades to come, particularly in the middle- and low-income countries. In India, Western influence and lifestyles due to rapid urbanization and globalization contribute towards the increased number of people suffering from these diseases. This shift in lifestyle is occurring in places with uncorrected poverty and increasing disparities in income, leaving the poor more vulnerable to these diseases. Underprivileged people are more likely to bear the maximum risk of these noncommunicable chronic diseases due to low income (increased consumption of high-calorie, low-priced food), lack of awareness, and poor access to health care.

## Future Trends and Economic Impact of Chronic Diseases

With increasing life expectancy, the percentage of the population older than 35 years is expected to rise from 28% in 1981 to 48% in 2021. Also, the percentage of people in urban areas, which presently is around 30%, is expected to rise to about 43% in 2021. A report from PricewaterhouseCoopers in conjunction with the World Economic Forum predicts that the percentage of deaths nationwide from long-term maladies will skyrocket from 53% in 2005 to nearly 67% by 2020 (PricewaterhouseCoopers, 2007b). The projected foregone national income for India due to heart disease, stroke, and diabetes during the period 2005–2015 is estimated to be about $237 billion (see Table 11-2). Between 2000 and 2030, India is likely to experience more deaths of people in the age group of 35–64 than the United States, China, or Russia. The report warns that over the next 25 years, chronic diseases will reduce the labor supply, savings, and investments and ultimately affect the capital markets and outline the business rationale for workplace health promotion programs.

**Table 11-2 Projected Foregone National Income Due to Heart Disease, Stroke, and Diabetes in Selected Countries, 2005–2015 (Billions of Constant 1998 International Dollars)**

| | Brazil | Canada | China | India | Russia | United Kingdom |
|---|---|---|---|---|---|---|
| Estimated income loss in 2005 | 2.7 | 0.5 | 18.3 | 8.7 | 11.1 | 1.6 |
| Estimated income loss in 2015 | 9.3 | 1.5 | 131.8 | 54.0 | 66.4 | 6.4 |
| Estimated accumulated loss (2005–2018) | 49.2 | 8.5 | 557.7 | 236.6 | 303.2 | 32.8 |

Source: Data from PAHO presentation, 2008: author.

Traditionally, the Indian healthcare system has been more focused on curative rather than preventive aspects of medicine. There are policies and guidelines available for communicable diseases, but noncommunicable chronic diseases have not been in focus so far. Owing to poor health literacy, knowledge about healthy practices is lacking, particularly among the poor and the uneducated classes in India despite continual media campaigns. Even the educated class in India tends to rely on home remedies and nonscientific methods of treatment. As such, there is an urgent need to develop awareness among people through repetitive messages and aggressive social marketing. Workplaces present captive audiences that are amenable to behavioral change interventions and can be easily motivated. Hence, there is a strong case for worksite health promotion (WHP) as a strategy to manage the chronic disease epidemic.

## Healthcare System

For a country as diverse as India, the organization and management of the healthcare system is very much centralized. Health administration in India is governed by the Ministry of Health and Family Welfare, which has three departments: the Department of Health, the Department of Family Welfare, and the Department of Ayurveda, Unani, Siddha, and Homeopathy. Centralized health planning in India is an integral part of the national socioeconomic planning (Park & Park, 1991). Dating back to 1946, the government of India has intermittently formed committees to review the existing health situation and recommend measures for action. Germane to the planning process are the five-year plans that are chalked out on a periodic basis (Ibid). An outcome of the last five-year plan was the National Rural Health Mission (2007–2012) that seeks to reform the rural healthcare infrastructure (ILEP-INDIA, 2008).

In the year 2005, the total expenditure on health was 6.1% of the GDP. As of 2007, the total value of the healthcare sector was 34 billion U.S. dollars, with per capita healthcare spending of just about $34. As can be seen in Table 11-3, India's total healthcare expenses as percentage of its GDP are much lower than the world's average of around 9%. The country's public expenditure on health as a percentage of the total health expenditure is lower than the countries of China, Pakistan, and Bangladesh, and far lower than the world's average.

Table 11-3 **Total Health Expenditure as Percentage of GDP and Public Expenditure on Health as a Percentage of Total Health Expenditure**

| Country | Per capita expenditure (U.S. $) | Total health expenditure as % of GDP | Public expenditure on health as a % of total health expenditure |
|---|---|---|---|
| World average | 482 | 9.3 | 58.1 |
| India | 23 | 6.1 | 20.7 |
| China | 45 | 5.8 | 33.7 |
| Pakistan | 18 | 3.2 | 34.9 |
| Bangladesh | 14 | 3.1 | 25.2 |

Source: Data from World Health Report, 2005; World Development Report, 2004.

India's healthcare expenditure by the private sector is one of the highest in the world, accounting for close to 81% of total healthcare spending. The share of government spending is close to 19%. The public health expenditure is close to 0.9% of the GDP, well below the average of 2.8% for low- and middle-income countries and the global average of 5.5% (Ministry of Health and Family Welfare, n.d.). The majority of the costs of treatment are met by out-of-pocket expenditures, estimated at 84.6% of total healthcare expenditure. This has serious consequences for the poor, who spend proportionally more on health care as compared to the rich.

About 75% of health infrastructure, medical manpower, and other health resources are concentrated in urban areas where 27% of the population lives (Patil, Somasundaram, & Goyal, 2002). The private healthcare sector has grown significantly since 2000. Focused primarily on the tertiary and secondary healthcare segment, it has seen major investments through multispecialty hospitals and nursing homes.

# Influence of Culture and Mentality

## Indian Culture

Culture is defined as the collective mental programming of the people in a given environment (Hofstede, 1980). It is not very amenable to change because it is shared by a group of people and is deeply ingrained in family structures, educational structures, and work organizations; it is also is reflected in legal systems and governments. India is a multicultural, multiethnic society. To make sweeping generalizations about the Indian way of life is close to impossible given the kaleidoscope of customs, values, beliefs, and traditions. Each region in India has its distinct language, cuisine, food customs and etiquette, and social norms.

Even though India is a multicultural society, there are some aspects of the Indian culture that are common across regions. *Collectivism* is one such component. It is defined as a social pattern wherein people see themselves as belonging to one or more collectives (e.g., family, coworkers, organization, religious group, etc.) (Triandis, 1995). *Verticalness* is another important component of Indian culture. Verticalness relates to the propensity of members of a culture to stand out from others in their significant circle of friends, associates, neighbors, etc. (Triandis, 1995). As such, the Indian culture may be labeled as *vertical collectivistic* (Triandis, 1998). It is not uncommon in the Indian context for people belonging to different social classes who are working in the same organization to be treated unequally. Also, one may find that power is unequally distributed among people at the workplace, reflecting the Indian social respect for a paternalistic, hierarchic authority. Another dimension of the Indian culture is that it is more *relationship based* than *rule based*; that is, an individual's behavior is largely regulated by members of one's clan, such as one's superiors, parents, or political leaders (Bhagat, Steverson, & Segovis, 2007). Another distinct aspect of the Indian culture is that it is more *affective* than *reasoning*, especially in rural India. It is not uncommon for people to express their emotions openly in the presence of their peers, coworkers, and supervisors without fear of embarrassment or rebuke. Understanding this Indian paradigm is important for the health promotion manager, as most of the models of health promotion have been developed in Western countries, primarily the United States, where the culture is individualistic, rule based, and reasoning.

With respect to design of worksite health promotion programs, a collectivist culture may be more receptive to interventions that are directed towards groups rather than individuals. As such, behavioral change interventions that involve competitions, teamwork, and social interaction may be more appealing to the employees.

## Language

Even though English is commonly accepted as the language of business in private companies and multinational organizations in larger cities, regional languages are more commonly used in government offices and institutions in smaller towns. Also, blue-collar workers are more likely to resort to the use of regional languages than white-collar workers, regardless of the location of the organization. From the perspective of health promotion managers, this poses a challenge because health communication materials may need to be translated into regional languages.

## Food Customs and Habits

The Indian Factories Act of 1948 requires that all companies with more than 250 employees provide access to quality and wholesome meals to their employees. Cafeterias and catering services are often subcontracted, and food prices are subsidized for employees. Despite access to cafeterias, the practice of carrying home-cooked meals is common. It is also a common practice to share food, and lunch time is often seen as an opportunity to socialize with colleagues. Food customs and dietary preferences vary widely across regions and also among different religious groups. Hindus, for instance, abstain from eating beef, and Muslims avoid pork. Certain sects among Hindus, like Jains, are strictly vegetarian and may have dietary restrictions with respect to root vegetables such as onions, potatoes, garlic, and tubers. Hindus are known to avoid eating meat and fish on certain days of the week that have religious significance. Also, the practice of fasting on certain days is not uncommon. Among Muslims, fasting and praying during the months of Ramadan forms an integral part of life. Since religion plays an important role in one's life, it is important for the health promotion manager to be acquainted with these customs and traditions. Religious sentiments and cultural preferences need to be kept in mind while designing cafeteria services and menu options.

## Spirituality

India has a rich tradition of yoga and Ayurveda, and spirituality is closely interwoven with the daily life. Yoga, derived from the Sanskrit word meaning "union," is a spiritual practice that uses the body, breath, and mind to energize and balance the whole person. This mind–body therapy involves physical postures, breathing exercises, and meditation to improve overall well-being. While the practice of yoga started nearly 6,000 years ago, the earliest written records documenting yoga as a health practice are recorded in *The Vedas*, texts from India dating back at least 3,000 years. Yoga is not only an excellent form of exercise, but a way of life. There is increasing evidence to show that yoga may be beneficial for managing stress, hypertension, and diabetes, and for promoting good physical and mental health. Recently, yoga has been popularized by spiritual leaders and gurus through mass workshops and TV channels. In 2009, the Indian government resolved to make yoga a compulsory subject in central board schools (TOI, 2009). The move has been applauded by health professionals who see yoga as instrumental in managing the chronic disease epidemic.

Ayurveda is an ancient branch of empirical medicine that combines physical, psychological, and spiritual therapies in an approach to good health and longevity. Ayurvedic medicines are primarily derived from herbs and natural products and have been shown to be effective in the treatment of many chronic conditions. However, in urban areas, allopathic medicine has more or less overshadowed Ayurveda, and it is not uncommon for practitioners of alternative medicine to prescribe allopathic drugs. There is a growing market for integrated treatment in the south, where alternative therapies combined with yoga are marketed through spas and retreats. Southern India, especially Kerala, is a growing hub for tourists seeking alternative remedies.

# Drivers of Worksite Health Promotion

Worksite health promotion in India is still in its nascent stage. Traditionally, employee health management in India has been synonymous with occupational health and safety and ergonomics. However, WHP is becoming increasingly popular. In this section we take a look at the various stakeholders and key players that are likely to have a major say as the industry comes of age.

## Corporate Hospitals and Diagnostic Labs

A visible trend is that of corporatization of hospitals and the growth of the diagnostic laboratory market (The U.S. Commercial Service in India at the American Center, n.d.). Corporate hospitals such as Apollo, Wockhardt, and Fortis have partnered with several large organizations to offer preventive health screenings for their employees. These screenings include preventive health checkups by physicians and laboratory screenings for diabetes, lipid profiles, and liver and kidney diseases. Among the pathology labs, the key players are SRL-Religare, Metropolis, Thyrocare, Piramal, Quest Diagnostics, and Lal Path Labs.

Competition in this sector has been instrumental in lowering the costs of health screenings. Corporations are able to avail themselves of bulk discounts, and the cost of a comprehensive health screening may range from Rs 1,500 to Rs 4,000 (U.S. $30 to $80). Given the fact that annual insurance premiums in India are still low (roughly Rs 4,000 for an insured sum of

Rs 500,000), the costs of these screenings are not covered by insurance. However, insurance companies may contribute 1–1.25% of the insured sum for the purpose of screenings in cases where the insured had at least 3 years with no insurance claims. As such, there is no strong incentive for insurance companies to pay for health screenings.

Even though health screenings may be beneficial in identifying potential risk factors and creating awareness, they should be seen as a precursor to a behavioral modification or disease management program. If screenings are not followed by effective counseling and health education with the aim to modify lifestyles, the whole purpose of the screening is defeated. Presently, it appears that health screening is seen as an end in itself and not as a means to an end.

## Insurance Companies

The extent of health insurance access is very limited. It is estimated that approximately 11% of the population has any form of health insurance. Less than 1% of the population has any form of private health insurance. Group insurance accounted for 35% of the total health insurance business (PricewaterhouseCoopers, 2007a). The government or state health insurance schemes include the Central Government Health Scheme and Employee State Insurance Scheme. In addition, there are several community-based insurance schemes run by nongovernment organizations in certain states; these may cover about 30 million people (Devadasan, Ranson, Van Damme, & Criel, 2004).

Health insurance in India is also known as medical insurance, and it is traditionally indemnity insurance that primarily covers hospitalizations and inpatient care. Insurance premiums are low and affordable, around Rs $130 per annum for a coverage of about $12,500 (Health Insurance India, 2010b). As of the time of writing, there is no health policy mandate that requires the employer in the private sector to provide health insurance for employees. Health insurance has been traditionally provided by organizations as an add-on benefit or perk to their employees. Until recently, the health insurance market in India was tightly regulated by the government with caps imposed on tariffs. Insurance companies were obliged to keep the premiums low despite rising claims and incurred losses. On January 1, 2007, the Insurance Regulatory and Development Authority (IRDA) eliminated the tariffs on general insurance (India Brand Equity Forum, 2009). From the perspective of employers, this is no longer good news because health insurance premiums are expected to rise.

Corporations can avail of discounts on health insurance premiums based on the number of subscriptions. The discounts range from 2.5% (for 101–500 employees) to 30% (greater than 50,000 employees). Insurance premiums are subject to appreciation or depreciation based on claims history. Discounts on insurance premiums may range anywhere from 5% to 40% in case of a low incurred claims ratio (Health Insurance India, 2010b). On the other hand, a high-incurred claims ratio may lead to loading of premiums up to 200%. Since for large organizations savings on health insurance premiums could be significant, there is a strong incentive for these organizations to keep the claims low. It is a known fact that high-risk people are likely to incur high healthcare costs, and thus there is a strong rationale for worksite health promotion.

## Health Professionals: Physicians and Corporate Hospitals

In the absence of organized vendors, occasionally independent physicians offer their services to corporations. These services include health education workshops, screenings, and outpatient services. Some of these physicians have training in occupational health, whereas others are family practitioners. Very recently, corporate hospitals like Apollo, Fortis, and Manipal have shown interest in setting up wellness clinics, which provide health promotion and disease prevention services in addition to traditional clinical care. The clinics have also targeted the worksite health promotion market.

## Wellness Industry

According to a joint Ernst and Young-FICCI report published in 2009, the wellness industry is expected to grow at a compound annual growth rate of 30–35% for the next 5 years (openPR, 2009). Growth is expected in seven core segments; namely, allopathy, alternative therapies, beauty treatments (e.g., cosmetics, plastic surgery, facial treatments), counseling, fitness/slimming, nutrition, and rejuvenation. As the wellness industry grows, some of the key players could evolve into prospective vendors for worksite health promotion programs.

## Government of India

The Indian Factories Act of 1948 regulates the health of workers in establishments. The act makes provisions to ensure safety in hazardous work environments and requires any factory with greater than 200 workers to have a full-time on-site physician trained in occupational health. The act was formulated to address the concerns of industrial workers and has not been amended since the globalization wave in the 1990s. Newer legislations and policies are needed to address the needs of workers in the service industry. Even though the National Rural Health Mission, as stated in its 10th and latest 5-year plan, articulates the need for worksite health promotion; a national worksite health promotion policy is yet to be formulated.

## Nongovernmental Organizations

Key nongovernmental organizations in India with regard to health promotion and occupational health are:

- The Indian Association of Occupational Health
- The Public Health Foundation of India
- Disease Management Association of India
- Chronic Care Foundation, India

These nongovernmental organizations aim at improving and stabilizing the Indian healthcare system in various settings by promoting awareness and education, and by strengthening research and policy development through resources, knowledge, and collaboration of all state holders.

## International Players

Given the rapid economic growth in India and the foray of multinational companies, international vendors have sensed an opportunity for growth. Healthways, Inc., a leading service provider in the United States, has been exploring the Indian market, and others are likely to follow. Some of these initiatives are very recent, and it would be too early to comment on what business model these companies adopt for India. Nevertheless, the influx of ideas and capital from the West, and strategic partnerships with stakeholders in India, will give a much-needed thrust to the industry.

## Employers

No stakeholder could have a greater incentive in promoting the health of their employees than the employers themselves. Health promotion has been found to have both tangible and intangible benefits, and several studies have shown positive return on investment (ROI) from programs. Some Indian companies have taken notice, and in the absence of vendors offering comprehensive services, they have developed their programs in-house, offering services through employee assistance programs and human resource departments. Companies like Infosys, Wipro, TATA, IBM, Cisco, and Johnson and Johnson all have some form of WHP initiative. Since these are highly respected companies and leaders in their respective fields, they are likely to set an example for other companies.

# Programs and Good Practices

Healthcare benefits, work–life balance, and perks are increasingly becoming important to keep employees happy and to attract new talent. In India, some major employers have long-standing and sophisticated health promotion programs. In this section, we will take a look at three cases: Wipro, Infosys, and TATA Chemicals.

### Wipro

Wipro runs a number of health promotion programs covering its employees from both the information technology and the business process outsourcing sectors. The programs include aspects such as nutrition consulting, arena (health centers), medical camps, monthly medical lectures, cafeterias (offering low-calorie food), employee well-being events, the Mitr (Friend) initiative to provide counseling for employees of the company, etc.

In the Mitr program, 28 employees, all volunteers, were trained to counsel fellow employees to manage stress. The term *Mitr* signifies to employees that they do have a friend in Wipro and that they should be able to confide and share their problems. "We at Mitr can help them cope with their problems," said Wipro's Anil Jalali, head of compensation and benefits. The key highlights of the program are:

- Chosen counselors work voluntarily, ensuring full commitment and buy-in from the employees.
- The counseling team goes through a careful selection process. This ensures that not only skills and requirements are met but that motivation is high amongst the selected.
- Rigorous training is given after the selection process.
- Awareness about the program is provided and widespread communication is available to as many people as possible to help them in personal and work-related problems, thereby spreading the message that there is a friend eager to be of help whenever required.
- Help is discontinued only when the employee feels confident enough to cope with issues himself/herself.
- Suggestions are accepted from the employees (i.e., both the counselors and counseled).
- The program is conducted in office premises and is for Wipro employees, by Wipro employees.

## Infosys Technologies

Infosys Technologies, which is a leading information technology service provider in India, has taken a holistic approach to promote a positive environment through collaborative care and health management among its employees. The initiative is seen as a catalyst to improve the health standards of the employees, thereby reducing absenteeism and increasing productivity.

Infosys has adopted a wellness initiative named Health Assessment Lifestyle Enrichment. The initiative has six broad components, namely, health, safety, leisure, stress, fun at work, and team building. Besides creating awareness about health and lifestyle issues, the program also incorporates fun and team-building exercises to ensure maximum participation. The approach is to build the program around the employees' interests, hobbies, and lifestyles. Central to the delivery of the program are the Health Assessment Lifestyle Enrichment online assessment tool and a 24-hour hotline to address the employees' concerns. Employees all across the country can call this help line to receive counseling services and expert opinions on health and lifestyle issues. The Health Assessment Lifestyle Enrichment online tool and the help line allows the human resource department to collect and track key indicators such as absenteeism and presenteeism and also monitor the effectiveness of the program as well as gains in productivity.

### *Key Elements of the Wellness Program*

- Provide an integrated approach to improve health and increased productivity on one hand and reduce absenteeism and control costs on the other
- Demonstrate that the company cares for its employees
- Ensure continuous in-house feedback
- Use the enterprise information portal for communication and dissemination of knowledge about the programs
- Interact with public health agencies such as the National Business Group on Health, the Wellness Council of America, and the European Network for Workplace Health Promotion, as well as nongovernmental orgainizations, hospitals, and psychologists
- Programs rolled out in India and Australia

### TATA Chemicals

Healthy, Wealthy & Wise is the worksite wellness program at Tata Chemicals Limited. It is a comprehensive program designed to help and support workers in establishing healthier lifestyles. The program attempts to address the key dimensions of well-being, which include physical, emotional, intellectual, spiritual, and financial components. Interventions are structured at three levels: generating awareness, competitions, and creating enabling environments and facilities. Some of the salient features of the program include:

- Identifying and appointing wellness coordinators at each of the site locations
- Daily emails titled, "An apple a day," that communicate health promotion messages
- Use of the company's intranet for communication and collection of data through health risk appraisals
- Health checkups offered by an on-site physician
- Awareness sessions and group discussion on health topics
- Ask-the-expert sessions: workshops with doctors, nutritionists, psychologists, fitness trainers, spiritual gurus, etc.
- Peer support: appointing mentors
- Competitions, games, and fun activities directed toward each of the wellness components

## Outcomes and Indicators

Worksite wellness programs are a very recent phenomenon in India. Even industry leaders have had such initiatives in place for fewer than 5 years, and some for fewer than 3 years. Given the fact that the programs are still in their infancy, it is too early to comment on ROI metrics and productivity gains. However, there are clear indications that corporations have the metrics in sight.

The Health Assessment Lifestyle Enrichment program offered at Infosys collects valuable data about program participation, presenteeism, absenteeism, and healthcare costs. As an information technology company, Infosys has systems in place such as an intranet that allows for self-reporting of data. Not every company, though, has such systems in place, and without them, collecting data is more tedious. Numerous scientifically validated survey and evaluation tools have been developed in the West to measure ROI and productivity gains, and it would be in the interest of Indian companies to make use of them to evaluate their programs.

## Existing Research

Just a handful of studies have been done in recent years in the worksite wellness field in India, and most of them have been assessments and evaluations of the magnitude of the problem and the scope of possible solutions. An operational study (Ahuja & Bhattacharya, 2007) done by the Confederation of Indian Industries (CII) in partnership with the World Health Organization, looked into employee health risks, workplace culture, organizational systems, and management practices. The study surveyed 1,000 workers from 10 industrial houses in 4 sectors—manufacturing, civil construction, software/consultancy, and drug/pharmaceutical—and found a high incidence of stress, hypertension, diabetes, and smoking among employee populations. The study also identified challenges with respect to convincing top management to adopt health promotion programs and regarding compliance issues. The study presented a strong case for worksite wellness in India and also set comprehensive guidelines for their successful implementation.

## Conclusion

WHP programs have evolved in the Western world over the last 4 decades and only recently have come of age. When we turn our focus to a country like India, we see an open playing field where health promotion is only just finding its roots. One would be tempted to apply the American model of health promotion to India, but doing so without a careful understanding the Indian paradigm may be a futile exercise. In India, health is still viewed in the context of the traditional biomedical models of preventive and social medicine. To introduce the concept of health promotion to the medical fraternity and allied health professionals would be to take a giant leap, bypassing the stages other countries have been through. But while on one hand the lack of understanding about health promotion is a challenge to overcome, at the same time it could represent a great opportunity. Countries such as India can learn from the mistakes made in other countries and adopt best practices. As the Indian system evolves to include WHP, it is likely to face challenges on three fronts:

1. Creating a knowledge base and policy framework for worksite health promotion
2. Building a human resource capacity for worksite health promotion
3. Creating organizational infrastructure for the delivery of services

## Creating a Knowledge Base and Policy Framework for Worksite Health Promotion

Existing behavior change theories need to be reviewed and validated in the context of the Indian paradigm, and empirical evidence from programs implemented in India is needed. Behavioral modification interventions and health communication messages will have to be customized based on the cultural sensitivities of different population subsets. There is also a need to generate health communication materials (brochures, media, websites, etc.), and to translate them into local languages.

From a policy perspective, various stakeholders need to be engaged to advocate an industry status for WHP. The government can be a facilitator by creating favorable policies and enabling an environment that will foster workplace health promotion. For example, Section 80-D of the Indian Income Tax Act provides tax deductions for medical insurance premiums up to 10,000 rupees per year. Policy reforms are needed to extend these deductions to preventive health screenings, so that there is a strong incentive for corporations to provide such screenings to their employees.

## Building a Human Resource Base for Worksite Health Promotion

Successful implementation of WHP in India will be challenging given the dearth of allied healthcare professionals. Unlike in the United States, where universities offer courses and programs in health education, health promotion, exercise physiology, and behavioral sciences, such disciplines are still not finding acceptance in Indian universities. Currently in India, health-related knowledge lies solely with physicians and nurses, and possibly, physiotherapists, occupational therapists, dieticians, and nutritionists. However, it would be safe to assume that health professionals are underprepared to engage with worksite health promotion. Even though the country produces close to 20,000 doctors every year, the percentage of these physicians who will choose to specialize in public health is woefully meager.

Until recently, the only option for medical graduates who wished to specialize in public health was to pursue a higher degree in preventive and social medicine. According to figures from the Medical Council of India, the annual intake of such graduates was around 450, a disappointing figure in a population of 1.1 billion. Even among public health professionals, knowledge of health promotion and behavioral change interventions is limited, as the system is fixated on the traditional model of occupational health and safety. There is an urgent need for a paradigm shift from the biomedical model of disease management to the sociopsychological model of health promotion and disease prevention. In addition, major reforms are needed in the medical education system to incorporate courses on health promotion, health communication, health psychology, patient counseling, organizational behavior, and human resources.

The future, however, is promising. Organizations such as the Public Health Foundation of India, the Disease Management Association of India, and the Chronic Care Foundation, India show potential and will be instrumental in catalyzing this transition. They have the institutional capacity to develop training modules, certification programs, and skill-building workshops for health professionals. Also, corporate hospitals such as Apollo, Manipal, and Fortis could offer certificate courses in workplace health promotion. The Public Health Foundation of India will provide the industry with close to 2,000 graduates in public health every year.

## Creating Organizational Infrastructure for Delivery of Services

As referenced in the section on drivers of WHP, there are several stakeholders in India with an interest in worksite health promotion. These include government, employers, insurance companies, physician groups, corporate hospitals, diagnostic labs, and wellness industry and international vendors. Though there have been several independent initiatives, there is not a single domestic or international vendor with the capacity to provide a comprehensive worksite health promotion program to a large organization. This presents a great opportunity for entrepreneurs to generate innovative business models for delivery. The sector is largely unorganized, and there is the potential for strategic partnerships among stakeholders. For instance, it would make good business sense for physician groups, wellness companies, and diagnostic labs to collaborate and offer a comprehensive WHP package in order to leverage their core competencies. It would also be advisable for insurance companies to recruit the services of physicians, not just for underwriting, but also to educate employees about judicious use of their insurance benefits, thereby keeping claims low. And lastly, employers should offer WHP services to their employees, thereby making an investment in long-term human capital.

Building a business case for worksite health promotion has always been a difficult proposition, given the long-term benefits and the problem of measuring productivity. It is likely to be even more challenging in India, given the lack of awareness about WHP and the novelty of the concept. Also, healthcare costs, though expected to rise in the future, are currently not a matter of great concern for employers. Insurance premiums are now low and affordable, but that might change soon. Lastly, India presents a large pool of talented youth for the service sector, and even though employers would like to retain their employees, the supply is usually greater than the demand. In such a situation, employers may be reluctant to make long-term investments in the health of their employees. As the WHP industry evolves, newer models may emerge that are suited to the Indian paradigm. The success of WHP in India calls for perseverance, ingenuity, and concerted efforts on the part of the various stakeholders.

# Summary

Due to globalization, rapid urbanization, and changing lifestyles, India is reeling under a demographic and epidemiologic shift. Noncommunicable diseases, which used to be limited to only the rich and those leading an urbanized lifestyle, have now trickled down to rural areas as well. India now faces a pandemic of chronic disease in the coming decades—diseases that are expected to cause losses in national income of $237 billion over the next 10 years. To meet these challenges, the healthcare system, now based on the traditional biomedical model of disease management, will need to evolve to the psychosocial model of health promotion and disease prevention. Since the workplace presents a captive audience that is amenable to behavioral change intervention, there is a strong case for worksite health promotion as a strategy for fighting the chronic disease epidemic. This has been repeatedly articulated in several government initiatives and also by nongovernment organizations such as the Public Health Foundation of India, the Disease Management Association of India, and the Chronic Care Foundation, India. Workplace health promotion also presents a strong business case for various stakeholders including the wellness industry, physician groups, corporate hospitals, insurance companies, and employers.

Successful implementation of programs, however, will not be without challenges. The novelty of the concept, the dearth of trained manpower, the gaps in scientific knowledge, the lack of policy framework, and poor organizational capacity are all likely to pose major hindrances to WHP. Surmounting these hurdles will require perseverance, ingenuity, a concerted effort on the part of the stakeholders, and an in-depth understanding of the Indian paradigm.

# Review Questions

1. Describe the demographics of the Indian workforce.
2. List the primary disease burdens of India. How is this burden changing over time?
3. What are the three departments within the Ministry of Health and Family Welfare?
4. How do India's healthcare expenditures compare with those of Bangladesh?
5. How does the Indian culture affect population health and workplace health promotion efforts?
6. Who are the stakeholders and key players who are likely to have a major role in India's workplace health promotion?
7. Compare and contrast the programs at Wipro, Infosys, and TATA Chemicals.

# References

Ahuja, R., & Bhattacharya, D. (2007). *Healthy workplace in corporate sector—India: An operational research.* Retrieved Dec 22, 2009, from http://www.whoindia.org/EN/Section20/Section29_1414.htm

Bhagat, R. S., Steverson, P. K., & Segovis, J. C. (2007). International and cultural variations in employee assistance programmes: Implications for managerial health and effectiveness. *Journal of Management Studies, 44*(2), 222–242.

Central Intelligence Agency (CIA). (2007). *The world factbook.* Retrieved July 9, 2010, from https://www.cia.gov/library/publications/the-world-factbook/geos/in.html

Central Intelligence Agency (CIA). (2010). *The world factbook.* Retrieved July 9, 2010, from https://www.cia.gov/library/publications/the-world-factbook/geos/in.html

Devadasan, N., Ranson, M. K., Van Damme, W., & Criel, B. (2004). Community health insurance in India: An overview. *Economic and Political Weekly, 39*, 3179–3183.

The Factories Act, 1948 [Act No. 63 of 1948]. Retrieved Feb 2, 2010 ,from http://indiacode.nic.in/fullact1.asp?tfnm=194863

Government of India. (2005). *Government hierarchy—health.* Retrieved March 12, 2009, from http://india.gov.in/citizen/health/govt_hierarchy.php

Gupta, R. (2008, January). A healthier future for India. *McKinsey Quarterly, January 2008.*

Health Insurance India. (2010a). Group health insurance policy for corporates/organization. Retrieved July 9, 2010, from http://www.healthinsuranceindia.org/group_health_insurance_india.asp

Health Insurance India. (2010b). Individual/Family health insurance products in India (single person). Retrieved July 14, 2010, from http://www.healthinsuranceindia.org/comparision_individual_health_insurance_policies.asp

Hofstede, G. (1980). Motivation, leadership and organisation: Do American theories apply abroad? *Organisational Dynamics, Summer,* 42–63.

ILEP-INDIA. (2008). National Rural Health Mission—an opportunity for National Leprocy Eradication Programme. Retrieved July 9, 2010, from http://nlep.nic.in/pdf/UpdateOct_2008.pdf

India Brand Equity Forum. (2009, January). *Healthcare.* Retrieved March 12, 2009, from http://www.ibef.org/artdispview.aspx?in=29&art_id=21509&cat_id=119&page=1

IndianExpress.com. (2006, March 29). PM launches Public Health Foundation. Retrieved March 12, 2009, from http://www.indianexpress.com/news/PM-launches-Public-Health- Foundation/1359/

Ministry of Health and Family Welfare, Government of India. (2007, March). Bulletin on rural health statistics in India. Retrieved March 12, 2009, from http://mohfw.nic.in/NRHM/BULLETIN%20ON.htm

Ministry of Health and Family Welfare, Government of India. (2008a). *National rural health mission*. Retrieved March 12, 2009, from http://mohfw.nic.in/NRHM/Documents/ NRHM%20Mission%20Document.pdf

Ministry of Health and Family Welfare, Government of India. (2008b). *National rural health mission, ASHA*. Retrieved March 12, 2009, from http://mohfw.nic.in/NRHM/asha.htm

Ministry of Health and Family Welfare. Government of India. (n.d.). *Task force on medical education for the National Rural Health Mission*. Retrieved July 9, 2010, from mohfw.nic.in/NRHM/Documents/Task_Group_Medical_Education.pdf

Misra, R., Chatterjee, R., & Rao, S. (2003). *India health report*. New Delhi, India: Oxford University Press.

National Health Profile 2007. (2007). *Human resources in health sector.* Retrieved March 12, 2009, from http://www.cbhidghs.nic.in/writereaddata/linkimages/Health%20Human%20Resources4484269844.pdf

OpenPR. (2009, April 20). *Indian wellness services market to grow at 30–35% CAGR, says FICCI-Ernst & Young report*. Retrieved February 2, 2010, from openpr.com/.../Indian-wellness-services-market-to-grow-at-30-35-CAGR-says-FICCI-Ernst-Young-Report.pdf

Park, J. E., & Park, K. (1991). *Text book of preventive and social medicine* (13th ed.). Jabalpur, India: Banarasidas Bhanot.

Patil, A. V., Somasundaram, K. V., & Goyal, R. C. (2002). Current health scenario in rural India. *Australian Journal of Rural Health, 10*, 129–135.

PricewaterhouseCoopers. (2007a). *Emerging market report: Health in India 2007.* Retrieved March 12, 2009, from http://www.pwc.com/extweb/pwcpublications.nsf/ docid/3100DC81746FA2308525734F007458DF/$File/emerging-market-report-hc-in-india.pdf

PricewaterhouseCoopers. (2007b). *Working towards wellness—an Indian perspective.* Retrieved July 9, 2010, from http://www.pwc.com/in/en/publications/india-publication-working-towards-wellness.jhtml

Shakthivel, S., & Joddar, P. (2006, May 27). Unorganised sector workforce in India. *Economic and Political Weekly*, 27 May.

TimesofIndia.com (TOI). (2009, August 27). NCERT wants yoga to be must in schools. Retrieved February 2, 2010, from http://timesofindia.indiatimes.com/india/NCERT-wants-yoga-to-be-must-in-schools/articleshow/4938837.cms

Triandis, H. C. (1995). *Individualism and collectivism.* Boulder, CO: Westview Press.

Triandis, H. C. (1998). Vertical and horizontal individualism and collectivism: Theory and research implications for international comparative management. In J. L. Cheng & R. B. Peterson (Eds.), *Advances in international comparative management.* Greenwich, CT: JAI Press.

The U.S. Commercial Service in India at the American Center. (n.d.). *Diagnostic laboratory market.* Retrieved July 9, 2010, from http://www.trade.gov/td/health/indiaivd05.pdf

World Bank. (2008). India country overview 2008. Retrieved March 12, 2009, from http://www.worldbank.org.in/WBSITE/EXTERNAL/COUNTRIES/SOUTHASIAEXT/INDIAEXTN/0,,contentMDK:20195738~menuPK:295591~pagePK:141137~piPK:141127~theSitePK:295584,00.html

World Health Organization, SEARO. (2009). Country health system profile: India. Retrieved March 12, 2009, from http://www.searo.who.int/EN/Section313/Section1519.htm

Chapter 12

# Israel

Peter Thomas Honeyman and Linda Kovler

After reading this chapter you should be able to:

- Identify core strategies that are the focus of Israel's workplace health promotion efforts
- Describe Israel's historical evolution of workplace health promotion
- Explain the different approaches employed by corporate health promotion efforts throughout Israel
- Review the central disease states and health issues driving Israel's health promotion needs
- Name the components of, and the associated funding sources for, Israel's healthcare system
- Discuss the impact of culture on Israel's health status and health promotion efforts

| Table 12-1 Select Key Demographic and Economic Indicators | |
|---|---|
| Nationality | Noun: Israeli(s)<br>Adjective: Israeli |
| Ethnic groups | Jewish 76.4% (of which Israel-born 67.1%, Europe/America-born 22.6%, Africa-born 5.9%, Asia-born 4.2%), non-Jewish 23.6% (mostly Arab) (2004) |
| Religion | Jewish 76.4%, Muslim 16%, Arab Christians 1.7%, other Christian 0.4%, Druze 1.6%, unspecified 3.9% (2004) |
| Language | Hebrew (official), Arabic used officially for Arab minority, English most commonly used foreign language |
| Literacy | Definition: age 15 and over can read and write<br>Total population: 97.1%<br>Male: 98.5%<br>Female: 95.9% (2004 est.) |
| Education expenditure | 6.9% of GDP (2004)<br>Country comparison to the world: 25 |
| Government type | Parliamentary democracy |

*continued*

| Table 12-1 Select Key Demographic and Economic Indicators, *continued* | |
|---|---|
| Environment | Limited arable land and natural fresh water resources pose serious constraints; desertification; air pollution from industrial and vehicle emissions; groundwater pollution from industrial and domestic waste, chemical fertilizers, and pesticides |
| Country mass | Total: 22,072 sq km<br>Country comparison to the world: 152<br>Land: 21,642 sq km<br>Water: 430 sq km |
| Population | 7,233,701<br>Country comparison to the world: 97 |
| Age structure | 0–14 years: 27.9% (male 1,031,629/female 984,230)<br>15–64 years: 62.3% (male 2,283,034/female 2,221,301)<br>65 years and over: 9.9% (male 311,218/female 402,289)<br>(2010 est.) |
| Median age | Total: 29.3 years<br>Male: 28.6 years<br>Female: 30 years (2010 est.) |
| Population growth rate | 1.671% (2010 est.)<br>Country comparison to the world: 79 |
| Birth rate | 19.77 births/1,000 population (2010 est.)<br>Country comparison to the world: 102 |
| Death rate | 5.43 deaths/1,000 population (July 2010 est.)<br>Country comparison to the world: 177 |
| Net migration rate | 2.37 migrant(s)/1,000 population (2010 est.)<br>Country comparison to the world: 36 |
| Urbanization | Urban population: 92% of total population (2008)<br>Rate of urbanization: 1.7% annual rate of change (2005–2010 est.) |
| Gender ratio | At birth: 1.05 male(s)/female<br>Under 15 years: 1.05 male(s)/female<br>15–64 years: 1.03 male(s)/female<br>65 years and over: 0.77 male(s)/female<br>Total population: 1 male(s)/female (2010 est.) |
| Infant mortality rate | Total: 4.22 deaths/1,000 live births<br>Country comparison to the world: 207<br>Male: 4.39 deaths/1,000 live births<br>Female: 4.05 deaths/1,000 live births (2010 est.) |
| Life expectancy | Total population: 80.73 years<br>Country comparison to the world: 12<br>Male: 78.62 years<br>Female: 82.95 years (2010 est.) |

*continued*

| Table 12-1 **Select Key Demographic and Economic Indicators,** *continued* | |
|---|---|
| Total fertility rate | 2.72 children born/woman (2010 est.)<br>Country comparison to the world: 83 |
| GDP—purchasing power parity | $205.8 billion (2009 est.)<br>Country comparison to the world: 51 |
| GDP—per capita | $28,400 (2009 est.)<br>Country comparison to the world: 48 |
| GDP—composition by sector | Agriculture: 2.6%<br>Industry: 32%<br>Services: 65.4% (2009 est.) |
| Agriculture—products | Citrus, vegetables, cotton, beef, poultry, dairy products |
| Industries | High-technology projects (including aviation, communications, computer-aided design and manufactures, medical electronics, fiber optics), wood and paper products, potash and phosphates, food, beverages, and tobacco, caustic soda, cement, construction, metal products, chemical products, plastics, diamond cutting, textiles, footwear |
| Labor force participation | 3.01 million (2009 est.)<br>Country comparison to the world: 103 |
| Unemployment rate | 7.6% (2009 est.)<br>Country comparison to the world: 74 |
| Industrial production growth rate | -1.5% (2009 est.)<br>Country comparison to the world: 82 |
| Distribution of family income (GINI index) | 39.2 (2008)<br>Country comparison to the world: 67 |
| Investment (gross fixed) | 16.4% of GDP (2009 est.)<br>Country comparison to the world: 128 |
| Public debt | 78.4% of GDP (2009 est.)<br>Country comparison to the world: 14 |
| Market value of publicly traded shares | $188.7 billion (December 31, 2008)<br>Country comparison to the world: 29 |
| Current account balance | $7.22 billion (2009 est.)<br>Country comparison to the world: 27 |
| Debt (external) | $84.69 billion (December 31, 2009 est.)<br>Country comparison to the world: 36 |
| Debt as a % of GDP | ——— |
| Exports | $45.76 billion (2009 est.)<br>Country comparison to the world: 48 |

*continued*

| Table 12-1 Select Key Demographic and Economic Indicators, *continued* | |
|---|---|
| Exports—commodities | Machinery and equipment, software, cut diamonds, agricultural products, chemicals, textiles, and apparel |
| Exports—partners | United States 35.05%, Hong Kong 6.02%, Belgium 4.95%, (2009) |
| Imports | $46.0 billion (2009 est.)<br>Country comparison to the world: 48 |
| Imports—commodities | Raw materials, military equipment, investment goods, rough diamonds, fuels, grain, consumer goods |
| Imports—partners | United States 12.35%, China 7.43%, Germany 7.1%, Switzerland 6.94%, Belgium 5.42%, Italy 4.49%, United Kingdom 4.03%, Netherlands 3.98% (2009) |
| Stock of direct foreign investment at | |
| Home | $58.7 billion (December 31, 2009 est.)<br>Country comparison to the world: 48 |
| Abroad | $55 billion (December 31, 2009 est.)<br>Country comparison to the world: 28 |

Source: CIA. (2010). *The world factbook.* Retrieved December 16, 2010, from https://www.cia.gov/library/publications/the-world-factbook/

# Introduction

Health includes physical, psychological, and social well-being. Israeli workplaces have a tradition of care for employees and their families and the promotion of social well-being.

The population of Israel is 7.2 million, of which 92% is urbanized. The median age is 29. Given that 28% of the population is under 15 and 10% are over 65 (CIA, 2009), age-related illnesses and disabilities are not the demographic problem experienced in other developed countries (World Health Organization, 2004).

Nearly 40% of the population was born outside of Israel (United Nations Development Program, 2009). The population is divided such that 76% are Jewish, of which 67.1% were born in Israel, 22.6% were born in Europe or the Americas, 5.9% were born in Africa, and 4.2% were born in Asia. Twenty-four percent are non-Jewish, mostly Arabic (CIA, 2009). Immigration has significantly slowed since 2000 (State of Israel Central Bureau of Statistics, 2009), but absorption and integration of new arrivals remains a societal priority.

The technologically advanced market economy has a per capita GDP of U.S. $26,000 (2007) (World Health Organization, Europe, 2004). In the current financial crisis, Israel has avoided recession, and the unemployment rate has risen from about 6% in 2007 to 8% in 2009. However, income inequality is a major issue, with a poverty rate of 20%, which is higher than in any Organisation for Economic Co-operation and Development (OECD) country. Poverty is strongly concentrated, present in about half of all Arabs and 60% of the ultrareligious Jewish population, caused by low labor market participation by Arab women and religious Jewish men (OECD, 2008).

Education presents a paradox in Israel. In all levels of education, there is below-average spending and below-average ranked achievement. However, there are much higher than average rates of college/university graduation (OECD, 2008). There are three official Israeli languages: Hebrew, Arabic, and English. Most signage is written in all three scripts. Pupils are educated in their family language of Hebrew or Arabic, and the additional teaching of both alternate languages is compulsory in state education.

An active movement for Jewish return to Palestine grew in the mid-19th century. This movement spurred the increased Jewish return to Palestine, which was further increased by the establishment of the State of Israel in 1949 and its subsequent development. These efforts, and the state of Israel, remain unfinished, without general recognition and security. Israel was built on land with few natural resources in hostile environment, with a traumatized population, and so the health of the society remains a key national priority (Avineri, 1981).

## Prevailing Health Issues and Risk Behaviors

Israeli life expectancy at birth is 80.7 years, which ranks 10th in the world (United Nations Development Program, 2009). Noncommunicable diseases account for 68% of deaths, with about one third from cardiovascular disease and one fourth from cancers.

The birth rate is the highest in the Eur A group (wealthier, developed economies), and near twice the average in this sector. In 2001, infant mortality was 11%, which is also higher than the Eur A group average (WHO, 2004).

The Israeli population is heterogeneous, which is reflected in many variables including household size, income, health behaviors, and health outcomes. The Jewish ultrareligious, the various immigrant groups, and the subgroups within the Arab population such as the Bedouin, are associated with significantly low socioeconomic status (Jaffe, Eisenbach, Neumark, & Manor, 2005). As an example of the variations caused by diversity, the non-Jewish male population has a life expectancy of 76 years, compared to Jewish male expectancy of 77 (State of Israel Central Bureau of Statistics, n.d.).

Surveys of Israelis aged 25–64 report that 90% of men and 87% of women perceive their health as good or very good. For comparison, the sample average for Eur A (not including Israel) was 73%. Despite these positive findings, mental health disability is above the Eur A group average (WHO, Europe, 2004). Smoking rates are 23% and have been falling since 2000 (State of Israel Ministry of Health, 2006). Per capita alcohol consumption is the lowest in the Eur A (WHO, Europe, 2004). Fourteen percent of the population have a BMI greater than 30 (State of Israel Ministry of Health, 2006). Approximately half of Israelis are physically inactive—activity defined as 20 minutes once a week—with the younger age groups (21–34 and 35–44) and females being less active on average (WHO, Europe, 2004).

The major challenges for health promotion policy, as set out in the *Healthy Israel 2020* initiative, are moving health promotion targeting to the use of evidenced-based interventions, achieving social justice, gaining public support, and balancing these goals with other budget demands (Rosenberg, Lev, Bin-Nun, McKee, & Rosen, 2008). In effect, this suggests targeting interventions on the disadvantaged, such as recent migrants, the ultrareligious, and sections of the Arab population. These are the groups who are also likely to be the least employed.

## Healthcare System

Israel has universal health insurance. Uniquely, individuals have the choice to join one of four competing, nonprofit health organizations, which deliver fairly similar services and plans (WHO, Europe, 2004). The largest organization, Kupot Holim Clalit, covers about 60% of the population.

Payment is through a wage proportional health tax, covering about 25% of costs, plus general taxation (45%) and further private funding (29%). The government adjusts payments to funds to match their membership numbers, weighted to formulas that recognize differing costs according to members' ages and disease burdens.

The Health Department has set levels for minimum service delivery levels, including for public health programs such as vaccination. Individuals can choose to increase their level of service by extra payment to their health organization. In addition, some employers choose to pay for private health insurance as a benefit. There is also universal national insurance, which covers unemployment, work sickness, and injury absences; disability from all causes; pregnancy leave; and retirement. It does not run prevention programs.

Primary care providers are usually linked to individual health organizations and are paid under varying salary or capitation models. Service is usually free and accessible within the same day. Specialist and hospital care is also generally accessible without much delay.

Health promotion from within the four health organizations is defined and its scope is minimal, related to screening and vaccination. The Health Department has maintained separate activities and programs related to health-related behaviors. It lobbied for legislation to have smoking banned from workplaces in early 2000 and to restrict smoking promotion, and it undertook public awareness campaigns, which have resulted in reduced rates of smoking. The Health Department also targets some migrant communities for additional surveillance. For example, infectious diseases such as TB are found in defined populations, and so programs are focused at these communities.

The society-building nature of Israel recognizes disadvantage and poverty and responds with diverse measures. For example, government policy recognizes areas of high unemployment and provides subsidies to industries that establish factories in the south of Israel. Communities with high concentrations of migrants or unemployed persons are targeted for support from government and nongovernment institutions. An example of this support is a volunteer program wherein many high-achieving children take a gap year between leaving school and joining the army to live in these communities, assisting in youth activities and helping low-achieving students with homework. Although these activities are not delivered by the health system, they are focused on delivering a healthier society.

## Influence of Culture and Mentality

The early core ideology of Israel was, and still remains, the building of a healthy society for its Jewish and other inhabitants (Avineri, 1981). The two initial strands were Jewish cultural values and an ideology of socialist utopia, the latter of which is in transition.

Jewish health beliefs derive from such cultural values as *tikun olam*—improving the society/world, and *gemilut chasadim*—charity, and are strongly influenced by the 10th century Jewish scholar/physician Moses Maimonides (or Rambam). These beliefs emphasize the importance of human life, care for one's body, and the care for the sick through professional health support and charitable hospital development in Jewish life.

The isolation of the Jewish communities during the Diaspora before the founding of the State of Israel gave rise to traditions around food and eating habits. The religious requirements for dietary restrictions (Kashrut) led to the development of a strong family and community culture with food—and not alcohol—at the center of every social and religious gathering. Alcohol is used in various religious ceremonies but usually in small quantities. Although drinking is on the rise among the younger population, alcohol consumption remains low in Israel today.

A culture of physical activity and affinity for the outdoors was almost unheard of in Jewish communities until the early 20th century. In the Diaspora, Jews were expelled throughout the ages from many countries in which they lived. They were not allowed to own land, and so Jewish parents encouraged academic as opposed to physical prowess. It was rare to see a Jewish sportsman. This emphasis began changing in the early 20th century in Palestine with the creation of the kibbutz movement based on socialist utopian idealism. The kibbutz pioneers put into practice concepts such as redemption through return to manual work on the land, job rotation, flat social structure, and equality between the sexes. Kibbutz membership is now about 6% of the Israel population (State of Israel Central Bureau of Statistics, n.d).

This revolutionary vision of the Jew, and later the Israeli, as physically fit and strong grew further in the aftermath of the Holocaust and with the need to form a national defense force. Through the present day, this need for national defense affects the way youth in Israel pursue sports and physical exercise during their teen years; at the age of 18, they are recruited into the IDF (Israel Defense Forces), with the fittest individuals getting into the most prestigious army units.

The largest healthcare provider, Kupot Holim Clalit, was established in Palestine under Turkish rule in 1911, as a mutual aid society for the Jewish population. The Histradut Jewish trade union, established in 1920 as another strand of the socialist utopian ideal, provided member benefits such as sick pay and health services and took over ownership and management of Kupot Holim Clalit. Even before the formation of the State of Israel, Jewish universities, hospitals, and a public health system were involved in control of infectious diseases, such as malaria. All of these organizations were staffed by skilled professionals who were fleeing German racial laws that barred Jews from professional roles in Germany.

The Histradut believed in the benefits of employment, becoming the largest employer in Israel until the 1980s. The Histradut included non-Jews from 1958 onward. At its peak in the 1980s, one third of Israeli citizens and 85% of employees were Histradut members. Many of the core industries in Israel are privatized former Histradut enterprises that keep the worker/family care as a core value. These workplaces remain unionized.

The IDF, through which most young men and women complete their national service, continue to be influential far beyond their defense role. Social integration, common language acquisition, and skilled training of diverse migrant groups occur during military service. The 19th century socialist utopian ideologues for the Jewish return had planned universal national service for community building, and while the defense component has subsumed the original intent, the IDF continues to have an important social role.

## Drivers of Workplace Health Promotion

The Israeli electoral system encourages temporary political coalitions, wherein government ministries are usually assigned for political expediency. The Health Ministry has in recent memory no long-term minister, and as such, policy direction is driven by budget constraints, professional input, and perceived populist demand.

The four Israeli health organizations have no incentive for any activity such as workplace health promotion (WHP) beyond meeting the service delivery levels for public health programs, set by the Department of Health. Workplaces have employees with mixed health organization memberships, which is a further disincentive for any health organization to enter the workplace.

Some health organizations have internal occupational health departments. The salaried physicians in these departments certify when employees are incapacitated and can obtain national insurance benefits. They also undertake worker surveillance for occupational hazards such as noise. In some workplaces they provide annual screenings distantly related to any real workplace hazards but provided as a dubious benefit. The physicians have little incentive to promote health. In addition, there is no recognized occupational nursing profession that might sit within the industry and play an advocacy role. A new development in some health organizations is the effort to charge employers for workplace health risk management programs as an extra revenue stream, but as yet, these programs are not widely used.

The Department of Health is in transition to refocus health promotion but will likely target disadvantaged groups, such as subgroups of migrants and minority sectors of society (Rosenberg et al., 2008). The national insurance acts to control costs, but not through prevention.

However, there are other bodies with union or government affiliation that act as advocates for employee health.

Employers receive no government incentives to promote health. Their activities in health and welfare are considered employee benefits, and in many cases are subject to taxation. Employers undertake such activities for their competitive advantage in hiring and retaining employees. The employer does not pay for national insurance, and any additional sickness insurance premiums the employer pays are not linked to individual company performance. Thus, employers have no incentive to promote health. In addition, the majority of Israeli employers are not advised by independent health consultants (occupational or otherwise) who would bring awareness of the internal costs of ill health. Finally, employers generally lack the management systems that would be a base for effective WHP.

The older enterprises, including many with prestate roots, remain focused on building a better society in line with Jewish and socialist ideals. They recognize the problems and associated social difficulties inherent in workforces comprised of migrants, and in line with cultural ideas they coordinate with workplace unions to support social well-being programs.

## Programs and Good Practices

Most Israeli employers implement social welfare activity. Where there are workplace unions, these activities are jointly managed. The elements of such social programs are both proactive and reactive.

The proactive social programs are wide ranging and varied. Nearly all workplaces with predominantly Jewish workforces follow the traditional Jewish holidays as a base for joint social activities. For example, during the Jewish New Year, employers usually give gifts to employees and frequently host social activities outside the workplace for employees and families. Many employers subsidize cultural activities and sports participation. These supports are seen as community-building activities that promote social well-being. Some employers support children's higher education, to encourage opportunity and family health. The union-run social support continues after retirement, with employees funding part of the retiree group activities.

Employers consider and support the importance of family life. An extreme example was seen during recent conflicts in which rocket fire closed schools. Some employers chose to convert their internal shelters to child-minding areas so that parents could bring their children to work, reducing parental worry and contributing to general morale.

Social welfare is managed by social workers, employed in the larger workplaces to help with families and illnesses. There are variations in organizational structure, with many social workers employed inside human resources departments; some are associated but independent. Workplace psychologists complement the efforts of social workers, and both groups may offer counseling. Other workplaces offer contracted services, as in the more traditional employee assistance programs.

The authors have not identified any published work on the issues presented to these social workers. Anecdotally, the major current issues for counseling appear to be marriage, family, and financial or legal problems. Given the high percentage of migrants and their higher rates of mental issues, industry support for these programs suggests that migrants' ongoing needs are not met by health services.

In addition, there are those Israelis who acquire disabilities from the ongoing conflicts. The state provides protections and benefits to enable these people to return to work. Employers and fellow employees are strongly supportive of their disabled colleagues continuing at work. Some employers also provide additional medical insurance to encourage employees to seek any necessary physiological support or private medical care, and to assist in chronic disease management.

Across Israeli workplaces, alcohol and work do not mix. Catered workplace functions are inevitably dry. There is no tradition of lunchtime, after work, special occasion, or birthday drinking. Toasts may be given in work to mark the frequent festivals, but grape juice is the norm.

Another common element in most workplaces is the provision of workplace meals. The style of food and dining probably has its origins in kibbutz dining rooms: there are no hierarchies and the social aspect of dining is emphasized. The food, judging from one author's experience of eating in workplace dining rooms around the world, is healthy thanks to the inclusion of salads and fruits of significant quantity and quality. Dietitian input on provided meals is the norm. The main meal in Israel is the midday meal, and so employees of differing food cultures are exposed to normative healthy eating.

All of these programs are larger and better supported in the advanced, knowledge-based industries than in less advanced industries. Here employers compete to attract and retain the best. In these workplaces, in-house gyms are more common. However, there is considerable variability with respect to support and encouragement for programs to encourage fitness. Around the year 2000, employers met with a disincentive to provide gyms. In order to prevent injuries, all such gyms were required to have a trained gym instructor. This has increased operating costs and so reduced opening hours.

## Intel Corp

Intel Corp is a leading employer in Israel and provides the most comprehensive example of WHP inside Israel. The aim of the Intel health promotion program, branded globally as Health for Life, is to create a culture of wellness throughout the workplace that will improve employee health and productivity. The program is multifaceted and includes a range of programs and tools from on-site physical health checks to work–life effectiveness tools. At the core of the Health for Life program is the 3 Step Wellness Check. This consists of a biometric health check, an on-line health risk assessment (HRA), and a meeting with a wellness coach. Ongoing coaching sessions are offered to all individuals who wish to participate. Aggregate data is collected from the annual HRA and the biometric checks, and the change over time in health outcomes is tracked. The HRA reports also give a breakdown of productivity and return on investment (ROI) data.

The Intel program has been designed globally but modified for the Israeli workforce. It is managed locally, and participation and satisfaction are tracked in a joint local and global team. The main challenges to the local customization have been language adaptation of the HRA and other materials; the hiring of wellness coaches in a market that is physician based and lacking in regulation of the coaching profession; incentivizing participation for the program—a concept that has not yet received buy-in from the local Israel management who are used to receiving free health care outside the workplace; and lastly, the prohibitive benefit tax imposed by the government on those employees participating in the wellness coaching. The first challenge around language was overcome by working with an international vendor on the creation of a specific Hebrew language version of the HRA. The second issue of wellness coaching was handled by the outsourcing the program to vendors who gave in-house training in wellness coaching to the nurses, dieticians, and exercise coaches involved. Local Intel management did not buy into the concept of financial incentives for participation in the program, but a small gift is being given for those who complete the program. The ideal solution to increase participation would be to collaborate on the program with Israel's national health organizations and to link Health for Life participation with a meaningful discount or additional service offering in employees' health insurance plan. The Intel Health for Life and employee benefits are designed on the global level but run alongside the more typical Israeli well-being programs, which are managed locally and focus on social events and quality of life.

There are other medium- and large-sized companies who invest in wellness programs such as nutritional workshops, health days, and on-site individual or group weight management. These are organized by the human resources/benefits department and measured, if at all, by participation alone and not by health outcomes.

## Other Employers

The aircraft industry and nuclear research institute have a solid occupational health program, focusing on diagnostic screening, emergency medicine, and improved employee access to health care. The police and army (IDF) remain the two large national institutions that have a structured employee health promotion plan. These plans cover smoking, nutritional awareness, weight management, physical exercise, some screening, and vaccinations.

The IDF introduced the smoke-free workplace (healthy bases program) prior to the Health Ministry initiatives in 2000. The IDF health educational program is largely delivered by peers. A comprehensive health educational curriculum, accessible as electronic files stored on computers, is given to all doing national service. The trainers are generally the more senior soldiers, and so the program may be delivered by peers 2 years more senior, rather than professionals. Topics range from pregnancy control to drugs and aids to infection control and understanding minority cultures.

## Outcomes and Indicators

The authors were unable to find any measure of performance of any element of workplace health promotion at the employer level, beyond the program imported by Intel.

Sickness absence is commonly tracked, however. The larger, better organized companies are aware of rates of long-term sickness absence. This is usually tracked in human resources, and the sick may be supported by social workers. Sickness is rarely managed through systems such as case management and return to alternate work. Although the employer picks up the cost of short-term, nonoccupational sickness absence, employers generally regard illness as a matter between the sick employee and his doctor.

The larger companies use employee surveys to judge the workplace environment or culture, looking at issues such as workplace attachment and conflict management. Competition to attract and retain skilled workers motivates these workplace assessments. Many high-tech companies participate in health-related benefit comparison; however, these comparisons exist to rank workplace benefits in attracting and retaining employees.

If the army is a workplace, then this is the place where program measurement takes place. For example, soldiers commonly travel home to their families on weekends. There were tragedies of soldiers dying on their weekends because of driving while tired. Recent programs appear to have markedly reduced such deaths. Soldiers undertaking national service are followed, from entrance through midpoints and to exiting the military for program measures such as rates of smoking and obesity. The measures are taken to improve program effectiveness, but the results, which are understood as positive, remain unpublished.

## Existing Research

The authors were unable to locate any research on workplace health promotion in Israel as distinct from occupational health and safety. The Workers Health Institute undertook health and safety research projects. However, the Institute was closed in 2005, and funding for possible research has stopped. Recently, Tel Aviv University has started a workplace health promotion course option within its occupational master's program, so there should be graduates with the skill to attempt programs going into the future. In addition, there have been recent unfunded doctoral and masters theses in the area.

## Conclusion

WHP in Israel combines the efforts of employers, employees, and society and addresses the prerequisites of health such as housing, food, security, access to medical care, income through employment, and quality working conditions. Currently, there is little of the WHP model, with its focus on health education and social marketing aiming to change behavioral risk factors.

Israeli workplace practices are unique in growing out of Jewish cultural beliefs and the 19th century ideology of Zionism, the return of Jews to a homeland, which incorporated society-building activities from its beginning. Health and, in particular, social health promotion are society- and belief-driven, rather than something flowing from health professionals or from attempts to control health costs. Work as a prerequisite to health was understood and pursued from the prestate period before modern research (Waddell & Burton, 2006). The current unemployment rates in Israel do not relate to lack of work, with Israel currently importing foreign labor to meet demands.

The higher rates of mental health issues may be explained by immigration, as studies in various countries indicate immigrants often have higher rates of mental illness than either the native-born population or the population in their countries of origin (Helman, 2002). This explanation is partial, seeing as how ongoing regional conflicts create casualties, both mental and physical.

Achieving a strong society built on refugees has been a societal focus. Workplaces have been one means to this end. Examples have been given of the normative effects of workplace practices. The gradual homogenization of people from diverse backgrounds occurs in work, from language acquisition to healthy eating and social care.

The government has had limited role in WHP, with the exception of smoking cessation policies. The Israel 2020 program suggests targeted focus on groups likely to be outside the workplace setting such as children, the unemployed, or the retired. Given the limits of government spending, removing taxation from employer benefits is unlikely to achieve the gains of other health-targeted spending. The inequalities in society continue to create health risks for the disadvantaged (Wilkinson & Pickett, 2009).

A major opportunity is the breakdown of the various health organizations' departments of occupational health and transfer of occupational health program payment to a cost covered by the employer. If these occupational health professionals leave their health bureaucracies and become industry-focused, they are likely to help employers understand the true costs of ill health in workplaces, and take on and expand programs currently being run by HR departments. Employers are likely to pay for these programs as they recognize that future success in a globalizing marketplace can only be achieved with a healthy, qualified, and motivated workforce. There is some risk that the original ideological motivation, and the shared nature of program control, might be lost in the pursuit of profits and science.

The further opportunity is likely to follow from the IDF programs. Their health promotion efforts are relatively recent, but given their usual excellence as reflected in their effect on industrial innovation inside Israel, we may see similar innovation in achieving measured results in health promotion. The pity is that so little of their programs is published.

The ultimate dream and challenge for WHP would be posed by regional peace. Prior to breakdown of the Madrid peace process, over 200,000 Palestinians worked inside Israel proper. The greatest chance for their societal well-being depends on rapid economic revival, which includes return of Palestinians to work inside Israel. Any WHP for this population would be complex to build, with participant input into the design acting as a major initial hurdle. Is it likely the designers of such programs would choose health education and social marketing focused on changing behavioral risk factors? It seems more likely that they would also choose programs similar to those that have contributed to Israel's health, namely focusing on renewing social well-being.

## Summary

Israel is a small, relatively poor country with good health outcomes. The unique features are that 40% of the population was born overseas, the median age is 29, university education rates are high, and the society is nonhomogeneous, with high rates of poverty and income disparity.

Patterns of health behaviors and health outcomes vary among population groups. Israel has higher than average rates of psychiatric problems as expected in a migrant society. Jewish culture, socialist utopian ideology, and the IDF have shaped most institutions inside Israel, including the nature of workplaces and the importance of personal health. The country lacks physical resources and is isolated in the region, so the economy is dependent on its human capital to grow by innovation. The economy remains strong and able to provide work. Given the mixed population, the defense forces and all workplaces play a central role in society building, including promotion of universal language acquisition, developing societal attachment, and setting standards for normative behavior including health practices. An example is that workplaces commonly provide meals that expose employees of varied food cultures to normative diets marked by increases in intakes of fruit and vegetables. Workplaces in Israel strongly promote social well-being and also provide services to help with psychological, personal, and family issues.

Being an open market for multinational companies, Israel imports best overseas models of workplace health promotion. The IDF, with universal conscription, has started health promotion, and based on history, they are likely to be the future innovators. There is no published work on IDF health promotion activities, however.

## Review Questions

1. Compare the health issues of Israel with the health statistics of Eur A.
2. Who funds the Israeli healthcare system and how are the health needs of the disadvantaged and impoverished addressed?
3. How does the IDF help or hinder health promotion efforts?
4. Describe the current status of Israel's workplace health promotion programs.

5. How have Israeli workplaces used health promotion to attract and retain the best employees?
6. What is Intel's method of collecting outcome indicators for workplace health promotion programs in Israel?

# References


Avineri, S. (1981). *The making of modern Zionism: The intellectual origins of the Jewish State.* New York, NY: Basic Books, Inc.

Central Intelligence Agency. (2009). *The World Fact Book: Israel.* Retrieved November 2009 from https://www.cia.gov/library/publications/the-world-factbook/geos/is.html

Helman, C. G. (2002). *Culture, health, and illness* (4th ed.). London, England: Arnold Publications.

Jaffe, D., Eisenbach, Z., Neumark, Y., & Manor, O. (2005). Individual household and neighborhood socioeconomic status and mortality: A study of absolute and relative deprivation. *Science and Social Medicine, 60,* 989–997.

Organisation for Economic Co-operation and Development. (2008). *Education at a glance.* Retrieved November 2009 from http://www.oecd.org/topicdocumentlist/0,3448,en_33873108_39418575_1_1_1_1_37455,00.html

Rosenberg, E., Lev, B., Bin-Nun, G., McKee, M., & Rosen, L. (2008). Healthy Israel 2020: A visionary health targeting initiative. *Public Health, 122,* 1217–1225.

Shai, I., Scwarzfuchs, D., Henkin, Y., & Shahar, D. R. (2008, July 17). Weight loss with low-carbohydrate, Mediterranean, or low-fat diet. *New England Journal of Medicine, 359,* 229–241.

State of Israel Central Bureau of Statistics. (n.d.). Retrieved November 2009 from http://www1.cbs.gov.il/reader/?MIval=cw_usr_view_SHTML&ID=719

State of Israel Ministry of Health. (2006). *Knowledge, attitudes, and health practices in Israel.* Jerusalem, Israel: Ministry of Health.

United Nations Development Program. (2009). *Human development report 2009: Israel.* Retrieved November 2009 from http://hdrstats.undp.org/en/countries/country_fact_sheets/cty_fs_ISR.html

Waddell, G., & Burton, K. (2006). *Is work good for your health and well-being?* London, England: TSO.

Wilkinson, R., & Pickett, K. (2009). *The spirit level: Why more equal societies almost always do better.* London, England: Penguin.

World Health Organization, Europe. (2004). *Highlights on health in Israel.* Retrieved in 2004 from http://www.euro.who.int/document/E88549.pdf

Chapter 13

# Italy

Giuseppe Masanotti

After reading this chapter you should be able to:

- Identify core strategies that are the focus of Italy's workplace health promotion efforts
- Describe Italy's historical evolution of workplace health promotion
- Explain the different approaches employed by corporate health promotion efforts throughout Italy
- Review the central disease states and health issues driving Italy's health promotion needs
- Name the components of, and the associated funding sources for, Italy's healthcare system
- Discuss the impact of culture on Italy's health status and health promotion efforts

Table 13-1 **Select Key Demographic and Economic Indicators**

| | |
|---|---|
| Nationality | Noun: Italian(s)<br>Adjective: Italians |
| Ethnic groups | Italian (includes small clusters of German-, French-, and Slovene-Italians in the north and Albanian-Italians and Greek-Italians in the south) |
| Religion | Roman Catholic 90% (approximately; about one third practicing), other 10% (includes mature Protestant and Jewish communities and a growing Muslim immigrant community) |
| Language | Italian (official), German (parts of Trentino-Alto Adige region are predominantly German speaking), French (small French-speaking minority in Valle d'Aosta region), Slovene (Slovene-speaking minority in the Trieste-Gorizia area) |
| Literacy | Definition: age 15 and over can read and write<br>Total population: 98.4%<br>Male: 98.8%<br>Female: 98% (2001 census) |
| Education expenditure | 4.5% of GDP (2005)<br>Country comparison to the world: 88 |

*continued*.

**Table 13-1 Select Key Demographic and Economic Indicators,** *continued*

| | |
|---|---|
| Government type | Republic |
| Environment | Air pollution from industrial emissions such as sulfur dioxide; coastal and inland rivers polluted from industrial and agricultural effluents; acid rain damaging lakes; inadequate industrial waste treatment and disposal facilities |
| Country mass | Total: 301,340 sq km<br>Country comparison to the world: 71<br>Land: 294,140 sq km<br>Water: 7,200 sq km<br>*Note:* includes Sardinia and Sicily |
| Population | 58,126,212 (July 2009 est.)<br>Country comparison to the world: 23 |
| Age structure | 0–14 years: 13.5% (male 4,056,156/female 3,814,070)<br>15–64 years: 66.3% (male 19,530,696/female 18,981,084)<br>65 years and over: 20.2% (male 4,903,762/female 6,840,444)<br>(2010 est.) |
| Median age | Total: 43.7 years<br>Male: 42.3 years<br>Female: 45.3 years (2010 est.) |
| Population growth rate | -0.047% (2010 est.)<br>Country comparison to the world: 207 |
| Birth rate | 8.18 births/1,000 population (2010 est.)<br>Country comparison to the world: 221 |
| Death rate | 10.72 deaths/1,000 population (July 2010 est.)<br>Country comparison to the world: 50 |
| Net migration rate | 2.06 migrant(s)/1,000 population (2010 est.)<br>Country comparison to the world: 41 |
| Urbanization | Urban population: 68% of total population (2008)<br>Rate of urbanization: 0.4% annual rate of change (2005–2010 est.) |
| Gender ratio | At birth: 1.07 male(s)/female<br>Under 15 years: 1.06 male(s)/female<br>15–64 years: 1.03 male(s)/female<br>65 years and over: 0.72 male(s)/female<br>Total population: 0.96 male(s)/female (2010 est.) |
| Infant mortality rate | Total: 5.51 deaths/1,000 live births<br>Country comparison to the world: 185<br>Male: 6.07 deaths/1,000 live births<br>Female: 4.91 deaths/1,000 live births (2010 est.) |

*continued*

| Table 13-1 **Select Key Demographic and Economic Indicators,** *continued* | |
|---|---|
| Life expectancy | Total population: 80.2 years<br>Comparison to the world: 18<br>Male: 77.26 years<br>Female: 83.33 years (2010 est.) |
| Total fertility rate | 1.32 children born/woman (2010 est.)<br>Country comparison to the world: 206 |
| GDP—purchasing power parity | $1.739 trillion (2009 est.)<br>Country comparison to the world: 11 |
| GDP—per capita | $29,900 (2009 est.)<br>Country comparison to the world: 46 |
| GDP—composition by sector | Agriculture: 1.8%<br>Industry: 25%<br>Services: 73.1% (2009 est.) |
| Agriculture—products | Fruits, vegetables, grapes, potatoes, sugar beets, soybeans, grain, olives, beef, dairy products, fish |
| Industries | Tourism, machinery, iron and steel, chemicals, food processing, textiles, motor vehicles, clothing, footwear, ceramics |
| Labor force participation | 24.97 million (2009 est.)<br>Country comparison to the world: 23 |
| Unemployment rate | 7.7% (2009 est.)<br>Country comparison to the world: 78 |
| Industrial production growth rate | -13.5% (2009 est.)<br>Country comparison to the world: 154 |
| Distribution of family income (GINI index) | 32 (2006)<br>Country comparison to the world: 101 |
| Investment (gross fixed) | 18.9% of GDP (2009 est.)<br>Country comparison to the world: 105 |
| Public debt | 115.2% of GDP (2009 est.)<br>Country comparison to the world: 6 |
| Market value of publicly traded shares | $NA (December 31, 2009)<br>Country comparison to the world: 16 |
| Current account balance | $-66.57 billion (2009 est.)<br>Country comparison to the world: 188 |
| Debt (external) | $NA (December 31, 2009 est.) |
| Debt as a % of GDP | ——— |
| Exports | $412.9 billion (2009 est.)<br>Country comparison to the world: 8 |

*continued*

| Table 13-1 Select Key Demographic and Economic Indicators, *continued* | |
|---|---|
| Exports—commodities | Engineering products, textiles and clothing, production machinery, motor vehicles, transport equipment, chemicals, food, beverages and tobacco; minerals, and nonferrous metals |
| Exports—partners | Germany 12.6%, France 11.57%, United States 5.92%, Spain 5.69%, United Kingdom 5.13%, Switzerland 4.69% (2009) |
| Imports | $410.2 billion (2009 est.)<br>Country comparison to the world: 8 |
| Imports—commodities | Engineering products, chemicals, transport equipment, energy products, minerals and nonferrous metals, textiles and clothing, food, beverages, and tobacco |
| Imports—partners | Germany 16.68%, France 8.82%, China 6.53%, Netherlands 5.63%, Spain 4.3%, Russia 4.12%, Belgium 4.08% (2009) |
| Stock of direct foreign investment at | |
| Home | $366.9 billion (December 31, 2009 est.)<br>Country comparison to the world: 12 |
| Abroad | $556.5 billion (December 31, 2009 est.)<br>Country comparison to the world: 12 |

Source: CIA. (2010). *The world factbook.* Retrieved December 16, 2010, from https://www.cia.gov/library/publications/the-world-factbook/

# Introduction

Italy is a peninsula located in the south of Europe and covers an area of 301,336 square kilometers, with a population about 60,000,000 (ISTAT, 2008). Foreign residents comprise 5.8% of the total population, a figure that confirms the growing trend of the previous years. During the period from 1950 to 2000, the population over 65 years of age increased, reaching about 20% of the total population (ISTAT, 2006). In 2008, the statistics with respect to old age showed a further increase, reaching a total increase of 142.6% (Allamani et al., 2007). Compared to the international data, the country of Italy is one of the most involved countries in the phenomenon of aging. This phenomenon creates obvious social and economic changes, particularly regarding labor market and economic growth (CNEL, 2009; ISTAT, 2005, 2006, 2007).

The lack of need for workers, in fact, was first addressed by enterprises, which responded by reducing the number of hours worked and overtime, increasing the use of part-time workers, and increasing layoffs and leave abandonment (CNEL, 2009). In this way, job cuts have been limited. The employment rate, therefore, remained essentially stable at 58.7% (CNEL, 2009). Moreover, the greater possibility of participating in the labor market helped to create a positive employment trend, especially for women, whose activity rate increased by almost two percentage points in 2008. This growth rate was similar to the annual growth observed the mid-1990s, when a series of sociocultural transformations (including the increase of education level in female population and the development of the service sector) facilitated the process. In 2008, the employment rate of women reached 51.6% (CNEL, 2009). Breaking a nearly decade-long declining trend in 2008, the unemployment rate grew, increasing to 6.8% in 2008 (CNEL, 2009). The increase in unemployment was widespread, a cross economic classes, geographic regions, and age groups.

At the end of the 20th century, Italy ranked among the top industrial countries in the world, especially in the northern hemisphere. Italian industries produce textiles, chemicals, vehicles, heavy machinery, electrical goods, and food. However, more than 30% of the land area was still devoted to crops, orchards, or vineyards. In 2008, the GDP reached the value of 1,272,852 million euros (ISTAT, 2009a). In Italy, the economic picture has since deteriorated, especially in the last quarter of 2008; in fact, there has been a decrease of GDP by 1 percentage point and a decrease in expenditure of resident households of 0.9%. Much graver is the decline of gross fixed investment (-3.0%) and foreign trade (exports down 3.7%, imports down 4.5%). Inflation due to the sudden rising energy prices, and then declining in the fall, has averaged 3.3% yearly (3.5% since the harmonized Eurostat).

With respect to the religious beliefs and practices of Italians, most are Catholic. The largest minority consists of recent Islamic immigrants. Also, the presence of the Vatican in Italy has a very strong role on the society's decisions (Cartocci, 2001; Inglehart, 1997).

The family remains the most important institution in most Italians' lives, although there are some changes occurring in this area (Cavalli, 2001). For many reasons, the Italian family now closely resembles the norms that prevail in the rest of Europe; as it has trended from a larger family to a smaller one caused by a declining birth rate (Cavalli, 2001). On the other hand, Italy's family structure remains distinctively Mediterranean rather than North European.

The average level of education has increased in the last 40 years. In 1951, 9.2% of the total population held a secondary degree, while in 2004 that percentage reached 62.9%. However, the percentage of the population with a tertiary level of education remains rather low—1% in 1951 and 8.6% in 2004 (ISTAT, 2005).

The Italian parliament consists of a senate and a chamber of deputies elected by popular election for 5-year terms. The president of the Italian Republic is elected for a 7-year term by a joint session of parliament and has the right to dissolve the senate and chamber of deputies at any time except during the last 6 months of his tenure. The actual running of the government is in the hands of the prime minister, who is chosen by the president and must have the confidence of the parliament.

Italy is divided into 20 regions and 2 autonomous provinces. Each region is governed by a governor and council elected directly by the resident population. The regional governments have considerable authority, and in particular, are responsible for the health of the population.

In Italy, workplace health promotion (WHP) is a very popular theme at a cultural level debate, but it is still not very popular in practice. Although there are examples of good practice (Briziarelli, 1996) in the implementation of processes to promote the health of employees, they are few compared to the total number of firms and workers. A significant step in the development of WHP started in 1996 with the establishment of the European Network for Workplace Health Promotion (ENWHP) (Kuhn, Henke, & Peters, 1999). In Italy, one of the founders of this network, the University of Perugia Department of Public Health, was the research leader for the network. Slowly, the promotion of health in the workplace is gaining consensus in Italy and becoming more and more familiar to companies in particular.

## Prevailing Health Issues and Risk Behaviors

Life expectancy at birth has definitively increased over the past 40 years. Thus, a female born in 2008 may expect to live more than 82 years and a male almost 77 years. The increase in life expectancy at birth and the reduction in births are well-established trends in Italy. This implies a significant increase in the elderly population. These demographic changes are affecting the determination of health needs, creating an epidemiological picture that reveals the prevalence of certain types of diseases that affect the older population, such as chronic degenerative diseases and cancer (Ministero della Salute, 2008).

In Italy, cardiovascular diseases are one of the most important public health problems, and in fact, are the leading cause of death and disability in the elderly population. The frequency of new coronary events a year in the age group 35–69 years is 5.7 per 1,000 men and 1.7 per 1,000 women. For cerebrovascular events, the incidence is 2.3 for 1,000 in men and 1.4 for 1,000 in women (Ministero del Lavoro, 2009). Another very common disorder is diabetes mellitus, which in Italy affects about 2.5 million people, with 30% of the patients affected by at least 1 complication (Ministero del Lavoro, 2009). Every year in Italy there are about 240,000 new cancer cases and 140,000 are mortal (28% mortality overall). It has been estimated that beginning in 2010 there will be about 270,000 new cases of cancer each year and 145,000 will be mortal. In data from the Italian Cancer Registries, lung cancer has the highest incidence, followed by breast cancer, then colon-rectum and stomach (Ministero del Lavoro, 2009). The incidence of these diseases is constantly increasing because of both the aging population and the growing exposure to risk factors such as smoking, alcohol, improper diet, and lack of physical inactivity.

In Italy, prevalence of new smokers is still too high, especially among the young and women. Smoking is particularly risky among women of childbearing age, with consequent health risks even for the unborn. Smoke exposure and passive smoking, especially in the workplace and at home, are responsible for the increase of respiratory diseases in children (e.g., bronchial asthma), and lung cancer and cardiovascular disease in adults.

Alcohol abuse is another important health focus in Italy. The reduction of health and social harm caused by alcohol has been recognized as one of the most important public health objectives. There are about 900,000 young people under 16 years of age who self-report that they drink alcohol at least once a day (ISTAT, 2008). A comparison between 1998 and 2005 shows that the percentage of consumers of alcohol among persons aged 14 and over remained stable at around 70%. In 2005, almost one third of the population 11 years of age and over (31%)

were daily consumers of alcohol. Alcohol was a factor in the cause of 30–50% of road accidents and the leading cause of death for young people aged 18–24 years of age. According to ISTAT, in 2007, alcohol-related traffic accidents resulted in 5,131 deaths from 230,871 road accidents, while 325,850 others suffered injuries of varying severity (ISTAT, 2007).

Diet contributes to unhealthy lifestyles, usually with a low intake of fruit and vegetables, excess consumption of fat, and low physical activity. The prevalence of obesity and overweight in the north of Italy is 19.3% and in south, 28.7%. The phenomenon of obesity in childhood is now an alarming issue. In Italy, one child in every four is affected by overweight or obesity (ISTAT, 2008).

Analysis of reports of occupational diseases since 2005 reveals that after an initial 3-year period (2004–2006), the numbers remained substantially stable, around 26,700 cases (INAIL, 2009). In 2008–2009, there was an increase of 3,000 registered cases (+11.7%) (INAIL, 2009). In 2008, INAIL registered 874,940 injuries, which is almost 37,500 cases less than in 2007. This represents a decrease of 4.1%, a significant improvement on the decrease of 1.7% registered in 2007. Even the statistics for fatal accidents in 2008 are numerically better: 1,120 died at work in 2008—a reduction of 7.2% compared to the 1,207 workplace deaths of the previous year.

## Healthcare System

Health care in Italy is provided by the National Health System (NHS), a government-funded institution that provides medical care to the entire population. It was introduced by Law n. 833 of December 27, 1978, which sought to implement the constitutional principle of health protection as a fundamental right of the individual and as a community interest (Article 32 of the Constitution). This public service is governed by the Ministry of Health and administered locally by local health units (today called agencies) intended for the protection of the health of citizens and workers by means of prevention, treatment, and rehabilitation (Caroppo & Turati, 2007). The four principles on which the law has been based are:

1. To guarantee health for all persons
2. To provide equal accessibility and distribution of health services
3. To provide a free service for Italian citizens
4. To protect and respect the dignity of all

The NHS is the shared responsibility of all: the national, regional, and local governments, with the active participation of the population.

The NHS is financed through the general taxation with the aim to guarantee equal levels of assistance for everyone. The individual contribution is independent from the risk of disease or the number of services used, but determined exclusively from the individuals' taxpaying capacity. Generally free, or with a small copayment, anyone can receive diagnostic procedures and treatment from a family doctor, pediatrician, district of the local health agency, or hospital. Primary and secondary prevention and rehabilitation services are accessed in the same way.

The current practice of occupational health is regulated by the Legislative Decree 81/2008, which is a collection of general regulations and indications for prevention in the workplace. This legislative decree indicates two levels of prevention. At the first level, the company level, the employer is obliged to guarantee the health and safety of his employees. To oversee health and occupational and environmental medicine, physicians collaborate with the employers to evaluate the risks present, who and which risks will face the single worker or freelancer and decide with him which preventive measures and controls will be necessary. The participation of the employees, a basic criterion for prevention in the workplace, is assured by an employee representative for prevention and safety within the company or group of companies. This person is required to take an active part in the application of prevention regulations, both by collaborating with others involved in prevention within the company, and also by informing and motivating the workers themselves, as they should be the recipients of prevention regulations. The second level of prevention as outlined in the decree involves the local health services. In particular, the legislation indicates that the Workplace Prevention and Safety Services located in the local department of prevention have the responsibility for checking and monitoring the application of laws related to health and safety.

Today, the law (dating from 2008) has added WHP and the necessity of evaluating psychosocial risk factors to its scope. The 1994 national health plan explicitly introduced health promotion in the repertoire of intervention strategies. It is known that promotion of well-being is best accomplished by implementing programs in a variety of settings, based on the population and the goals of specific interventions. The school and the workplace are among the main settings in Italy, and the workplace has been gaining importance as a focal point for health promotion interventions. In addition, recent studies and interventions have addressed issues related to the quality of life in various neighborhoods. These interventions are generally aimed at the improvement of relationships between citizens and social structures, such as schools, the local health agencies, and the local government, in order to create better living environments.

Health expenditure accounts for about 7% of GDP; furthermore, over the last decades, it has been growing significantly faster than income (ISTAT, 2009b). Given the projected aging of the population and, with that, associated medical costs, it seems likely that expenditure will continue to increase. Recent projections published by the Economic Policy Committee and the Organization for Economic Cooperation and Development (OECD) confirm these trends, with health expenses expected to have a high growth rate among age-related expenditures. The actual growth rate of public health expenditure over the period 1996–2006 was on average 4.7%, more than 1.5 times the annual growth rate registered in the previous decade (Francese & Romanelli, 2009).

Pharmaceuticals were the main drivers of the strong rising trend observed between 1996 and 2006 (OSMED, 2008), with nominal prices having increased on average by 8.6% per year and consumption 7.3%. In 2007, the increasing ratio of public health expenditure to GDP seemed to stop. According to the annual statistics, 2005, the capacity of the NHS was 103,658 doctors working in hospitals; 230,251 nurses in hospitals; 47,022 MMG, and 1,222 structures (public/private 214,225/51,130 beds).

## Influence of Culture and Mentality

Italy is a country of rich tradition and heritage. A part of this heritage has been the role of alcohol and drinking in daily life. Alcohol, especially wine, has been present in Italy from ancient times. The Mediterranean countries are wine producers, and for most of them, wine production and marketing are important economic issues (Osservatorio Permanente Alcool e Giovani, 2007). Drinking wine is part of daily life, and values and traditions related to alcoholic beverages are different than in northern Europe. Trends in consumption and alcohol-related mortality, as well as changes in patterns of drinking, appear specific to southern European countries as opposed to northern Europe (Österberg & Karlsson, 2002).

The consumption of alcohol is not a topic of primary interest. In fact, southern Europeans do not equate alcohol with wine, but rather with spirits, while they may identify beer with soft drinks.

A study in 2007 investigated the relationship between changes in the dietary habits of Italians and the food culture of the country (De Rita, 2007). This study discovered that Italians are traditionalists, being the last in Europe in the ranking of changes in dietary habits (15% versus 22%). Italians are rediscovering the pleasure of breakfast (+11.7% in the period 1995–2005), which includes food and milk, not just coffee. The working rhythm and working hours influence the Italian meal habits. For many, dinner is becoming the main meal of the day. The increased focus on work has left less time for cooking, and therefore, increased the consumption of ready foods.

Globalization has had an impact on food customs and has led to the emergence of some fears resulting from the national mass marketing of fast foods. Unlike in other countries, in Italy the industrialization of food production has not been imposed on the existing culture, by inventing and imposing new products, but rather was integrated into the traditional culture. Food culture, in recent years, has become one of the Italians' increased interests. The adoption of a Western lifestyle has had a strong negative effect on consumption of food, nutrition, and eating habits in Italy (Raine et al., 2008). Furthermore, since cars have become more popular, the population has become less inclined to be physically active.

## Drivers of Workplace Health Promotion

Towards the end of the 1970s in Italy, Law 833 transferred the control for workers' health to local structures of the NHS. This move was aimed at providing more equality of services focusing on the health of the worker, although in reality, the differences did not disappear completely. The reason for this is that the preexisting laws regulating the technical aspects of prevention and safety were not adjusted in accordance with the cultural and sociopolitical changes that led to the creation of the NHS. Also, the laws governing working environment enacted after this date maintained this double standard. Typical examples are the regulations applying to noise and asbestos. These are completely different in the ways in which they apply to living conditions, on the one hand, and working environments, on the other, in terms of threshold levels, methods for ascertaining the existence of the hazard, and prevention regulations.

More recently, directives of the European Union have made the situation more complex by restating the central importance of business needs. In countries such as Italy, where the creation of the NHS placed the protection of workers' health under the wing of public services, this has created some difficulties.

In the last two national health plans and in several regional ones, health promotion and education are clearly indicated as the most important strategies that health professionals can bring to the table. To summarize, Italy did not create a national institute for health promotion first and then focus on health promotion afterwards; instead, the principles of health promotion were and are present in the local and regional levels. In fact, at regional and local levels, the NHS gave itself a clear structure for health promotion.

In countries such as Italy, in which control of workers' health is in the hands of the NHS, the right to a healthy life is constrained by a number of factors, including economic background, the views of employers, and the so-called rules of the labor market and market forces.

In 1996, Italy joined the European Network for Workplace Health Promotion. The network aims to increase awareness of the promotion of health in the workplace (WHP) among businesses, especially small and medium-sized enterprises, and to raise awareness, encouraging them to adopt a policy of developing human resources for WHP and overcome an attitude of passive compliance with the standards and legislation. An analysis of case studies in Italy shows that the adoption of a correct strategy for social responsibility has an inherent assumption that the implementation of programs in the promotion of health labor and the union of WHP and correct strategy for social responibility can significantly improve business performance, while reducing accidents and occupational diseases of workers. For these reasons, Istituto Superiore Prevenzione e Sicurezza sul Lavoro (Institute for Prevention and Safety at Work) (in collaboration with the Department of Medical Surgical Specialties and Public Health of the University of Perugia for the European Network for Workplace Health Promotion Italy) ensures the dissemination of models of good practice in small, medium, and large companies in Italy and Europe, encouraging action, studies, and research. Today as a result of the new organization of the state and the evolution of the law on health and safety, the scenario has changed significantly. Today, the main drivers for WHP are the regional governments, mayors, and/or the companies themselves. Due to the reorganization of the state of Italy and the new equilibrium between regional and central government, the responsibility for the health of the population falls directly under the regional governments. The central government, in collaboration with the regions, set the minimum level of services that the government must provide; the rest depends on regional funds and know-how. The second drivers are the companies that have already integrated the WHP philosophy; their success is more and more a cause for interest to other companies and the mass media. We continue to focus increasing attention on the successful aspects of those programs, even as the number of companies that utilize health education programs continues to grow.

## Programs and Good Practices

*Azienda sana* is a contest organized by the Veneto region in collaboration with all stakeholders at the regional level. It is open to all of the region's public and private companies, with the aim of recognizing and rewarding those companies' projects and initiatives that were developed with standards of quality with respect to the following: information and training on health and safety, implementation of systems for managing health and safety, promotion of health, and corporate social responsibility. The competition is also an instrument for conveying company guidelines and standards of reference for regional, national, and European levels; for working with quality standards in training and management systems for health and safety at work; and for promoting corporate social responsibility. It also provides an occasion to raise awareness of workplace health, to enhance the commitment and investment of companies dedicated to the improvement of working conditions and health, and to facilitate, circulate, and export the most significant and valuable contributions to other manufacturers. Today, all the companies that participated (around 400) have created a regional network of healthy companies that work in collaboration with local health services and researchers to document evidence of successful programs and to try to continue to improve their management systems.

In Italy, the research group of the Department of Public Health at the University of Perugia has identified many models of good practice drawn from different branches of companies of various sizes (Briziarelli, Masanotti, Notargiacomo, & Perticaroli, 2000; ENWHP, 1999). Two models of good practices are Acroplastica s.r.l., Caserta, and Brunello Cucinelli S.p.A.

### Acroplastica s.r.l., Caserta

Acroplastica s.r.l. is a thermoplastic and thermosetting industry that today employs over 150 workers, up from 69 when the company began. A management team at Acroplastica composed of representatives of the human resources department, the staff, the safety department, and occupational medical services jointly developed written guidelines on workplace health promotion. Those guidelines were designed to ensure the safety and protection of all employees at the workplace, to provide a healthy lifestyle, and to prevent environmental hazards.

With respect to management responsibilities, the executive team is responsible for all health and safety activities. The staff representatives are responsible for detecting risks and developing appropriate preventive actions. Staff surveys focused on work requirements and staff needs are undertaken twice a year and provide statistics with respect to days lost due to illness and industrial accidents and occupational medical reports. These surveys provide valuable information that is used for planning workplace health promotion activities. On average, every employee spends 40 hours a year taking training courses on quality management and health and safety issues. The need for future training is reviewed regularly. Employees are also involved in planning new jobs and work processes. These measures are assisted by working groups that deal with quality issues on health and safety matters. The company also provides rest and break rooms and organizes drug support programs and various sport and leisure time events.

Since the company adopted this strategy in 1995, employees are more satisfied with their working conditions, with the executive team, and with the working atmosphere. This has been evaluated with anonymous questionnaires, and the results obtained in only 5 years are amazing; worker satisfaction is over 97%, the number of smokers dropped to a significant 24%, and the absenteeism rate fell to 2%. The number of accidents registered in the period 1998–2000 was less than one per year, and since then, no accidents have been registered.

These processes have also had a positive impact on business (+39% in the last 3 years), consolidating the position of the company on the European market. These strategies have contributed to a series of other positive economic results for the company—the consumption of electricity and the production of refusals decreased respectively by 9% and 46%, while the number of employees increased by 26%.

## Brunello Cucinelli S.p.A.

Brunello Cucinelli, Perugia, was founded in 1978, and has three plants manufacturing cashmere garments for men and women. The workforce is very young, with an average age of 33.8. Nobody works part time and there are no night shifts. The company was founded with 5 workers, and today it has 456 employees.

The company believes that equality and informality help to bring out the best in its employees. The same democratic policy is applied at all three sites, and everyone is on a first-name basis. This employee-centered culture allows individuals to express themselves in a way that is not possible in a strictly hierarchical environment. The management team is eager to allow each employee to use his or her personal skills. In fact, when new employees are hired, the company takes a very close look at the positive benefits that each individual brings with him or her. Personality is also considered to be an important factor in terms of staff relationships; as a happy working environment is enjoyed at all sites, the managers do not want a new employee to upset this balance by bringing a difficult personality into the equation.

Emphasis is also placed on developing skills via practical, ongoing training. Employees are actively involved in the planning and decision-making processes and are encouraged to voice their opinions. Twice-yearly meetings are arranged so that any problems within the organization can be discussed and resolved. When a problem is identified, action is taken immediately to make corrections. The situation is then reviewed 2 months later to see if the steps taken are working. Staff are also able to have input into this process. Very often these meetings are not necessary, as the channels of communication are such that staff can discuss problems with management at any time.

Employees have control over their working lives, and the flexibility encouraged by the company means that they can arrange their working hours to fit in with family commitments. In fact, no formal permission is required if a staff member has to leave work early for family reasons. Employee and customer satisfaction are also evaluated regularly.

Management places the highest priority on the health and safety of the workforce. However, every person in the company is expected to take active responsibility for health and safety. The management team regularly reviews health promotion activities and periodically assesses the health of individual workers. Resources are set aside specifically for health and training purposes; however, no definite sum is allocated because activities depend on the requests submitted by the staff. If a staff member is on sick leave for a long time, efforts are made to reinstate that person gradually, so that physical and psychological adjustments can be made.

Every year 40 employees (25% of the total workforce) are able to attend external courses on a wide range of subjects, including ergonomics, correct posture and lifting techniques, fire safety, and first aid. Air conditioning systems have been installed and new computer monitors introduced. More comfortable desks and chairs have also been purchased following consultation with staff.

Employees are always consulted before the company makes any changes or installs new equipment. Management is keenly aware that the impact of change in the workplace is felt most acutely by the employees, and takes steps to ensure that staff are happy with each and every development.

The business is run along the lines of a family. Staff relationships are excellent, and at the end of the year, incentive bonuses are distributed equally regardless of the seniority of employees—a decision reached by staff members themselves. The atmosphere at work is extremely informal, yet highly professional.

Efforts are made to give staff as much time off as possible, and at traditional holiday times such as Christmas and Easter, the company closes 2 days earlier than other organizations. Staff members have access to break and rest rooms, a work medical service, and a canteen where special meals can be prepared upon request.

Brunello Cucinelli and the community are strongly interlinked. Almost every family in the area has at least one member working there. The company is very much aware that it is located in a beautiful part of Italy and is concerned with maintaining the highest possible environmental standards. It has also donated money for a community soccer field and has financed the restoration of a number of medieval buildings in the region. One building in particular, on a former farm, has been turned into an attractive community center where many cultural events are held and which has a cafe where local people enjoy meeting.

## Outcomes and Indicators

Monitoring and evaluation should be an integral part of the process of goal-setting and development of a workplace health promotion program. It is essential to identify and employ, from the outset, a set of criteria and indicators essential to a system of managing health and environment in the workplace (U.S. Department of Health and Human Services, 1991). The skills for measuring indicators and evaluating the management of health, environment, and safety are very valuable.

In developing procedures and evaluation indicators, it is necessary to take into account the difficulties encountered when collecting statistics to determine the health-related effects of employment and environmental workplace factors such as lifestyle and social behaviors. The indicators must be relevant and meaningful for improving human health. They must allow the demonstration of the improvements achieved within the company or group of companies, using the same system of assessment of health, environment, and security (Van Dijk, Hulshof, & Verbeek, 1999).

The output is a direct result of various health, environment, and safety management processes. In general, the output indicators are criteria used for the assessment of the extent or the intensity of the work done by the system management of health, environment, and safety at the enterprise level (HESME). Therefore, these indicators can be used to evaluate the performance of the HESME system, but not necessarily to evaluate the final result. The output indicators are related to the final results of HESME, although some factors that are not controllable by the HESME system can influence the value of performance indicators such as the rate of absenteeism due to illness. Other output indicators might be:

- Mortality rate for accidents at work
- Incidence of serious nonfatal accidents
- Accident rate (more than 3 days of leave for health reasons)
- Incidence and prevalence of occupational diseases compensated for cause, age, sex, and occupation
- Estimated rate of work-related illnesses, including incidence, prevalence, and mortality
- Rate of morbidity due to age, sex, and occupation
- Absence from work due to illness, age, and occupation
- Percentage of smokers by age, gender, and occupation
- Production of an annual report on the performance HESME
- Presence of harmful factors (by type of factors, including physical, chemical, biological, and mental health impairing)
- Test of HESME policy development, which should include the involvement of workers
- Test of the implementation of the system for managing health, environment, and security, with the participation of workers
- Energy use in production units or units of income gross
- Total water use
- Total volume of waste generated (reused, recycled, incinerated, or deposited) and generation of solid waste
- Generation of hazardous waste

- Emission of exhaust gases into the atmosphere
- Discharge of waste water

The choice of indicators, the monitoring system, and the dissemination of results inside and outside the company are of fundamental importance in ensuring the success of various initiatives and a high standard of quality (Masanotti, 2001). The indicators can be short-, medium-, and long-term, based on objectives. The achievement of these objectives is essential because when WHP activities and objectives are fulfilled, employers tend to expect financial success from these activities. Employers hope for economic benefits from a decrease in absenteeism and a decreased number of injuries, including greater efficiency, higher quality products, improved business, and better customer satisfaction. Employees, meanwhile, expect to improve their quality of life through increased satisfaction at work, stress reduction, improvement in their working environment, and the reduction of diseases linked to work.

## Existing Research

Current research priorities include a better understanding of the following issues: the specific dimensions of healthy and unhealthy jobs; the ways in which healthy working conditions and productivity can go together and can be in conflict; gender-specific work conditions and health linkages, especially with respect to physical and psychosocial hazards in the workplace; and the costs of unhealthy working conditions for business and society in general. Today, research in the field of health and safety is in line with indications coming from the EU community and conducted within the relevant networks present in Europe. Italy is a part of several networks, including the European Agency for Safety and Health at Work, the European Network for Workplace Health Promotion, the Network on Prevention and Promotion of Healthy Lifestyles, EPODE, the European Network Education and Training in Occupational Safety and Health, and the European Occupational Safety and Health Network. The research commissioned from these networks focuses on concerns ranging from standardization to guidelines, from research to evaluation, from safety to health promotion. In the last period, the health-related priorities for the European community were lifestyle concerns (e.g., diet, physical activity, and smoking) and mental health in general and specifically in the workplace.

## Conclusion

Workplace health promotion (WHP) is a process of awareness and change that directly involves all stakeholders (both workers and employers) and promotes well-being and the adoption of healthy lifestyles. Currently the demand for WHP is still low because companies are concerned almost exclusively with ensuring compliance with regulatory obligations imposed by D.Lg.81/08. This new law introduced the terms *health promotion, psychosocial, risks/evalua-*

*tion,* etc. The implementation of health management systems must not be limited to safety prescriptions and the mitigation of risk factors, but must also promote employee well-being. Therefore, it is desirable and expected that companies support an increase in WHP activities to better satisfy the new law and the market's need for quality products and services. In this way, there will be a transition from a static view (risk management) to a more dynamic emphasis (management of one's own health and welfare). It is clear that work must be done to advance a health-promoting culture. Only by working at that level will it be possible to make the new regulations effective. Paying greater attention to safety, health, and the environment can also have a positive effect on the community.

Under a recently established initiative, WHP also has been clearly recognized as an essential component for the evaluation of management of occupational health and safety equipment systems. Each firm must move from a culture of mere technical and organizational adaptation to a common culture of prevention based on clear information and training. A common expression is that a global company is reluctant to face safety problems with courage and determination, but for the most part the business world knows that the compatibility of production, safety, environment, and health are fundamental, as is the population's strong acceptance of their importance. But laws alone are not enough. The culture must change. Safety must be taught in school, so that it may enter in the conscience of future workers and future business owners. Safety education must be instilled in our set of personal values, not just as rules to be followed, not just as obligations to be fulfilled, but in the full awareness that working in safety not only protects human lives but also increases a country's wealth, reduces social costs at the root, and provides a stimulus for healthy economic competition. Along with laws and controls to ensure that the laws are observed, there must be a common commitment particularly in the schools and in the workplace in order to spread the culture for health.

## Summary

Italy is a peninsula located in the south of Europe and is demographically in transition from very young to one of the oldest countries in the world. Health education is one of the fundamental principles of the National Health System, but only since the late 1990s have health education and promotion been part of a clear strategy for future investments by the national government. The workplace is a key setting for this strategy, mainly due to the high level of accidents that take place each year in Italy. In this chapter, the author has highlighted the context, strengths, and weaknesses of the Italian system, the state of development and implementation of the promotion of health and safety in the workplace, and initiatives that might spur a change in today's trends.

## Review Questions

1. What is the significance of aging to Italy's health promotion efforts?
2. Name three lifestyle habits of the Italian population that contribute to poor health. Describe their impact on health promotion.
3. What are the components of the Italian healthcare system, and how are they funded? Regulated? Managed?
4. How does the Italian culture of food and alcohol consumption affect population health and health promotion efforts?
5. What are some of the factors constraining a healthy life for Italian workers?
6. Describe the mission, benefits, and challenges of the Azienda sana program.
7. Review the case study describing the Brunello Cucinelli workplace. How does this culture impact employee health?
8. List five output indicators of health, environment, and safety management processes and their purpose within workplace health promotion programs.
9. What are the future priorities for workplace health promotion research?

## References

Allamani, A., Anav, S., Cipriani, F., Rossi, D., & Voller, F. (2007). Osservatorio permanente sui giovani e l'alcool, *Quaderni dell'osservatorio 19, Italy and Alcohol: a country profile.* Rome, Italy: Litos.

Briziarelli, L. (1996). Practice of workplace health promotion in Italy. In *Conference Proceedings. ENWHP.* Dortmund, Germany.

Briziarelli, L., Masanotti, G., Notargiacomo, A., & Perticaroli, S. (2000). Workplace health promotion: The implementation. *Prevenzione oggi, (3),* 3–13.

Caroppo, M. S., & Turati, G. (2007). *I sistemi sanitari regionali in Italia.* Milan, Italy: Vita e Pensiero.

Cartocci, R. (2001). *Senso civico, identità italiana e identità Europea tra i giovani Italiani.* Bologna, Italy: Il Mulino.

Cavalli, A. (2001). Reflections on political culture and the "Italian national character." *Daedalus, 3* (130), 119–137.

Consiglio Nazionale dell'Economia e del Lavora (CNEL). (2009). *Mercato del Lavoro 2009–2010.* Retrieved November 2009 from www.portalecnel.it/.../

De Rita, G. (2007, November 16). L'evoluzione delle abitudini alimentari degli Italiani tra nuove tendenze e solide tradizioni. In atti del festeggiamenti per i cinquant'anni della delegazione locale dell'. Parma, Italy: AIC.

Economic Policy Committee and European Commission. (2006). *The impact of ageing on public expenditure: Projections for the EU-25 Member States on pensions, health care, long-term care, education and Unemployment Transfers (2004–2050).* Retrieved from http://ec.europa.eu/economy_finance/publications/publication_summary6656_en.htm

ENWHP. (1999). *Healthy employees in healthy organisations: Models of good practices.* Essen, Germany: BKK.

Francese, M. E., & Romanelli, M. (2009). *Health care in Italy: The national health system, expenditure determinants and regional differentials.* Rome, Italy: Banca D. Italia.

INAIL. (2009). *Rapporto annuale inail: Analisi dell. Fandamento Infortunistico 2008.* Milan, Italy: INAIL.

Inglehart, R. (1997). *Modernization and post-modernization: Cultural, economic, and political change in 43 societies.* Princeton, NJ: Princeton University Press.

ISTAT. (2005). *Bilancio demografico nazionale—Periodo di riferimento: Anno 2004.* Annuario statistico italiano 2005.

ISTAT. (2006). *Bilancio demografico nazionale—Periodo di riferimento: Anno 2005.* Annuario statistico italiano 2006.

ISTAT. (2007). *Health for All.* Rome, Italy.

ISTAT. (2008). *Conti Economici Regionali 2008.* Rome, Italy.

ISTAT. (2008, 2009). *Rilevaziones sulle forze de lavoro.* Rome, Italy.

ISTAT. (2009a). *Annuario ISTAT 2008: sanità e salute in Italia.* Rome, Italy: ISTAT

ISTAT. (2009b). *Bilancio demografico nazionale—Periodo di riferimento: Anno 2008.* Annuario statistico italiano 2009.

Kuhn, K., Henke, H., & Peters, V. (1999). *ENWHP, final report 1998.* Dortmund, Germany: Bundesanstalt fur Arbeitsschutz und Arbeitsmedizin Hauptsitiz.

Masanotti, G. (2002, April). Modello teorico e presentazione della banca dati dei modelli di buona pratica. In *Atti della Conferenza Nazionale sulla Salute e Sicurezza nei luoghi di lavoro—Symposium Europeo Sulla Promozione Della Salute Nei Paesi Del Sud Europa. Italia, Siracusa 5-6-7.* Rome, Italy: Rondomedia.

Ministero del Lavoro, della Salute e delle Politiche Sociali. (2009). Relazione sullo Stato Sanitario del Paese 2007–2008. Rome, Italy: Ministero del Lavoro, della Salute e delle Politiche Sociali.

Ministero della Salute. (2007). *Rapporto nazionale di monitoraggio dei livelli essenziali di assistenza—Anno 2004.* Rome, Italy.

Ministero della Salute. (2008). Piano sanitario nazionale 2006–2008. Rome, Italy: Ministero.

OECD. (2006). Future budget pressures arising from spending on health and long-term care. *Economic Outlook, 2006 1*(79).

Osservatorio Nazionale sull'Imiego dei Medicinali. (2008). *L'uso dei Farmaci in Italia. Rapporto Nazionale 2007.* Rome, Italy.

Osservatorio Permanente Alcool e Giovani. (2007). *Italians and alcohol.* Rome, Italy: Casa Editrice Litos

Österberg, E., & Karlsson, T. (2002). Alcohol policies in EU member states and Norway. In *A collection of country reports.* Helsinki, Finland: Stakes.

Raine, K, Spence, J. C., Church, J., Boulé, N., Slater, L., Marko, J., … (2008). *State of the evidence review on urban health and healthy weights.* Ottawa, Canada: CIHI.

U.S. Department of Health and Human Services. (1991). *Healthy people 2000: National health promotion and disease prevention objectives.* Washington, DC: ODPHP Communication Support Centre.

Van Dijk, V. J. H., Hulshof, C. T. J., & Verbeek, J. H. A. M. (1999). Good occupational health practice: Concepts and criteria. In *Good occupational health practice and evaluation of occupational health services.* Research Reports 24. Helsinki, Finland: Finnish Institute of Occupational Health.

Chapter 14

# Japan

Takashi Muto

After reading this chapter you should be able to:

- Identify core strategies that are the focus of Japan's workplace health promotion efforts
- Describe Japan's historical evolution of workplace health promotion
- Explain the different approaches employed by corporate health promotion efforts throughout Japan
- Review the central disease states and health issues driving Japan's health promotion needs
- Name the components of, and the associated funding sources for, Japan's healthcare system
- Discuss the impact of culture on Japan's health status and health promotion efforts

Table 14-1 **Select Key Demographic and Economic Indicators**

| | |
|---|---|
| Nationality | Noun: Japanese (singular and plural)<br>Adjective: Japanese |
| Ethnic groups | Japanese 98.5%, Koreans 0.5%, Chinese 0.4%, other 0.6%<br>*Note:* up to 230,000 Brazilians of Japanese origin migrated to Japan in the 1990s to work in industries; some have returned to Brazil (2004) |
| Religion | Shintoism 83.9%, Buddhism 71.4%, Christianity 2%, other 7.8%<br>*Note:* total adherence exceeds 100% because many people belong to both Shintoism and Buddhism (2005) |
| Language | Japanese |
| Literacy | Definition: age 15 and over can read and write<br>Total population: 99%<br>Male: 99%<br>Female: 99% (2002) |
| Education expenditure | 3.5% of GDP (2005)<br>Country comparison to the world: 128 |

*continued*

| Table 14-1 **Select Key Demographic and Economic Indicators,** *continued* | |
|---|---|
| Government type | A parliamentary government with a constitutional monarchy |
| Environment | Air pollution from power plant emissions results in acid rain; acidification of lakes and reservoirs degrading water quality and threatening aquatic life; Japan is one of the largest consumers of fish and tropical timber, contributing to the depletion of these resources in Asia and elsewhere |
| Country mass | Total: 377,915 sq km<br>Country comparison to the world: 61<br>Land: 364,485 sq km<br>Water: 13,430 sq km<br>*Note:* includes Bonin Islands (Ogasawara-gunto), Daito-shoto, Minami-jima, Okino-tori-shima, Ryukyu Islands (Nansei-shoto), and Volcano Islands (Kazan-retto) |
| Population | 127,078,679 (July 2009 est.)<br>Country comparison to the world: 10 |
| Age structure | 0–14 years: 13.5% (male 8,804,465/female 8,344,800)<br>15–64 years: 64.3% (male 41,187,425/female 40,533,876)<br>65 years and over: 22.2% (male 11,964,694/female 009 est.) |
| Median age | Total: 44.6 years<br>Male: 42.9 years<br>Female: 46.5 years (2010 est.) |
| Population growth rate | -0.191% (2010 est.)<br>Country comparison to the world: 217 |
| Birth rate | 7.64 births/1,000 population (2010 est.)<br>Country comparison to the world: 222 |
| Death rate | 9.54 deaths/1,000 population (July 2010 est.)<br>Country comparison to the world: 69 |
| Net migration rate | NA (2009 est.) |
| Urbanization | Urban population: 66% of total population (2008)<br>Rate of urbanization: 0.2% annual rate of change (2005–2010 est.) |
| Gender ratio | At birth: 1.06 male(s)/female<br>Under 15 years: 1.06 male(s)/female<br>15–64 years: 1.02 male(s)/female<br>65 years and over: 0.74 male(s)/female<br>Total population: 0.95 male(s)/female (2010 est.) |
| Infant mortality rate | Total: 2.79 deaths/1,000 live births<br>Country comparison to the world: 221<br>Male: 2.99 deaths/1,000 live births<br>Female: 2.58 deaths/1,000 live births (2010 est.) |

*continued*

| Table 14-1 **Select Key Demographic and Economic Indicators,** *continued* | |
|---|---|
| Life expectancy | Total population: 82.12 years<br>Country comparison to the world: 3<br>Male: 78.8 years<br>Female: 85.62 years (2010 est.) |
| Total fertility rate | 1.21 children born/woman (2010 est.)<br>Country comparison to the world: 218 |
| GDP—purchasing power parity | $4.15 trillion (2009 est.)<br>Country comparison to the world: 4 |
| GDP—per capita | $32,700 (2009 est.)<br>Country comparison to the world: 40 |
| GDP—composition by sector | Agriculture: 1.6%<br>Industry: 21.9%<br>Services: 76.5% (2009 est.) |
| Agriculture—products | Rice, sugar beets, vegetables, fruit, pork, poultry, dairy products, eggs, fish |
| Industries | Among world's largest and most technologically advanced producers of motor vehicles, electronic equipment, machine tools, steel and nonferrous metals, ships, chemicals, textiles, processed foods |
| Labor force participation | 65.93 million (2009 est.)<br>Country comparison to the world: 9 |
| Unemployment rate | 5.1% (2009 est.)<br>Country comparison to the world: 46 |
| Industrial production growth rate | -17% (2009 est.)<br>Country comparison to the world: 159 |
| Distribution of family income (GINI index) | 38.1 (2002)<br>Country comparison to the world: 74 |
| Investment (gross fixed) | 20.6% of GDP (2009 est.)<br>Country comparison to the world: 86 |
| Public debt | 189.3% of GDP (2009 est.)<br>Country comparison to the world: 2 |
| Market value of publicly traded shares | $NA (December 31, 2009)<br>Country comparison to the world: 3 |
| Current account balance | $140.6 billion (2009 est.)<br>Country comparison to the world: 2 |
| Debt (external) | $2.132 trillion (June 30, 2009 est.)<br>Country comparison to the world: 8 |
| Debt as a % of GDP | ——— |

*continued*

| Table 14-1 Select Key Demographic and Economic Indicators, *continued* | |
|---|---|
| Exports | $542.3 billion (2009 est.)<br>Country comparison to the world: 5 |
| Exports—commodities | Transport equipment, motor vehicles, semiconductors, electrical machinery, chemicals |
| Export—partners | China 18.88%, United States 16.42%, South Korea 8.13%, Taiwan 6.27%, Hong Kong 5.49% (2009) |
| Imports | $499.7 billion (2009 est.)<br>Country comparison to the world: 6 |
| Import—commodities | Machinery and equipment, fuels, foodstuffs, chemicals, textiles, raw materials |
| Import—partners | China 22.2%, United States 10.96%, Australia 6.29%, Saudi Arabia 5.29%, United Arab Emirates 4.12%, S. Korea, 3.98%, Indonesia 3.95% (2008) |
| Stock of direct foreign investment | |
| Home | $151.5 billion (December 31, 2009 est.)<br>Country comparison to the world: 25 |
| Abroad | $747.1 billion (December 31, 2009 est.)<br>Country comparison to the world: 8 |

Source: CIA. (2010). *The world factbook.* Retrieved December 16, 2010, from https://www.cia.gov/library/publications/the-world-factbook/

# Introduction

## Key Demographics

Japan is an island nation situated off the eastern seaboard of the Eurasian continent in the northern hemisphere. It consists of the main islands of Hokkaido, Honshu, Shikoku, Kyushu, and Okinawa. Its surface area totals approximately 380,000 square kilometers, which is 0.3% of the global land mass (*The World Factbook*, 2010). Forests, farmland, and residential land account for 66%, 13%, and 5% of the national land, respectively.

In 2008, Japan had a total population of 127.69 million. Japan's population in 2001 was the ninth largest in the world, equivalent to 2.1% of the global total. Its population density measured 341 persons per square kilometer, making it fourth among countries with a population of 10 million or more. After World War II, Japan's economy achieved high growth, becoming the economy with the second largest GDP in the world since 1967. It has remained the world's second largest economy.

The number of foreign residents in Japan is approximately 2 million (1.5% of the total population). Korea accounts for 32% of foreign residents, followed by China (24%), Brazil (14%), Philippines (10%), Peru (3%), and the United States (3%).

Japan's primary and mid-level education is based on a 6–3–3 system. Six years of elementary school and three years of junior high school are mandatory. Children enter elementary school at the age of six and graduate from junior high school at fifteen. There are no fees for tuition or textbooks for compulsory education at public schools. Almost 100% of junior high school graduates proceed to high schools, and approximately 50% of high school graduates go to universities or junior colleges.

In 2008, Japan's labor force was 66.48 million. The unemployment rate was 4.1%. The postwar Japanese employment system characterized by lifetime employment and seniority-based wage levels changed rather dramatically in the late 1980s and early 1990s as the economy underwent a severe and prolonged slump in a globalized business environment. The recent employment situation in Japan has been tough. The unemployment rate is high among young people because they do not seek jobs and are categorized as NEET (not in employment, education, or training). The unemployment rate is also high among middle-aged people because their ages surpass the employers' desired age limit.

## General Trends (Social, Political, Cultural, and Work)

Recently, socioeconomic environments surrounding Japanese companies have undergone drastic changes (Nariai, 2002). Severe competition due to globalization of the economy, the development of information technology, the aging of the workforce amid low birth rates, and the change in people's attitudes towards working life, such as a growing tendency to emphasize family and other interests over work, have in combination led to significant reform of all aspects of business operations and working patterns (Sasajima, 2003; Seike, 1997). These developments include changes in organizational structure and management style and the diversification of working patterns, such as temporary, flexible, and part-time work; telework; and small office or home office.

## Current National Issues

Declining birth rate and aging population are current national issues. In 2008, the total fertility rate (the average number of children to be born to a woman over the course of her lifetime) was 1.37. Population of the elderly (65 years and over) was 28.22 million and constituted 22.1% of the total population. The younger population (0–14 years) was 17.18 million, which was 13.5% of the total population. The population at productive age (15–64 years) totaled 82.30 million, accounting for 64.5% of the entire population (Okamoto, 1994; Haub, 2010).

The increase in national medical care expenditures is also a current national issue. The rapid progress of the aging population has resulted in a rise in medical costs for the elderly, and it is a major reason for the uptrend in national medical care expenditures. In the 2007 fiscal year, national medical care expenditure totaled about 31 trillion yen, or approximately 9% of GDP. Of these, medical costs for treating the elderly were about one third of total medical expenditure.

An increase in the number of suicide cases has become a national issue. The number of suicide cases has been more than 30,000 per year since 1998. The suicide rate is high for men in their 20s, 30s, and 40s, i.e., the working age population. Severe competition among companies brought about by economic globalization and information technology is considered to be the main reason for the increase.

### Significance of Workplace Health Promotion in Society

Interest in corporate social responsibility has been increasing in Japanese companies (Okamoto, 2004). Although corporate social responsibility is often mentioned and discussed in terms of environmental protection and in the compliance to laws and regulations, it should also be discussed in the field of occupational safety and health. The maintenance and promotion of employees' health through the prevention of occupational injuries and diseases should be an important corporate responsibility. However, as of yet, very few Japanese companies have documented corporate social responsibility incorporating occupational safety and health (Kawashita, Taniyama, Fujisaki, & Mori, 2005; Taniyama, Kawashita, So, & Mori, 2005). Corporate social responsibility and the occupational safety and health management system (OSHMS) share a common approach in that both are voluntary and do not depend on laws and regulation. Namely, both ideas are based on ethics, which should be discussed more in the field of occupational safety and health (Westerholm, Nilstun, & Ovretveit, 2004).

## Prevailing Health Issues and Risk Behaviors

### Life Expectancy

The average life expectancy in Japan was 86.05 years for women and 79.29 years for men in 2008. Japan has one of the highest average life expectancies in the world (*The World Factbook*, 2010). Along with improvements in living standards and better nutrition, the health insurance system has contributed to achieving levels of average life expectancy for the Japanese people.

### Disease Trends

The mortality rate was 8.2 per 1,000 persons, and the infant mortality rate was 2.8 per 1,000 live births in 2004. The major causes of death per 100,000 persons were malignant neoplasm (253.9), heart diseases (126.4), and cerebrovascular diseases (102.2). These three causes accounted for approximately 60% of all deaths. Malignant neoplasm became the leading cause of death in 1981, and has continued to increase, accounting for approximately 30% of all deaths.

## Health Status

Figure 14-1 shows the trend of the number of occupational injuries that needed 4 or more absence days (Japan Industrial Safety and Health Association [JISHA], 2004). The number of injuries decreased from more than 300,000 in the late 1970s to about 130,000 in 2003. Figure 14-1 also shows the trend of the number of worker deaths caused by occupational accidents. The number of deaths decreased from more than 3,000 in the late 1970s to less than 2,000 in 2003. Figure 14-2 shows the trend of the number of occupational diseases. The number of occupational diseases also has a decreasing tendency. Figure 14-3 shows the trend of abnormal rates at annual health checkups for workers. Approximately half of workers have at least one abnormality in health checkup items. Figure 14-4 shows the percentage of workers feeling severe stress at workplaces. The percentage has increased gradually, and about 60% of workers felt severe stress over the past 10 years.

## Health or Risk Behaviors

The trend of proportion of habitual exercisers who exercise for more than 30 minutes per day, more than twice per week, and for more than 1 year by age groups can be seen in Figure 14-5. The percentage is approximately 20% during 10 years, with no remarkable improvement. Figure 14-6 shows the trend of nutrition balance over 50 years. Intake of fat has gradually increased, and currently it is about 25%. The trend of salt intake per day is decreasing every year, but is still more than 10 g/day (Figure 14-7). Figure 14-8 shows the trend in the smoking rate. In men, it has decreased dramatically from 60% in the 1980s to 37% in 2008, but it was still high compared to the United States, United Kingdom, and Canada.

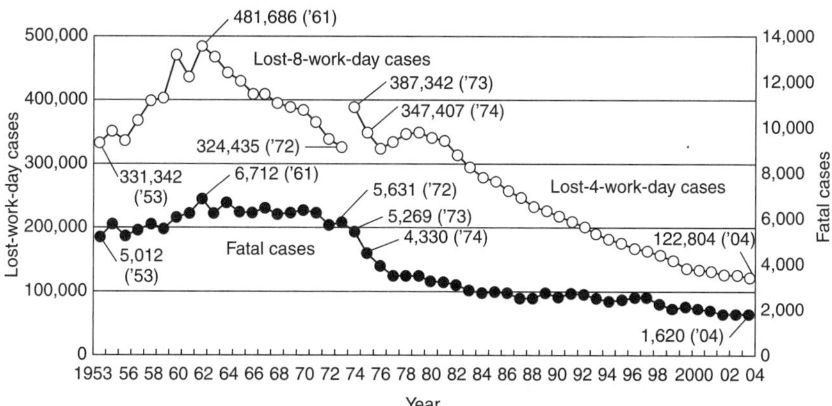

Figure 14-1 Trend of lost work days and fatal cases in Japan.
Source: Japan Industrial Safety and Health Association. (JISHA) (2004).

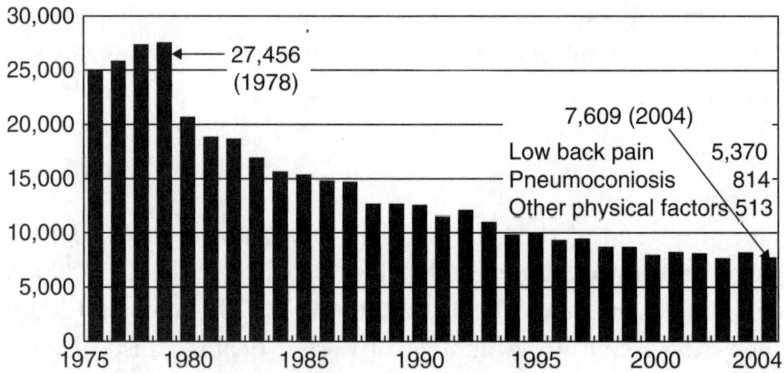


Figure 14-2 Trend of number of occupational diseases in Japan.
Source: Ministry of Health, Labour, and Welfare.

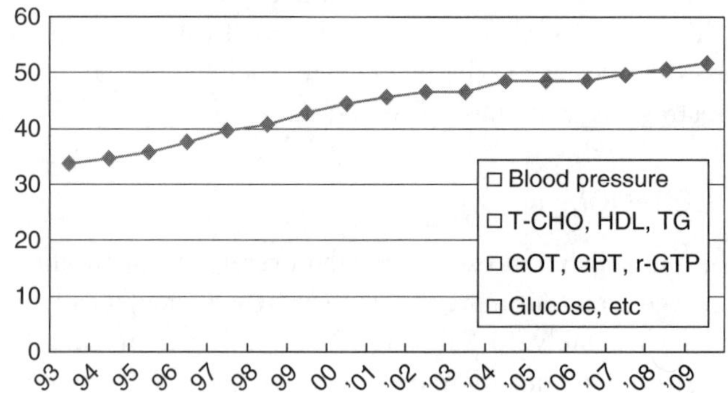


Figure 14-3 Trend of abnormal rates at workers' annual health checkups.
Source: Ministry of Health, Labour, and Welfare.

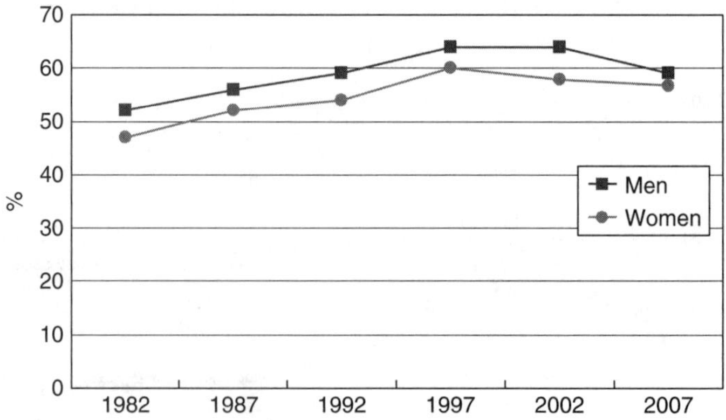


Figure 14-4 Workers with severe stress at workplace.
Source: Ministry of Health, Labour, and Welfare.

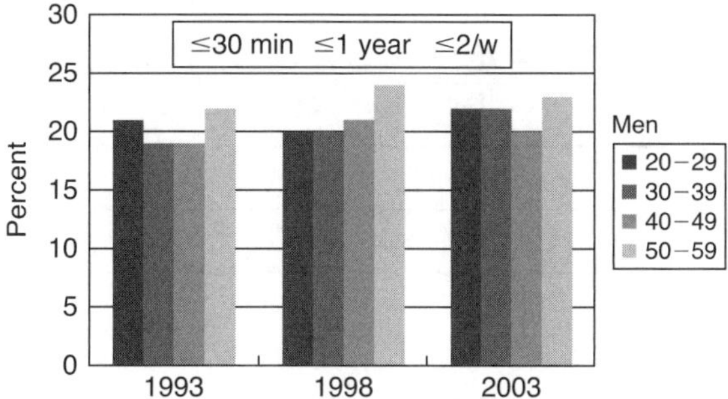


Figure 14-5 Trend of physical activities.
Source: Ministry of Health, Labour, and Welfare.

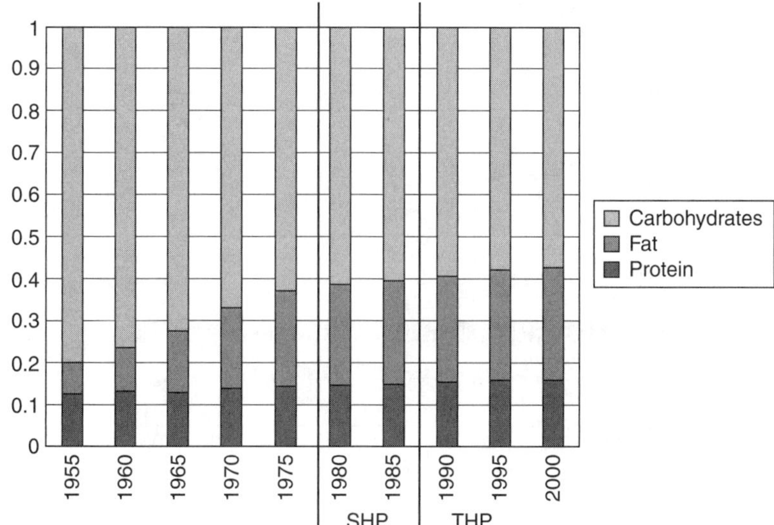


Figure 14-6 Trend of nutrition balance.
SHP: Silver Health Plan
THP: Total Health Promotion Plan
Source: Ministry of Health, Labour, and Welfare.

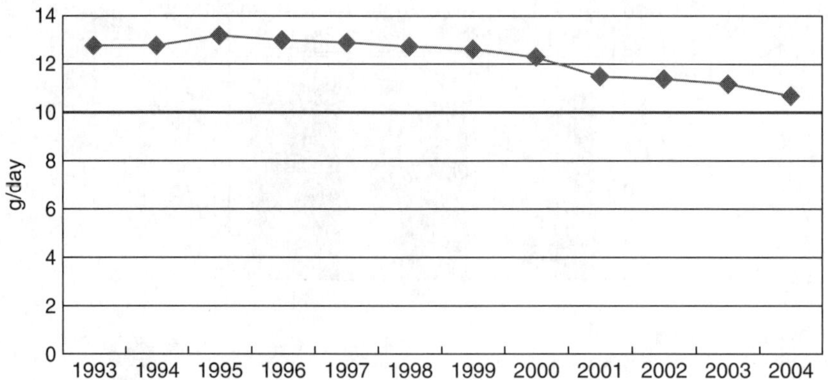


Figure 14-7 Trend of salt intake.
Source: Ministry of Health, Labour, and Welfare.

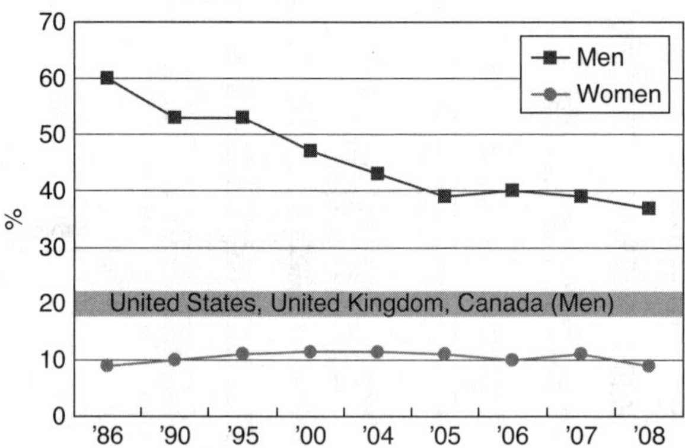


Figure 14-8 Trend of smoking rate.
Source: Ministry of Health, Labour, and Welfare.

## Major Challenges Now and for the Future

### *Prevention of* Karoshi

In Japan, *karoshi* (death brought on by overwork or job-related exhaustion) has become a serious problem in recent years. Figure 14-9 shows the trend of *karoshi* acknowledged by the Labor Standard Office. In order to prevent *karoshi*, the Ministry of Health issued a notification on the comprehensive measures to prevent ill health due to overwork in 2002. Employers were required to reduce overtime work and to provide health guidance by occupational physicians to workers who engaged in more than 100 hours per month of overtime or more than 80 hours during the previous 2–6 months. In 2005, the Industrial Safety and Health ISH Law was amended to reflect the 2002 notification, requiring employers to implement interviews of overloaded workers by occupational physicians and to ask for recommendations and health advice from them.

## Prevention of Mental Health Disorders

The number of workers who are absent from work due to mental disorders is increasing, and the word *karo-jisatsu* (suicide brought on by overwork or job-related exhaustion) has been coined recently. Figure 14-10 shows the trend of karo-jisatsu and mental disorders acknowledged by the Labor Standard Office. In 2000, the Ministry of Health, Labour, and Welfare issued guidelines on mental health promotion in the workplace to promote early detection, treatment, and return to work of those with depression (Ministry of Health, Labour, and Welfare, 2003). Employers are required to make a mental health promotion plan with specific reference to how the system will work, how it will be implemented and staffed, and privacy policy that will be followed. They are also required to implement the plan through four methods of care: employee's self-care, line care conducted by managers and supervisors, care by the company's healthcare staff, and care by external healthcare staff.

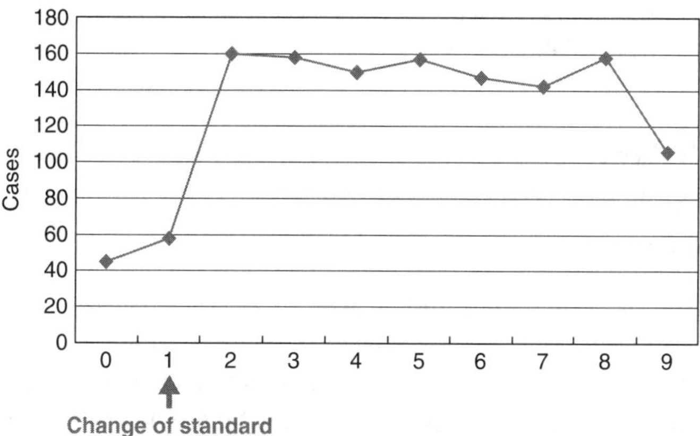


Figure 14-9 Trend of *Karoshi* acknowledged by Labor Standard Office.
**Source: Ministry of Health, Labour, and Welfare.**

## Smoking Measures

In 1996, the Ministry of Health, Labour, and Welfare issued guidelines on smoking measures in the workplace to protect nonsmokers from tobacco smoke and to create comfortable working environments. Although the number of workplaces grappling with smoking issues in the workplace has increased, additional effort has been deemed necessary due to the high interest in the adverse effects of secondhand smoke and WHO initiatives on a framework for a smoking policy. A notification was issued in 2000 concerning an outline of an educational program for promoting smoking measures in the workplace. In 2003, the Ministry of Health, Labour, and Welfare issued new guidelines on smoking measures in the workplace, reflecting the Health Promotion Law enforced in 2003 that obligated employers to take appropriate measures to protect nonsmokers from environmental smoking.

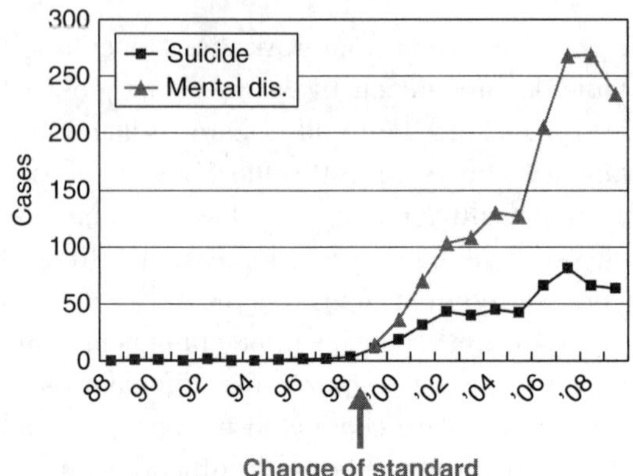


Figure 14-10 Trend of karo-suicide and mental disorders acknowledged by Labor Standard Office.
Source: Ministry of Health, Labour, and Welfare.

## Healthcare System

### Organizational Form

Public health centers or community health centers do not provide occupational health services (OHS) in Japan. Most hospitals do not have a section or department that provides OHS, although some physicians employed by public or private hospitals and general practitioners work as occupational physicians on a part-time basis. Some in-house OHS providers provide employees with medical curative services, but most other OHS providers do not provide such services.

The principal law regarding OHS is the Industrial Safety and Health (ISH) law, stipulated in 1972 (Hatakenaka, 2003). The purpose of the ISH law is to "secure the safety and health of workers in workplaces, as well as to facilitate the establishment of a comfortable working environment, by promoting comprehensive and systematic countermeasures concerning the prevention of industrial accidents and occupational diseases." Employers are required to take working environment measurements at workplaces where there is exposure to the harmful conditions, and to provide workers exposed to hazardous jobs with biannual health examinations. They are also required to provide workers engaging in nonhazardous jobs with annual health examinations.

The ISH law stipulates that companies employing 50 or more workers must establish a health committee, appoint an occupational physician, and appoint at least 1 health officer from among their employees. Large companies with more than 1,000 employees (500 employees in hazardous workplaces) must appoint at least 1 full-time occupational physician. A health committee meeting is held every month by the attending occupational physician to discuss occupational health issues in the workplace and to propose measures to the company. The health officers are in charge of implementing the measures proposed by the health committee with the advice from occupational physicians.

## Financing

Japan has adopted a national health insurance system, which covers all Japanese people. Under this system, every citizen belongs to a public health insurance program such as a group health insurance scheme or a national health insurance program and can obtain necessary medical treatment. Under the medical insurance scheme, patients pay 30% of all service fees.

The primary law concerning the compensation of workers for occupational injuries and diseases in Japan is the Workers' Accident Compensation Insurance Law (Araki, 2002; Miyatake, 2002; Muto, Sakurai, Hsieh, & Shimada, 1999; Nakane, 2003), which is a compulsory state-run insurance program. The government collects insurance premiums from employers and provides insurance benefits to injured workers or their survivors. Contributions are based on the total pay of the insured workers and are paid exclusively by employers. Contribution rates are determined for each specific industry on the basis of accident rates and other performance data for the preceding 3 years and range from a minimum of 0.6% to a maximum of 1.44%. The Workers' Accident Compensation Insurance covers employees in all workplaces in industry and commerce.

The Ministry of Health, Labour, and Welfare initiated the policy of subsidizing occupational health and safety activities conducted in small-scale enterprises (SSEs) in the early 1960s. Activities to be subsidized include the primary and secondary prevention of occupational injuries and diseases, as well as health promotion activities. The amount of subsidy is limited from one third to two thirds of costs used for the preventive activities. The long history of financial assistance for SSEs and the increasing amount of subsidies suggest that the Ministry recognizes the importance of financial assistance in promoting occupational health activities in SSEs (Muto & Takata, 2001).

## Health Resources

Japan has 260,000 physicians (206 per 100,000 persons) (Toyabe, 2009). The number of nurses and hospital beds are 822,000 and 1.6 million, respectively, and its ratio per 10,000 persons is 62 and 129, respectively (Nomura, 2007).

The number of occupational physicians certified by Japan Medical Association and acknowledged by the Ministry of Health, Labour, and Welfare was 70,000 as of June 2009. The number of certified occupational physicians certified by the Japan Society for Occupational Health was 357 as of 2005. The problem is that certified occupational physicians are not acknowledged by the ministry as occupational physicians in spite of their high level of occupational health expertise. There are about 1,500 health nurses and several thousand other nurses working in occupational health settings. The revised ISH law stipulated the functions of health nurses, such that health nurses are to provide health guidance for employees requiring assistance to maintain their health.

Nothing is stipulated concerning ergonomists, industrial hygienists, or psychologists in the ISH law. However, the functions of occupational health consultants are stipulated in the ISH law. Occupational health consultants, mostly experienced occupational physicians, health officers, or health nurses who hold a license issued by the ministry can consult about the health of a workplace at the request of an employer. The ISH law stipulates that workers who handle acid should be examined by a dentist.

## Service Delivery

Large companies with more than 1,000 employees usually organize their own in-house OHS providers by employing occupational physicians and nurses, and they conduct health examinations. Companies with 300 to 999 employees mostly employ nurses on a full-time or part-time basis, depending on the needs of the company, and also occupational physicians on a part-time basis. In such companies, and also some large companies, health examinations are conducted by external OHS providers. It is difficult for most companies with fewer than 300 employees to employ nurses due to financial constraints, so external OHS providers provide the necessary occupational health services, including health examinations. As it is usually difficult for SSEs to develop and implement preventive programs by themselves, external OHS providers are expected to play a key role in the development and implementation of preventive activities in SSEs.

## Social Determinants of Health

Workplaces with fewer than 50 employees are not required to appoint an occupational physician nor to organize a health committee. Considering the key roles of the occupational physician and health committee in occupational health activities, it is difficult for these workplaces to be covered by appropriate and effective OHS providers. Such small workplaces comprise 97% of all workplaces and 60% of the employed workforce. Figure 14-11 shows that the implementation rate of the annual general health examination, which is required by the ISH law, is lower in SSEs (Ministry of Health, Labour, and Welfare, 2004). Figure 14-12 shows that the implementation rate of workplace health promotion (WHP) and Total Health Promotion (THP) Plan is also lower in SSEs. These facts show that the size of the company determines the condition for maintaining and promoting health, and it is a social determinant of health.

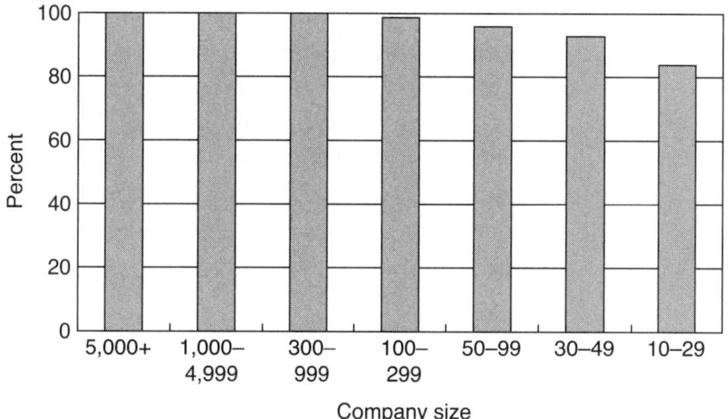


Figure 14-11 Implementation rates of annual health checkups by company size.
**Source: Ministry of Health, Labour, and Welfare, 2002.**

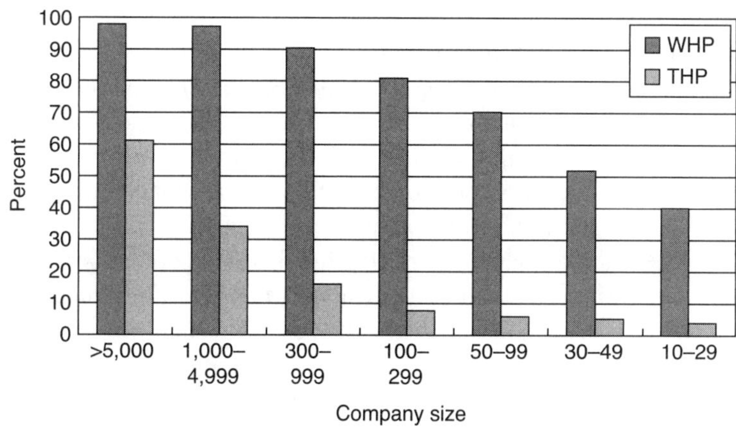


Figure 14-12 Implementation rates of WHP and THP by company size (2002).
**Source: Ministry of Health, Labour, and Welfare.**

## Prevention and Health Promotion

The revised ISH law in 1988 stipulates that the employer shall make continuous and systematic efforts for the maintenance and promotion of workers' health by taking appropriate measures, such as providing health education, health counseling, and other services to the workers. It also stipulates that the minister of health, labour, and welfare shall announce the guidelines for the measures to be taken by the employer for the maintenance and promotion of workers' health in order for such measures of the employer to be enforced appropriately and effectively.

Guidance on the Total Health Promotion Plan, which is an administrative measure based on the ISH law, covers concrete aspects of workplace health promotion. The objective of workplace health promotion is the prevention of lifestyle-related diseases, such as hypertension, diabetes, hyperlipidemia, and obesity. Thus, the targets are workers' lifestyles: nutrition, physical activity, smoking, alcohol use, and stress management. Under this measure, personnel involved in health promotion programs include health educators, mental health advisors, dieticians, and healthcare trainers. These are newly created professions in order to implement health promotion programs in the workplace.

## Outlook

In 1999, the Ministry of Health, Labour, and Welfare adopted guidelines on the occupational safety and health management system. In 2000, the ministry launched a project to promote OSHMS implementation in companies. In 2001, a notification was issued to the effect that the Japanese guidelines included all elements of the OSHMS guidelines adopted by the International Labor Organization. International trends in adopting the OSHMS, the aging working population, the prevention of health hazards caused by new chemicals, and fears concerning the inadequate communication of information regarding safety and health to the younger generation were cited as reasons for adopting the OSHMS. Rather than detailing specific measures, these guidelines encourage employers to engage in sustained and voluntary activities by establishing the OSHMS. Although no reference is made to the services of OHS providers in the Japanese version of OSHMS, occupational health professionals are expected to play a key role in the development and implementation of the OSHMS.

Small-scale workplaces are exempted from the requirements of ISH law, such as the assignment of occupational physicians and the establishment of a health committee. Considering the key roles of occupational physicians and the health committee in the occupational health activities, it is difficult for these workplaces to be covered with appropriate OHSs. There is a proposal that the lower limit of employees should be 30 instead of 50, or that an occupational physician works for a certain number of hours required to provide sufficient occupational health care for workers (Higashi, 2006; Muto, 1999). Regional occupational health centers (ROHCs) are highly regarded as the first systematic approach to OHSs in small companies, but there remain many problems to be solved, such as the low utilization rate, deficiency of manpower, and the relationship between the existing OHS providers and ROHCs (Muto, Mizoue, Terada, & Harabuchi, 1998). Among others, the low utilization rate is a big problem, and the possibility of collaboration between ROHCs and community health centers is examined and discussed (Muto, 2004). While external OHS providers offer their services at the market price, the services rendered by ROHCs are free.

## Influence of Culture and Mentality

Japanese workers are generally considered to be very diligent, hardworking, or workaholic. These mental traits influence nonabsence from work and workers' health status. Japanese workers' working time is very long (1,970 hours per year) (Sasajima, 2003), and work–life balance is very poor. The average worker is entitled to 18 paid vacation days a year, but uses just 9 days. The low utilization rate is due to the desire to save up the vacation days in case of sickness or other unforeseeable circumstances as well as the lack of an established mechanism for taking long vacations. These attitudes of workers are one of the causes of work-related diseases *karoshi* and *karo-jisatsu*.

In Japan, it was a tradition to think that women should engage in housekeeping while men work for companies. Therefore, women were expected to quit working when they got married or when they had a child. The female labor force participation rate (rate of the labor force for persons aged 15 years old and over) shows an *M*-shaped curve in terms of age. This curve indicates that young women work until they get married, leave the labor force upon the birth of a child, and then rejoin the workforce after their children have grown up and the burden of child rearing is reduced.

## Drivers of Workplace Health Promotion

### Who Is Most Active in the Field of Workplace Health Promotion?

Japanese workplace health promotion has a relatively long history of over 30 years. WHP emerged in Japan against the backdrop of fears over low productivity due to the rising number of older workers. WHP initiatives first appeared in Japan in 1979 as the Silver Health Plan (SHP), as a policy of the Ministry of Labour. It intended to promote the physical health of middle-aged employees by improving their levels of physical activity (Muto et al., 1996). This initiative predated by 7 years the 1986 declaration of the Ottawa Charter for Health Promotion. The Silver Health Plan was revised in 1988 as the Total Health Promotion (THP) Plan intended to promote the physical and mental health of all employees. The foundation of the THP plan is in the Industrial Safety and Health Law that stipulates health promotion is an employer's obligation. WHP is not defined explicitly, but due to the revised Industrial Safety and Health Law of 1988, it is the employers' continuous and systematic responsibility to maintain and promote the health of workers, as well as it is the workers' responsibility to maintain and promote their health. In this respect, it is the Ministry of Labour that is most active in the field of WHP.

## Who Has a Major Interest in WHP and Why?

The Ministry of Labour has a major interest in WHP because the productivity of Japanese companies will improve if it is successful. On the contrary, companies do not seem to be interested in the implementation of THP. Figure 14-13 shows the trend of implementation rate of WHP and THP. As of 2007, the implementation rate of THP was still below 10%. One of the reasons may be that companies do not perceive the effectiveness of THP in terms of decrease in sickness absence and medical expenses and increase in productivity, as shown in Figure 14-14. The diligent nature of Japanese workers may be the reason for the low impact on sickness absence. Costs of health insurance are covered by employers and employees on a fifty-fifty basis, so companies may not feel the importance of lowering medical costs by implementing WHP.

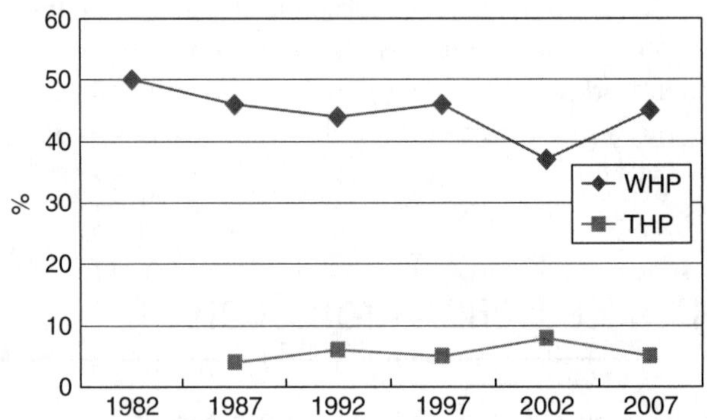


Figure 14-13 Trend of implementation rate of WHP and THP.
**Source: Ministry of Health, Labour, and Welfare.**

## What Role Does the Government Play?

In Japan, health promotion is specified in the Industrial Safety and Health Law as part of an employer's obligations (Hatakenaka, 2003). The role of the state is explicitly set forth. Under the law, several concrete guidelines have been issued by the Ministry of Labour. These include:

- Establishment of a health promotion committee in the workplace
- Annual health checkups for all employees
- Fitness evaluations
- Creation of more comfortable workplaces
- Smoking guidelines
- Mental health promotion measures

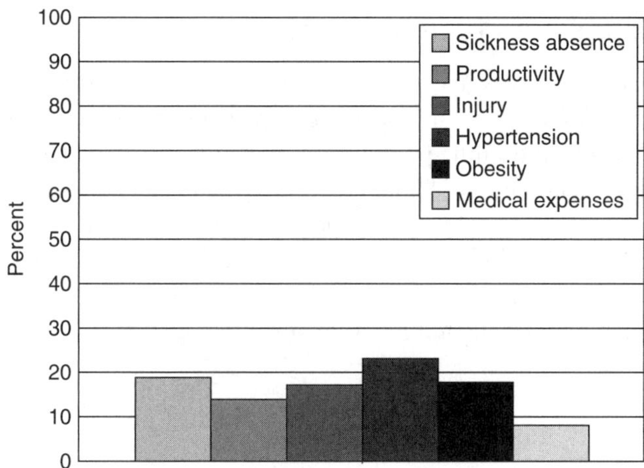


Figure 14-14 Perceived effectiveness of THP (1997).
**Source: Ministry of Health, Labour, and Welfare.**

Financial assistance for enterprises implementing WHP is also a characteristic of Japanese WHP (Muto, Sakurai, Hsieh, & Shimada, 1999; Muto & Takata, 2001). In accordance with law, subsidies are provided for companies that implement health promotion programs. Two thirds of the costs of operating WHP programs over a period of 3 years are reimbursed by the Ministry of Health, Labour, and Welfare. From 1999, only small- and medium-sized enterprises with fewer than 300 employees have been eligible to apply for the subsidy program, indicating the administrative body's recognition of the importance of WHP within small- and medium-sized enterprises.

## Are These Dynamics Currently Changing?

Workplace health promotion (WHP) has recently attracted attention in Japan for several reasons. First, the Health Promotion Act promulgated in 2003 recognizes the importance of WHP to prevent lifestyle-related diseases among Japanese people, and it stresses the collaboration of WHP and community health promotion. Second, due to increased competition among companies caused by globalization of economy, there are many workers who have to work longer hours, and the overwork has caused *karoshi*. In addition, many workers report psychological stress related to their work, and mental health problems, especially suicide due to depression (*karo-jisatsu*), have become a major occupational health issue. Companies are afraid of being sued if they have incidences of *karoshi* or *karo-jisatsu*. Thus, from the standpoint of risk management, companies have become interested in prevention activities including WHP.

### Who Are the Vendors or Program Providers?

The major factors affecting workers' health were thought to be workers' personal lifestyles in Japan. Consequently, WHP in Japan has emphasized intervention in personal lifestyles. In order to cope with this need, training programs for personnel in charge of health promotion programs have been developed and implemented. Six types of specialists in charge of WHP have been developed: occupational physicians responsible for health assessment, healthcare trainers responsible for developing individual exercise regimens, healthcare leaders responsible for exercise training, occupational health educators responsible for health education, mental health advisors responsible for mental health counseling, and occupational dieticians responsible for nutrition education.

## Programs and Good Practices

### What Types of Programs Exist?

Table 14-2 shows the trend in percentages of workplaces covered by different WHP programs. There was no particular trend in the implementation rate of any WHP, comprehensive health checkups, or mental-health programs. The implementation rate of health counseling and smoking measures showed an increase. THP was implemented in less than 10% of all workplaces for the 25 years studied.

**Table 14-2 Trend in Percentage of Workplaces Covered by Different Workplace Health Promotion Programs**

| Contents | 1982 | 1987 | 1992 | 1997 | 2002 | 2007 |
|---|---|---|---|---|---|---|
| Any health promotion program | 50.1 | 45.8 | 43.9 | 46.4 | 37.4 | 45.2 |
| Health counseling | ——— | ——— | 35.3 | 43.1 | 51.7 | 46.1 |
| Smoking measures | ——— | 29.4 | 34.1 | 47.7 | 59.1 | 75.5 |
| Health checkups[1] | ——— | 79.2 | 85.7 | 84.8 | 87.1 | 86.2 |
| Health checkups[2] | 31.2 | 47.1 | 31.7 | 35.7 | 28.5 | 27.7 |
| Mental health | 34.5 | 30.3 | 22.7 | 26.5 | 23.5 | 33.6 |
| Fitness assessment | 6.9 | 12.7 | 11.4 | 7.9 | 7.3 | 3.1 |
| Total Health Promotion | ——— | 3.6[3] | 6.1 | 4.9 | 8.0 | 5.0 |

Source: Ministry of Labour. Survey on state of employees' health.

[1] Mandatory health checkups stipulated in the Industrial Safety and Health Law.

[2] Comprehensive health checkups not stipulated in the Industrial Safety and Health Law.

[3] Silver Health Plan

## Example of Good Practices

### WHP at Osaka Gas Company

Osaka Gas Company was established in 1905. The number of employees is approximately 15,000. Main lines of business of the company are natural gas import, distribution and sale, production and sale of gas appliances and related construction works, and heat supply service. With the higher average age of employees brought about by advancing the compulsory retirement age, health care in enterprises has become an increasingly important issue. Helping employees stay well means improving their morale, increasing productivity, and reducing absenteeism due to illness. To attain these objectives, the physical fitness program as well as the regular medical checkups have very important roles to play. The company set up a healthcare system in 1976 and has engaged in improving health and physical fitness capabilities of its employees.

In addition to annual medical checks, the examination for the purpose of health promotion is held for employees aged 35 or more during working hours every 2 years. First, examinees input the information of their lifestyle, past illnesses, and abnormal symptoms. Then they take laboratory blood tests, including total blood cell count, hemoglobin, total cholesterol, HDL-cholesterol, triglyceride, liver function, uric acid, and glucose; physical characteristics (height, body weight, waist and hip circumferences), bone density check, pulmonary function testing, oral examination by dentist, exercise testing, and physical fitness testing. Based on the results of these checks, they are given a health diagnosis by a physician.

After the health diagnosis, employees are given an individual health program by healthcare staff. Individual counseling and seminars are held in subjects concerning nutrition, alcohol, tobacco, salt, daily physical activity, stress, and other health risk factors. Furthermore, follow-up services, such as nutrition, exercise programs, and health counseling, are given by physicians, nurses, fitness trainers, and other medical staff. Psychiatric interviews by a psychiatrist are also available.

The health promotion program for employees has brought results of increased productivity, increased morale, improved lifestyle (decreased prevalence of employees with smoking, increased physical activity), and decreased mortality of employees. Purchasing health management and fitness requires understanding and firm policy on the part of top management. The management's positive attitude toward health and fitness helps create the employees' trust and confidence in the company.

## Outcomes and Indicators

Table 14-3 shows the indicators and the percentages for perceived effectiveness of the THP plan. Indicators include productivity, health status, lifestyles, and attitudes. The most well-perceived effectiveness was increased interest in health promotion, followed by increased activation of the workplace atmosphere and increased participation in health checkups. Effectiveness in terms of health status was generally not as well perceived.

Table 14-3 **Perceived Effectiveness of the Total Health Promotion Plan**

| Indicators | Effective | Not decided | Not effective |
|---|---|---|---|
| **Productivity** | | | |
| Decreased absence due to illness | 19.2% | 64.0% | 16.8% |
| Increased productivity | 13.8% | 73.4% | 12.8% |
| **Health status** | | | |
| Decreased injuries | 17.4% | 70.9% | 11.7% |
| Decreased hypertension | 22.8% | 61.6% | 15.6% |
| Decreased obesity | 17.7% | 52.4% | 29.9% |
| Decreased medical care costs | 8.3% | 74.0% | 17.7% |
| **Lifestyles** | | | |
| Increased participation in health checkups | 50.7% | 40.1% | 9.2% |
| Increased exercise habit | 35.5% | 40.8% | 23.7% |
| Increased smoking cessation | 7.6% | 35.2% | 57.2% |
| **Attitudes** | | | |
| Increased interest in health promotion | 79.0% | 15.8% | 5.2% |
| Positive increase in workplace atmosphere | 49.5% | 43.1% | 7.4% |

Source: Ministry of Health, Labour, and Welfare (1999).

# Existing Research

Table 14-4 shows several results of WHP programs conducted in Japan and reported in professional journals with peer review. Physical exercise programs improved blood pressure (Hayashi et al., 1999), and HDL cholesterol (Naito et al., 2008). Exercise and nutrition programs improved medical parameters (Irie et al., 1996). Multi-component programs were effective in improving obesity and total cholesterol (Muto and Yamauchi, 2001), and blood pressure and LDL cholesterol (Arao et al., 2007), but THP was not effective (Furuki, Honda, Jahng, Ikeda, & Okubo, 1999). Mental health programs were either effective (Tsutsumi et al., 2005) or not effective (Kawakami, Takao, Kobayashi, & Tsutusmi, 2006). A smoking cessation program was moderately effective (Muto, Nakamura, & Oshima, 1998). An oral health program proved to be cost effective (Ichihashi, Muto, & Shibuya, 2007). In interpreting these results, we must consider the publishing bias.

Table 14-4 **Results of Workplace Health Promotion Programs Conducted in Japan**

| Author | Program contents | Study design | No. of subjects | Intervention period | Main findings |
|---|---|---|---|---|---|
| Hayashi | Walking | QE[1] | 6,104 | 10 years | Reduction in hypertension |
| Irie | Exercise, nutrition | PP[2] | 24 | 12 weeks | Improvement in medical parameters |
| Muto | Smoking cessation | QE | 70 | 6 months | Net quit rate: 17.2% |
| Furuki | Total Health Promotion | QE | 1,014 | 4 years | No improvement in medical parameters |
| Muto | Multicomponent program | RCT[3] | 400 | 1 year | Improvement in BMI, total cholesterol (TCHO) |
| Kawakami | Mental health program | RCT | 189 | 3 months | No effect on job stressors |
| Ichihashi | Oral health | QE | 357 | 20 minutes | Cost-beneficial |
| Arao | Multicomponent | QE | 177 | 6 months | Improvement in systolic blood pressure, LDL cholesterol |
| Naito | Exercise | QE | 2,929 | 4 years | Improvement in HDL cholesterol |

[1] Quasi-experimental, [2] Pre-post comparison, [3] Randomized controlled trial.

# Conclusion

The concept of Japanese WHP, targeting only employees' personal lifestyles, is narrower than that in Europe. However, if the guidelines on comfortable workplaces published in 1992 and on mental-health promotion published in 2000 are considered as supplementary policy for WHP, the concept of Japanese WHP can be thought of as expanding. This is due to the fact that these guidelines include interventions to the working environment and attitudes toward work.

The issue of coverage is important not only in improving health on the national level, but also in ensuring equity in health. Due to the limited resources of small-scale enterprises, it is particularly difficult to carry out health promotion activities in such small organizations, in spite of the declining health status of workers there. Regarding coverage in the Japanese WHP, the target should be small-scale enterprises.

The low percentage in perceived effectiveness on health outcomes and increase in the rate of workers with poor self-rated health, along with the prevalence of chronic diseases, seem to indicate that WHP has had no effect on the national level, in spite of the existence of some effective WHP programs. Thus, one could conclude that the overall effectiveness of WHP has yet to be demonstrated. The future tasks of WHP in Japan may include reconceptualizing current practices and defining WHP, incorporating it into the management system, and evaluation of programs.

## Summary

Workplace health promotion (WHP) initiatives first appeared in Japan in 1979 as a policy of the Ministry of Labour. The policy intended to promote the physical health of middle-aged employees by improving their levels of physical activity. The policy was revised in 1988 as the Total Health Promotion (THP) Plan, intended to promote the physical and mental health of all employees. The concept of THP, targeting only employees' personal lifestyles, is narrower than that in Europe. However, if the guidelines on comfortable workplaces are considered as supplementary policy for WHP, the concept of Japanese WHP can be thought of as expanding.

Japan is very unique in that health promotion is stipulated in the Industrial Safety and Health Law as employer's obligations, and several concrete guidelines have been issued by the Ministry of Health, Labour, and Welfare. In spite of these regulations and guidelines, implementation rate of health promotion programs is not very high, particularly in small scale enterprises. The low percentage in perceived effectiveness on health outcomes and the increase in the rate of workers with poor self-rated health, along with the prevalence of chronic diseases, seem to indicate that WHP has been of no effect on the national level, in spite of the existence of some effective WHP programs. The information provided in this chapter has clarified the fact that the overall effectiveness of WHP has yet to be demonstrated. The future tasks of WHP in Japan may include reconceptualizing current practices and defining WHP, incorporating it into the management system, and the evaluation of the programs.

## Review Questions

1. What are the central national issues affecting the health of Japan's corporate economy?
2. Explain corporate social responsibility as it applies to Japanese companies.
3. What is *karoshi* and why it is significant to corporate culture in Japan?
4. Describe the ISH law and its role in workplace health promotion programs.
5. Discuss the variation among OHS providers and describe their occupational roles in workplace health.
6. How is workplace health promotion affected by Japanese culture?
7. What have studies shown in regard to Japan's workplace health promotion programs?

## References

Araki, T. (2002). *Labor and employment law in Japan.* Tokyo, Japan: The Japan Institute of Labor.

Arao, T., Oida, Y., Maruyama, C., Muto, T., Sawada, S., Matsuzuki, H., & Nakanishi, Y. (2007). Impact on lifestyle intervention on physical activity and diet of Japanese workers. *Preventive Medicine, 45*, 146–152.

CIA. (2010). *The world factbook.* Retrieved December 16, 2010, from https://www.cia.gov/library/publications/the-world-factbook/

Furuki, K., Honda, S., Jahng, D., Ikeda, M., & Okubo, T. (1999). The effects of a health promotion program on body mass index. *Journal of Occupational Health, 41*, 19–26.

Hatakenaka, N. (2003). *The occupational safety and health law of Japan.* Tokyo, Japan: The Japan Institute of Labor.

Haub, C. (2010, May) *Population reference bureau.* Retrieved August 2009 from http://www.prb.org/Articles/2010/japandemography.aspx

Hayashi, T., Tsumura, K., Suematsu, C., Okada, K., Fujii, S., & Endo, G. (1999). Walking to work and the risk for hypertension in men: The Osaka health survey. *Annals of Internal Medicine, 130*, 21–26.

Higashi, T. (2006). Future challenges of occupational health services in a changing working world. In T. Muto, T. Higashi, & J. Verbeek (Eds.), *Evidence-based occupational health.* Amsterdam, Netherlands: Elsevier Publishing Co.

Ichihashi, T., Muto, T., & Shibuya, K. (2007). Cost-benefit analysis of a worksite oral health promotion program. *Industrial Health, 45*, 32–36.

Irie, M., Mishima, N., Nagata, S., Himeno, E., Nanri, H., Ikeda, M., . . . Nishino, T. (1996). Psychosomatic effect of a health program on obese employees. [in Japanese with English abstract] *San Ei Shi, 38*, 11–16.

Japan Industrial Safety and Health Association (JISHA). (2004). *Present status of Japanese industrial safety and health*. Tokyo, Japan: JISHA.

Kawakami, N., Takao, S., Kobayashi, Y., & Tsutusmi, A. (2006). Effects of web-based supervisory training on job stressors and psychological distress among workers: A workplace-based randomized controlled trial. *Journal of Occupational Health, 48*, 28–34.

Kawashita, F., Taniyama, Y., Fujisaki, J., & Mori, K. (2005). Industrial safety and health aspect in CSR (corporate social responsibility): Publication of CSR-related reports and the contents by TSE first section listed companies. *Journal of Occupational Health, 47*, 561. [In Japanese]

Ministry of Health, Labour, and Welfare. (2003). *Guidelines of workers' mental health promotion in the workplaces.* Tokyo, Japan: Ministry of Health.

Ministry of Health, Labour, and Welfare. (2004). *Survey of state of employees' health.* Tokyo, Japan: Romu Gyosei.

Miyatake, G. (2002). *Social security in Japan.* Tokyo, Japan: The Foreign Press Center.

Muto, T. (1999). International comparison highlights the standards of OHS: The Japanese case. In E. Menckel & P. Westerholm (Eds.), *Evaluation in occupational health practice* (pp. 100–111). Oxford, England: Butterworth-Heinemann.

Muto, T. (2004). Collaboration between occupational health and community health for promoting workers' health in small-scale enterprises. *International Symposium on Occupational Health in Small-scale Enterprises and the Informal Sector,* 86.

Muto, T., Kikuchi, S., Tomita, M., Fujita, Y., Kurita, M., & Ozawa, K. (1996). Status of health promotion implementation and future tasks in Japanese companies. *Industrial Health, 34*, 101–111.

Muto, T., Mizoue, T., Terada, H., & Harabuchi, I. (1998). Current problems and future tasks of occupational health centers for small-scale enterprises in Japan. In S. Lehtinen, A. Vartio, & J. Rantanen, (Eds.), *From protection to promotion: Occupational health and safety in small-scale enterprises* (pp. 6–39). Helsinki, Finland: Finnish Institute of Occupational Health.

Muto, T., Nakamura, M., & Oshima, A. (1998). Evaluation of a smoking cessation program implemented in the workplace. *Industrial Health, 36*, 369–371.

Muto, T., Sakurai, Y., Hsieh, S. D., & Shimada, N. (1999). Evaluation of financing methods for occupational injuries and diseases in Japan. In J. F. Caillard & P. Westerholm (Eds.), *Social security systems and health insurance: Financing and implication in occupational health* (pp. 221–229). Toulouse, France: Octares.

Muto, T., & Takata, T. (2001). Financial assistance in promoting occupational health services for small-scale enterprises in Japan. *International Journal of Occupational Medicine and Environmental Health, 14*, 143–150.

Muto, T., & Yamauchi, K. (2001). Evaluation of a multi-component workplace health promotion program conducted in Japan for improving employees' cardiovascular disease risk factors. *Preventive Medicine, 35*, 571–577.

Naito, M., Nakayama, T., Okamura, T., Miura, K., Yanagita, Y., Fujieda, Y., … Ueshima, H. (2008). Effect of a 4-year workplace-based physical activity intervention program on the blood lipid profiles of participating employees: The high-risk and population strategy for occupational health promotion (HIPOP-OHP) study. *Atherosclerosis, 1972*, 784–790.

Nakane, F. (2003). *Workmen's accident compensation insurance law*. Tokyo, Japan: Eibun-Horei-Sha, Inc.

Nariai, O. (2002). *The modern Japanese economy.* Tokyo, Japan: Foreign Press Center.

Nomura, Y. (2007). Current status of nursing in Japan. Highlights from ICN Conference and CNR 2007 Yokohama lectures, *4*, 75-78.

Okamoto, K. (1994, September). *Current issues and future challenges facing Japan's health care–How Japan will cope with an aging society*. Paper presented at the First U.K.–Japan Health Policy Conference.

Okamoto, K. (2004). *ABC of CSR: What is corporate social responsibility?* Tokyo, Japan: Nihon Keizai Shimbunsha.

Sasajima, Y. (2003). *Labor in Japan.* Tokyo, Japan: Foreign Press Center.

Seike, A. (1997). *New trends in Japan's labor market: Changes in employment practices.* Tokyo, Japan: The Foreign Press Center.

Taniyama, Y., Kawashita, F., So, Y., & Mori, K. (2005). Industrial safety and health in corporate social responsibility: Description on industrial safety and health in corporate social responsibility related reports about mental health in particular [in Japanese]. *Journal of Occupational Health, 47*, 562.

Toyabe, S. (2009, March 3). Trend in geographic distribution of physicians in Japan. *International Journal for Equity in Health.*

Tsutsumi, A., Takao, S., Mineyama, S., Nishiuchi, K., Komatsu, H., & Kawakami, N. (2005). Effects of a supervisory education for positive mental health in the workplace: A quasi-experimental study. *Journal of Occupational Health, 47*, 226–235.

Westerholm, P., Nilstun, T., & Ovretveit, J. (2004). *Practical ethics in occupational health.* Oxford, England: Radcliffe Medical Press.

Chapter 15

# Norway

Dieter Lagerstrøm

After reading this chapter you should be able to:

- Identify core strategies that are the focus of workplace health promotion efforts in Norway
- Describe the historical evolution of Norway's workplace health promotion efforts
- Explain the different approaches employed by corporate health promotion throughout Norway
- Review the central disease states and health issues driving workplace health promotion in Norway
- Name the components of, and the associated funding sources for, the Norwegian health-care system
- Discuss the impact of culture on the health status and health promotion efforts within Norway

Table 15-1 **Select Key Demographic and Economic Indicators**

| | |
|---|---|
| Nationality | Noun: Norwegian(s)<br>Adjective: Norwegian |
| Ethnic groups | Norwegian 94.4% (includes Sami, about 60,000), other European 3.6%, other 2% (2007 estimate) |
| Religion | Church of Norway 85.7%, Pentecostal 1%, Roman Catholic 1%, other Christian 2.4%, Muslim 1.8%, other 8.1% (2004) |
| Language | Bokmal Norwegian (official), Nynorsk Norwegian (official), small Sami- and Finnish-speaking minorities;<br>*Note:* Sami is official in six municipalities |
| Literacy | Definition: age 15 and over can read and write<br>Total population: 100%<br>Male: 100%<br>Female: 100% |
| Education expenditure | 7.2% of GDP (2005)<br>Country comparison to the world: 20 |

*continued*

| Table 15-1 Select Key Demographic and Economic Indicators, *continued* | |
|---|---|
| Government type | Constitutional monarchy |
| Environment | Water pollution; acid rain damaging forests and adversely affecting lakes, threatening fish stocks; air pollution from vehicle emissions |
| Country mass | Total: 323,802 sq km<br>Country comparison to the world: 67<br>Land: 304,282 sq km<br>Water: 19,520 sq km |
| Population | 4,660,539 (July 2010 est.)<br>Country comparison to the world: 116 |
| Age structure | 0–14 years: 18.5% (male 441,508/female 422,050)<br>15–64 years: 66.2% (male 1,564,482/female 1,522,519)<br>65 years and over: 15.2% (male 305,120/female 404,860)<br>(2010 est.) |
| Median age | Total: 39.7 years<br>Male: 38.8 years<br>Female: 40.5 years (2010 est.) |
| Population growth rate | 0.341% (2010 est.)<br>Country comparison to the world: 170 |
| Birth rate | 10.99 births/1,000 population (2010 est.)<br>Country comparison to the world: 179 |
| Death rate | 9.29 deaths/1,000 population (July 2010 est.)<br>Country comparison to the world: 74 |
| Net migration rate | 1.71 migrant(s)/1,000 population (2010 est.)<br>Country comparison to the world: 45 |
| Urbanization | Urban population: 77% of total population (2008)<br>Rate of urbanization: 0.7% annual rate of change (2005–2010 est.) |
| Gender ratio | At birth: 1.05 male(s)/female<br>Under 15 years: 1.05 male(s)/female<br>15–64 years: 1.03 male(s)/female<br>65 years and over: 0.75 male(s)/female<br>Total population: 0.98 male(s)/female (2009 est.) |
| Infant mortality rate | Total: 3.58 deaths/1,000 live births<br>Country comparison to the world: 214<br>Male: 3.92 deaths/1,000 live births<br>Female: 3.22 deaths/1,000 live births (2010 est.) |

*continued*

| Table 15-1 **Select Key Demographic and Economic Indicators,** *continued* | |
|---|---|
| Life expectancy | Total population: 79.95 years<br>Country comparison to the world: 23<br>Male: 77.29 years<br>Female: 82.74 years (2010 est.) |
| Total fertility rate | 1.77 children born/woman (2010 est.)<br>Country comparison to the world: 163 |
| GDP—purchasing power parity | $267.4 billion (2009 est.)<br>Country comparison to the world: 41 |
| GDP—per capita | $57,400 (2009 est.)<br>Country comparison to the world: 5 |
| GDP—composition by sector | Agriculture: 2.1%<br>Industry: 39.5%<br>Services: 58.3% (2009 est.) |
| Agriculture—products | Barley, wheat, potatoes, pork, beef, veal, milk, fish |
| Industries | Petroleum and gas, food processing, shipbuilding, pulp and paper products, metals, chemicals, timber, mining, textiles, fishing |
| Labor force participation | 2.59 million (2009 est.)<br>Country comparison to the world: 110 |
| Unemployment rate | 3.2% (2009 est.)<br>Country comparison to the world: 26 |
| Industrial production growth rate | -2.9% (2009 est.)<br>Growth rate country comparison to the world: 97 |
| Distribution of family income (GINI index) | 25 (2008)<br>Income (GINI index) country comparison to the world: 133 |
| Investment (gross fixed) | 21.4% of GDP (2009 est.)<br>Country comparison to the world: 74 |
| Public debt | 60.6% of GDP (2009 est.)<br>Country comparison to the world: 29 |
| Market value of publicly traded shares | $142.5 billion (December 31, 2008)<br>Country comparison to the world: 32 |
| Current account balance | $55.32 billion (2009 est.)<br>Country comparison to the world: 4 |
| Debt (external) | $548.1 billion (June 30, 2009 est.)<br>Country comparison to the world: 18 |
| Debt as a % of GDP | ——— |

*continued*

| Table 15-1 Select Key Demographic and Economic Indicators, *continued* | |
|---|---|
| Exports | $122.8 billion (2009 est.)<br>Country comparison to the world: 30 |
| Exports—commodities | Petroleum and petroleum products, machinery and equipment, metals, chemicals, ships, fish |
| Export—partners | United Kingdom 24.28%, Germany 13.4%, Netherlands 10.87%, France 8.55%, Sweden 5.76%, United States 4.82% (2009) |
| Imports | $65.84 billion (2009 est.)<br>Country comparison to the world: 37 |
| Import—commodities | Machinery and equipment, chemicals, metals, foodstuffs |
| Import—partners | Sweden 13.86%, Germany 12.89%, China 7.8%, Denmark 6.78%, United States 6.16%, United Kngdom 6.01% (2009) |
| Stock of direct foreign investment at | |
| Home | $123.3 billion (December 31, 2009 est.)<br>Country comparison to the world: 28 |
| Abroad | $174.7 billion (December 31, 2009 est.)<br>Country comparison to the world: 17 |

Source: CIA. (2010). *The world factbook.* Retrieved December 16, 2010, from https://www.cia.gov/library/publications/the-world-factbook/

## Introduction

Located at the northernmost part of Europe, Norway has a total area of 386,975 square kilometers and a population of 4.8 million. Because of the Gulf Stream, it is inhabited and cultivated up to the North Cape, which is located at the 71st degree of latitude. Although one third of the Norwegian population lives in the greater area of Oslo, the government is promoting a decentralizing settlement and industrial policy.

Until the 20th century, Norway was a poor country, making a living from farming and fishing. The discovery of huge oil deposits and the development of Norwegian offshore technology started a fabulous economic miracle in the 1960s. With an annual national budget surplus of several hundreds of billions Norwegian kroner (NOK) (in 2009 a surplus of 300 billion NOK was expected), Norway ranks amongst the wealthiest and most modern industrialized countries in the world. Within the last few years it received awards by the United Nations Development Program for providing the best living conditions (www.norwegen.no).

Due to the economic boom and resulting social developments, there is a need for highly qualified personnel, for example engineers and physicians, but there is also a need for workers in community services and the service sector. This situation, coupled with social and economical conditions and Norwegian politics, have led to immigration, causing changes within social structures.

Despite a strong economy and ongoing social changes, Norwegian politics are characterized by a strong humanistic attitude and a concerned sensibility for natural and environmental concerns. The basic Norwegian lifestyle is distinguished by an affinity for nature. This is reflected in Norway being the first country in the world to establish a Department of the Environment in 1972, and in Norway passing the *Allmannsretten*—the everyman's right—50 years ago. This law grants everybody the freedom to roam in nature and to use natural resources (with limitations on hunting) for personal use. Thus, the law established the right and the premise for maintaining the traditional Norwegian *Friluftsliv*—being and living in and with nature—that is the basis of the Norwegian philosophy of life. *Friluftsliv,* therefore, is an inherent part of kindergartens, a mandatory subject in school, and a subject of study at universities.

National identification and affinity for nature not only have influence on the Norwegian way of life, but when regarded from a global point of view, have also led to an astonishing symbiosis of ecology and economy. In order to determine the effects of workplace health promotion (WHP) programs in Norway, evaluations not only should include an assessment of economic benefits or the prevalence of evidence-based data, but also should be measured by the basic factors of health, happiness, and contentedness, and the ecological balance.

If there is no reaction to the overexploitation of natural resources and increasing environmental pollution, which are still widely spread for short-term profit maximization, these factors will have a dramatic influence on air, water, and light, so that basic requirements for constant good health will not be available anymore. Therefore, the Norwegian symbiosis of ecology and economy, as well as the Norwegian attitude toward way of life, can be a fruitful approach for WHP work. Since health can derive only from the reciprocal interaction among humans, their environment, and natural elements (such as air, water, light, etc.), a holistic view is required when evaluating WHP.

## Prevailing Health Issues and Risk Behaviors

Contemporary living conditions and ongoing societal development have led Norway to top the life expectancy and satisfaction rankings. However, new social conditions and modern, comfortable lifestyles have led to widespread diseases of civilization. Respiratory diseases, cardiovascular and metabolic problems, cancer, musculoskeletal disorders, and psychological problems represent major causes of death, while physical inactivity, poor diet, and stress cause major health problems (Bahr, 2008).

About 7.7% of absences from work are due to illness, which equals 25–30 million lost workdays a year (www.nov.no). Initiatives organized by the government, employers, labor unions, and nongovernmental organizations are trying to counteract this trend. There is documentation of causes of absenteeism and promising initiatives, including healthy cafeteria food, activity and work–life balance programs, fruit and water at work, and allocated sick days for employees to take at their own discretion (12 days/year; 24 days/year in companies taking part in the IA-program that attempts to achieve an inclusive working life by reducing sickness absence rate, making more jobs available for disabled employees, and increasing the retirement age) (www.nav.no; Olsen, 2003.)

In Norway, the major future challenge is the containment of chronic diseases. Existing laws, regulations, and framework conditions seem to be sufficient to meet this challenge. Considerable progress has been made with regard to smoking prevalence, with an impressive reduction from 32% in 2005 to 24% in 2006 (World Health Organization [WHO], 2009), due to comprehensive tobacco control measures, mainly smoke-free policies and cessation programs, and aggressive enforcement with high fines. Norway continues to fight the battle against tobacco use with multiple strategies. One of them is the National Strategy for Tobacco Control, which has set the long-term goal of a smoke-free society (Norwegian Ministry of Health and Care Services, 2007).

Another contributing risk factor is the prevalence rate of obesity, which is higher among the male population. The percentage with obesity rose from 9–10% in 1985 to 13–22% around 2000, except for women under 30, for whom the rate is lower. Although the obesity rate in Norway is very low compared to some other countries such as the United States where obesity prevalence is over 30%, it is nevertheless a contributing factor toward the difference in the life expectancy gap between men and women (Norwegian Institute of Public Health, 2009).

## Healthcare System

The Norwegian social and healthcare system is run by the state. All citizens have social and health insurance independent of age, social status, or occupation. Medical treatment is provided by a primary care physician who, if necessary, refers patients to specialized physicians. For every visit to the doctor, the patient must pay 15€. The annual limit is set at 1,780 NOK, which equals 180€. In case of an emergency, there is a nationwide emergency service. Hospitals are state run and organized regionally.

There has been an increase in the number of private insurances, hospitals, outpatient medical facilities, and healthcare providers for the internal labor market. *Arbeitstilsynet*, a state-run office of the Department of Employment, controls this sector and watches over approximately 240,000 businesses. Its work is based on the EU framework directive (Council Directive 89/39/EEC, from June 12, 1989), as well as on follow-up directives.

The exact cost of state expenses for the healthcare system cannot be easily determined, as the budget is distributed across several budget areas. Estimated numbers for 2009 are: 276 billion NOK (~34 billion euros) are spent on pensions and sick pay, 240 billion NOK (~30 billion euros) on retirement arrangements, and 240 billion NOK as financial support for health and educational facilities and child allowances. In addition, there are municipal and county (*Fylke*) contributions. Therefore, more than 50% of the national budget (overall amount in 2009: 848 billion NOK) goes to the healthcare and social system.

## Influence of Culture and Mentality

To this day, geography, climate, low population density (approximately 12 inhabitants per square kilometer), and close contact with nature have influenced Norwegian mentality and attitudes toward the way of life. These influences helped to shape the search for identity after gaining independence from Denmark in 1814. The relationship with nature developed into an astonishing nationwide spread of romanticism, possibly due to the lack of other identifying cultural characteristics.

The development of a national identity was intensified by the success of humanists, natural scientists, adventurers like Nansen and Amundsen, and the Norwegian Marine Corps' conquest of the world's oceans. In addition, the worldwide establishment of professional and amateur skiing by Norwegian students and emigrants (approximately 2 million descendants of Norwegian emigrants are living in the United States today) also contributed to Norwegian cultural identity.

German literary critic and author Enzensberger describes *Norwegian anachronism* as the feat of Norwegians defining their self-conception through nature and movement in nature. He refers to contact with nature still being predominant in a modern, rich, industrialized country and still being of more importance than the economic blessing of oil. Norwegians are still able to live in proximity to nature without neglecting technical progress and factors of civilization (Isaksen, n.d.).

The importance of nature and its cultural establishment is documented in the few words Norway has contributed to globally used vocabulary: words like *fjord*, *fjell*, *ski*, *slalom*, or the cultural phenomenon of *friluftsliv* are emotionally rooted and connected to experience. They cannot be looked up in a dictionary but—as Czech philosopher Konupek puts it—can only be understood by accompanying Norwegians in the cross-country ski trail or hiking. Considering this background, it is not a surprise that the most important Norwegian philosopher, Arne Naess (who died in 2009), was a devoted hiker and fan of *Friluftsliv,* which he described as "a rich life with simple means" (Naess, 1999).

More evidence of how strongly rooted nature is in Norwegian souls and lifestyle can be found in more than 400,000 private summer houses (*Hytten*), more than 20,000 kilometers of hiking trails and approximately 7,000 kilometers of cross-country ski trails listed by the Norwegian tourism association (www.dnt.no). Here you find more than 450 *Hytten* that can be used by anybody. In every municipality, there are countless leisure activities connected to nature. The fact that many companies run recreational facilities and vacation homes in the mountains or by the sea shows that near-natural activities and recreation play an important role in the context of WHP (Lagerstrom, 2007).

Influences on Norwegian values, attitudes, and behavior patterns include globalization and industrialization and an increasing number of immigrants and temporary employees. Besides these influences, humanism is another important shaping characteristic of the general atmosphere at workplaces. This is not only reflected in a distinctive, social break culture, i.e., Norwegians take regular coffee or social breaks during the workday, but can also be seen in the community spirit and the willingness to help others.

Only the future can reveal if this attitude and the good economic and social structures (that, for example, do not cause the need for multiple jobs) will be able to halt the ambition to increase material wealth and counteract encroaching laziness and sedentary ways of life.

## Drivers of Workplace Health Promotion

Sociocultural framework conditions, laws (www.aml.no), and working conditions ensure a good foundation for a healthy workplace. They not only consider protection and safety, ergonomic and spatial parameters, and working and recreation times, but are also based on a humanistic view in which individual needs, social concerns, and environmental aspects constitute central elements.

Due to the characteristics of Norwegian welfare, state organizations and institutions of the tradition-rich labor movement have a strong influence on the creation of framework conditions, their implementation, and control. The *Landsorganisasjonen i Norge*, the biggest workers' organization in the country with 860,000 members from 24 different private and public organizations, plays a leading role in the creation of humane, healthy, and safe workplaces (www.lo.no). It has tremendous influence on safety, health, and workplace regulations.

The AOF (www.aof.no), or Workers' Educational Association of Norway, plays an important role in the development of individual expertise of employees—including in regard to health. The AOF was founded in 1931 and consists of 36 technical, political, social, and cultural organizations within the labor movement.

The health, environment, and safety at workplaces (HMS) policy holds an exceptional position, with the responsibility for the organization, implementation, and in-company control of applicable measures (www.hms.no). Companies have to develop and document their own WHP system with a special focus. HMS policies allocate a lot of responsibility to the side of employers in order to ensure and improve health, milieu, and safety at workplaces.

To control regulations and the policy at workplaces, the *Arbeits-og Inkluderingdepartement*—the Department of Employment—established the Arbeitstilsynet, which has seven offices. These offices supervise the implementation of the *Arbeitsmiljoloven* (www.aml.to), which is health promotion policy based on EU framework directives (Council Directive 89/39/EEC, from June 2nd, 1989) and follow-up directives.

Despite high standard regulations and framework conditions concerning workplaces, there is a threatening increase of health problems such as smoking, stress, and obesity caused by lifestyle and behavior. This in turn influences social services, pension concerns, and absenteeism. To call a halt to this development, the work and welfare office was established on July 1, 2006 (www.nav.no), to coordinate state and municipal services. This department has 457 offices all over the country.

Besides the massive efforts of state-run offices, organizations, and institutions, there are many associations that support their work, including the *Norges Bedriftidrettsforbund* (NBIF)—the Norwegian Association of Company Sports—with more than 300,000 members in 4,500 clubs (www.bedriftsidrett.no). Because lifestyle-related health problems pose an increasing threat at the workplace, WHP activities during the last several years focused on topics like movement, nutrition, stress management, and other lifestyle concerns. Insurance companies contribute a great deal to company programs and to activities organized by the NBIF.

During the last few years, more private providers and international companies also became involved in the area of WHP. An example is the Danish company Falk, an Employee Assistance Program provider that cares for more than 1.7 million employees all over Europe.

## Programs

Norwegian laws and regulations at workplaces (for example HMS), as well as their supervision by the state (Arbeitstilsynet), guarantee a high level of protection and safety at workplaces. In addition, there are regular health controls and checkups, exemplified by smoking prohibition at workplaces and regulations for break time and break rooms.

A second typical characteristic for the WHP in Norway is the well-organized cooperation among institutions, organizations, offices, unions, and private institutions. This can be seen in campaigns and projects focused on employee commuting, nutrition programs, and scientific evaluations of WHP needs and necessities. The latest evaluation done by the Norwegian Sports University of Oslo in cooperation with NBIF and the Department of Health showed why it is problematic to motivate people to do more physical exercise (Ommundsen & Aadland, 2009).

Physically active people tend to make use of WHP programs more often than physically inactive people. Fifty-nine percent of people who exercise regularly are likely to understand the benefit of these offers, 48% of people with a positive attitude toward exercise understand these offers to be beneficial, and only 26% of those who do not exercise at all realize the benefit of the offer. The NBIF communication manager, Tim Gundersen, assesses the success rate with physically active people at 20% (www.nbif.no). Due to changes in disease patterns, increasing numbers of chronic diseases, and the insight that physically inactive people are hard to motivate to participate in sports and fitness programs, the NBIF not only extended its offers of physical activities and sports, but also broke new ground with its project *Aktiv Bedrift* (active company). The NBIF has recognized that in order to tackle the chronic disease problem, programs beyond physical activity and sports have to be offered. The concept, available to all Norwegian businesses, is divided into four phases (workplace analysis, action plan, measures, and evaluation) and conducted by a specifically trained consultant. Aktiv Bedrift aims at all employees, but focuses on less active staff.

The in-company home page plays an essential role. This is where all activities, programs, and teams are listed and kept up to date. Smaller companies share a home page and create a communication platform within their sector. The four phases of Aktiv Bedrift are addressed on the company web page as follows:

1. *Workplace analysis.* Along with the HMS data, a survey tool developed by the NBIF and the Department of Health is used to gather the staff's wishes and needs regarding physical and social activities.
2. *Action plan.* On the basis of the workplace analysis, i.e. the staff's registered wishes and needs, the company receives a document with specific proposals for initiatives and activities. The consultant is available to support organization, implementation, and further development.
3. *Measures.* The company is responsible for the creation of necessary framework conditions as well as for the implementation of proposed measures. The action plan determines if these measures are team competitions, workplace related activities, environmental measures, or campaigns like "use the stairs."
4. *Evaluation.* In order to document the health-related results, the company gathers data in cooperation with the consultant and issues a net-based evaluation of effects on health.

Although physical activity is a mainstay in the Aktiv Bedrift concept, the overall results show that there are more diverse and positive effects.

An increasing number of companies is using internal as well as commercially offered intensive programs (www.vital.no) by running advertisements like "Forti, Fett, Fertig" (forty, fat, burned out), and through media outlets, such as Frifagbevegelsen (www.frifagbevegelsen.no), information and communication are intensified in order to achieve changes.

Since physical activity, movement, sports, and of course, the cultural phenomenon of *Friluftsliv* are held in high esteem, such activities and programs have taken a central position in WHP ever since the first organized workers' initiatives in the 19th century (Larsen, n.d.). The oil industry in the North Sea, for example, placed great value on the establishment of fitness training centers on oil platforms (Damsgaard & Fjeld, 1978). In addition, many companies offer incentives, leisure time in vacation homes owned by the company, or cooperate with fitness studios, physiotherapists, or commercial providers specialized in WHP like Redcord (www.redcord.no) or TimeoutX—Nordic Energy (www.timeoutx.no).

## Good Practices

One of the companies that has implemented a comprehensive psychosocial risk management system is Statoil, a leading energy company in oil and gas production with about 30,000 employees.

Statoil focuses on the management of work-related stress through prevention while promoting a good work environment. The goal is to manage psychosocial risks in terms of organizational management, learning and development, social responsibility, and the promotion of good health at the workplace. Statoil cooperated with an international project initiated by the European commission (www.PRIMA-EF) in order to implement and develop a framework for psychosocial risk management at the workplace. The first step was the implementation of the psychosocial risk management approach, which identifies hazards, analyzes and manages risks, and protects workers. The second step was to develop a guideline presenting the basic principles and practical methods in a comprehensive but concise manner.

In an effort to gain a more comprehensive understanding of the psychosocial risks, Statoil has developed a psychosocial risk indicator and planned to begin administering it by 2010. This will identify factors such as job demand, job control, and social support. The system was designed to document and follow up psychosocial risks across the organization and be part of a comprehensive system, combing thorough care identification of major psychosocial hazards followed up by in-depth risk assessment and implementation of appropriate risk management measures.

Another workplace health promotion program that can be labeled as a model of good practice is implemented at the Department of Youth Affairs in Oslo, Norway (European Network for Workplace Health Promotion, 2004). In cooperation with the Centre for Health Promotion in Settings (CHPS), it has implemented a tool, known as the CHPS model, that focuses on empowering employees with resources and knowledge on how to manage stress-related change. The goal of the tool is to promote the health of workers by making their work tasks more manageable and comprehensible, and by giving the employees a sense of control over their work. Employees and managers can ease the process of organizational change by identifying and solving conflict and tension and by allowing a two-way communication of expectations. As a result, employees should be able to manage stress more efficiently, which should reflect in their overall subjective well-being and their productivity.

## Outcomes and Indicators

The classic inspection of regulations stands in the foreground of WHP because of the traditional linkage of protection, safety, and environment issues to the health of workers. Furthermore, continuous documentation of accidents and absenteeism due to illness reflect the coherence of HMS and questions coming up in its context. In-company HMS work helps to assess satisfaction and the general environment at workplaces, so that there is good overall information about health-related questions at workplaces. WHP, therefore, is driven more by state regulations and controls than by financial or scientific factors. Nevertheless, there are university research approaches and many interesting scientific issues in relation to health, attitude, and behavioral parameters, which are not at least caused by increasing focus on quality management. Therefore, holistic concepts and research approaches have gained more importance in Norway.

## Existing Research

From a historic point of view, Norwegian WHP focused on the development of safe working conditions. Research aspects related to WHP gained more importance because of changes in society and workplace-related framework conditions; chronic diseases; and the development of independent university research facilities. Besides safety and environment issues, studying of solutions related to diseases of the musculoskeletal and cardiovascular systems as well as psychological ailments, which currently cause two thirds of absent work days and premature pension, became a core theme.

A process-oriented, interdisciplinary pilot project was conducted with long-term unemployed individuals with diffuse musculoskeletal and mental problems, who represent a major problem group in Norway. This project documented that, next to work-related framework conditions and motivation, the type of intervention is of crucial significance for success. Fifteen out of 80 long-term unemployed workers took part in an 18-month physical and psychological training program. By the end of the 4-month introductory, intensive phase, 5 out of 8 participants who were clinically classified as being depressive could be reclassified as normal. On average, aerobic capacity increased by 29% and muscular strength by 57% (cervical and deltoid) and 24% (lumbar). Except for 3 people who only partly participated in the program, most participants went back to work (part or full time) in the course of the intervention phase (Kogstad, 1996).

Besides informational health seminars, individual counseling, and a fitness training concept aiming at competence and self-responsibility (part or full time), the Redcord training tool was a major part of the whole program. Redcord was developed in Norway and is estimated to be responsible for an 80% reduction of sick notes due to muscular issues since the 1990s (Moe & Thom, 1997; Falla, Jull, Hodges, & Vicenzino 2006).

Regarding sick notes that cannot be explained only by sickness, environment and motivation issues must be considered (Ose, Jensberg, Reinersten, Sandsmund, & Dyrstad, 2006). The discussion about work structure and organization has started anew due to a new study on motivation in workplaces (Kuvaas, 2009). Among 800 employees of different municipalities and areas of operation, it was determined that the New Public Management characterized by supervision and rapport encourages less motivation and commitment to work than a work structure based on self-determination and cooperation (Kuvaas, 2009). This finding leads to the conclusion that self-determination and self-responsibility can be central aspects of WHP.

Physical fitness, movement, and sports have a long tradition in Norway, which is reflected in company contexts. This does not refer only to classical sports initiated by companies, which have become more health-oriented in recent years, but also to the establishment of training centers across industries, like the ones established on oil platforms in the North Sea.

A survey done when the first training centers were established on oil platforms revealed that only 50% of the employees were motivated to use them (Damsgaard & Fjeld, 1978). This in turn led to a discussion about the extent and variety of offerings, and ways they might be implemented, which certainly is one reason why interesting and effective WHP activities in Norway are now more diverse and efficient. Many interesting WHP activities have already begun, and new research results are expected in the coming years.

The Aktiv Bedrift project of the NBIF, which has existed for several years, features a number of encouraging results. Not only is the increased level of in-company activity astonishing, but companies have also seen more and more detectable improvements in milieu and communication behavior, as well as an increase in community spirit (www.aktivlivsstiel.com).

At the large Norwegian shipyard Aker Kverner Pusnes, the following effects can be noticed (Sunde, 2010):

- participation of 80% of the staff
- creation of new activities
- cross-departmental community activities
- absence due to illness decreased to 2%
- increasing inclusion of local activity options
- increasing workplace attractiveness

A number of other companies report similar results. Remarkable are the project's recurring positive effects on workplace milieu, employee satisfaction, and physical fitness, which lead to a decrease in days of illness. Another reason for the success of Aktiv Bedrift is its focus on milieu and satisfaction instead of reduction of days of illness. Due to its establishment among companies' management and staff, its holistic approach, and its process-oriented implementation, the program seems to represent a promising approach for WHP activities.

It must be kept in mind that the concept has been developed on the basis of already existing, state-approved regulations and measures for a safe and healthy workplace. That is why Aktiv Bedrift is more a supplement and extension of experiences and activities than a new or competing concept.

# Conclusion

Due to the discovery of oil, Norway has developed in just a few centuries from a poor country that had been making its living from farming and fishing into one of the wealthiest and most modern countries in the world. Nevertheless, the self-conception and identity of Norwegians still reflect a close relationship with nature, one in which environmental and ecologic issues play a central role. This is reflected not only in legislation such as *Allemannretten* and in workplace regulations, but also in social contexts at workplaces. Workplace design, safety, and milieu issues are characterized by a humanistic approach. Norwegians' appreciation for autonomous action is demonstrated in employees' being allowed to call in sick for up to 24 days per year without a doctor's note.

Although framework conditions such as the economy and workplace design are outstanding, negative consequences of a prosperous society are increasingly felt. Chronic diseases are already a leading cause of death, and musculoskeletal problems are the main cause of a relatively high rate of absences due to illness (7.7%). In the context of WHP interventions, emphasis is placed on behavioral aspects in order to halt this development. In addition to government and nongovernment providers of WHP activities, there is an increasing number of commercial providers as well.

Beyond workplace-related programs related to body posture, nutrition, and stress, more emphasis is placed on programs that intend to compensate for an inactive way of life, as exemplified by countrywide campaigns for a more active way to work, activities of daily living, and recreational activities performed outdoors.

The challenge for promising WHP activities can be seen in the context of behavioral aspects, rather than in the context of employment relationships. Only the fostering of self-responsibility for a health-oriented lifestyle, in a way that leads to lasting effects, might make it possible to eliminate the main causes for health problems in workplaces.

## Summary

Due to the discovery of oil and the resulting economic development, Norway became one of the wealthiest and most modern countries in the world in a few centuries. In addition to a strong economy and the resulting social changes, Norwegian politics and society are still characterized by a humanistic attitude and a high sensibility for issues related to nature and the environment.

The Norwegian lifestyle and the symbiosis of ecology and economy shape Norwegian WHP as well. This is why the labor movement placed such emphasis on milieu, safety, and health, as well as on development of employees' competence. Additionally, state-run organizations and regulations—for example, regulations for health, environment, and safety (HMS)—and state controls at workplaces have led to a framework of high standards for workplace conditions.

As in most modern industrial societies, behavioral and lifestyle-related health problems pose a major challenge in Norway. In addition to a traditionally strong emphasis on physical activities, *Friluftsliv,* and sports—such as the efforts made by the Norwegian Association of Company Sports—WHP activities are characterized by networking and cooperating with institutions, organizations, unions, and private providers. As the rate of absence from work due to illness, stress, and mental disorders increases, WHP focuses on psychosocial factors and health programs, as well as on the investigation, development, and implementation of programs related to the working environment.

## Review Questions

1. Where does Norway rank internationally with regard to life expectancy and satisfaction?
2. What are the major future challenges to Norway's national health status?
3. What are the components of the Norwegian healthcare system and how are they funded? Regulated? Managed?
4. How did Norwegian philosopher Arne Naess define the cultural phenomenon *Friluftsliv*? How is this related to Norwegian culture?
5. Explain the role of *Landsorganisasjonen i Norge* in Norway's workplace health promotion programs.
6. How is Norway working to improve outcome indicators of workplace health promotion programs?
7. Describe one of the successful Norwegian workplace health promotion programs. What is the program, what are its components, and why has it been effective?

## References


Bahr, R. (2008). *Aktivitetshandboken—Fysisk aktivitet i furebygging og behandling*. Oslo, Norway: Helsedirektoratet.

Damsgaard, K., & Fjeld, J. (1978). *I form på plattform*. Oslo, Norway: Universitetsforlaget.

European Network for Workplace Health Promotion (2004). ENWHP toolbox. Woerden, The Netherlands: NIGZ Work & Health.

Falla, D., Jull, G., Hodges, P., & Vicenzino, B. (2006). An endurance-strength training regime is effective in reducing myoelectric manifestations of cervical flexor muscle fatigue in females with chronic neck pain. *Clinical Neuropsychology, 117*(4), 828–837.

Isaksen, J. (n.d.). *Mensch in Landschaft oder Norwegen bewegt- Erleben ist mehr als Verstehen- In IPN (Red), Schul- und Studienfahrten nach Sørlandet*. Kristiansand, Norway: Vest-Agder Fykeskommune.

Kogstad, O. (1996). Prosjektet aktiv helse. Fylkestrygdekontoret i Vest-Agder. Høgskolen i Agder, Kristiansand.

Kuvaas, B. (2009). A text of hypotheses derived from self-determination theory among public sector employees. *Employee Relations, 31*(1), 39–56.

Lagerstrom, D. (2007). *Friluftsliv-Entwicklung, bedeutung und perspektiven.* Achen, Germany: Meyer & Meyer.

Larsen, P. (n.d.). Hele folket i idrett. *Norges bedriftsdrettsforbund.* Oslo, Norway.

Moe, H., & Thom, E. (1997). Musculoskeletal disorders and physical activity: Result of a long-term study. *Den norske lægeforeningen, 29*, 4258–4261.

Naess, A. (1999). "Truth" as conceived by those who are not professional philosophers. Oslo, Norway.

Norwegian Institute of Public Health. (2009). Overweight and obesity in Norway — factsheet. Oslo, Norway.

Norwegian Labour and Welfare Organisation. (2010). Homepage. Retrieved February 15, 2011, from http://www.nav.no

Norwegian Ministry of Health and Care Services. (2007). *Norway's national strategy for tobacco control 2006–2010.* Oslo, Norway: Minstry of Health and Care Services.

Olsen, L. (2003). *Inclusive workplace—Norway's tripartite agreement.* Bureau for Workers' Activities. Geneva, Switzerland: ILO.

Ommundsen, Y., & Aadland, A. (2009). Fysisk inaktivitet hos voksne i Norge. Hvem er de og hva motiverer til fysisk aktivitet? Oslo, Norway: Helsedirektoratet.

Ose, S., Jensberg, H., Reinersten, R., Sandsmund, M., & Dyrstad, J. (2006). *Sykefravær-Kunnskapsstatus og problemstillinger.* Oslo, Norway: SINTEF.

Sunde, A. (2010) *Aker kværner pusnes.* Retrieved from http://www.aktivbedrift.no

World Health Organization (WHO). (2009). *WHO report on the global tobacco epidemic, 2009.* Geneva, Switzerland: WHO.

Chapter 16

# Russia

Rimma A. Potemkina

After reading this chapter you should be able to:

- Identify core strategies that are the focus of workplace health promotion efforts in Russia
- Describe the historical evolution of Russia's workplace health promotion efforts
- Explain the different approaches employed by corporate health promotion efforts throughout Russia
- Review the central disease states and health issues driving workplace health promotion in Russia
- Name the components of, and the associated funding sources for, the Russian healthcare system
- Discuss the impact of culture on the health status and health promotion efforts within Russia

Table 16-1 **Select Key Demographic and Economic Indicators**

| | |
|---|---|
| Nationality | Noun: Russian(s)<br>Adjective: Russian |
| Ethnic groups | Russian 79.8%, Tatar 3.8%, Ukrainian 2%, Bashkir 1.2%, Chuvash 1.1%, other or unspecified 12.1% (2002 census) |
| Religion | Russian Orthodox 15–20%, Muslim 10–15%, other Christian 2% (2006 est.)<br>*Note:* estimates are of practicing worshipers; Russia has large populations of nonpracticing believers and nonbelievers, a legacy of over 7 decades of Soviet rule |
| Language | Russian, many minority languages |
| Literacy | Definition: age 15 and over can read and write<br>Total population: 99.4%<br>Male: 99.7%<br>Female: 99.2% (2002 census) |
| Education expenditure | 3.8% of GDP (2005)<br>Country comparison to the world: 116 |

*continued*

| Table 16-1 Select Key Demographic and Economic Indicators, *continued* | |
|---|---|
| Government type | Federation |
| Environment | Air pollution from heavy industry, emissions of coal-fired electric plants, and transportation in major cities; industrial, municipal, and agricultural pollution of inland waterways and seacoasts; deforestation; soil erosion; soil contamination from improper application of agricultural chemicals; scattered areas of sometimes intense radioactive contamination; groundwater contamination from toxic waste; urban solid waste management; abandoned stocks of obsolete pesticides |
| Country mass | Total: 17,098,242 sq km<br>Country comparison to the world: 1<br>Land: 16,377,742 sq km<br>Water: 720,500 sq km |
| Population | 140,041,247 (July 2010 est.)<br>Country comparison to the world: 9 |
| Age structure | 0–14 years: 14.8% (male 10,644,833/female 10,095,011)<br>15–64 years: 71.5% (male 48,004,040/female 52,142,313)<br>65 years and over: 13.7% (male 5,880,877/female 13,274,173)<br>(2010 est.) |
| Median age | Total: 38.5 years<br>Male: 35.3 years<br>Female: 41.7 years (2010 est.) |
| Population growth rate | -0.467% (2010 est.)<br>Country comparison to the world: 224 |
| Birth rate | 11.1 births/1,000 population (2010 est.)<br>Country comparison to the world: 178 |
| Death rate | 16.06 deaths/1,000 population (July 2010 est.)<br>Country comparison to the world: 12 |
| Net migration rate | 0.28 migrant(s)/1,000 population (2010 est.)<br>Country comparison to the world: 69 |
| Urbanization | Urban population: 73% of total population (2008)<br>Rate of urbanization: -0.5% annual rate of change (2005–2010 est.) |
| Gender ratio | At birth: 1.06 male(s)/female<br>Under 15 years: 1.05 male(s)/female<br>15–64 years: 0.92 male(s)/female<br>65 years and over: 0.44 male(s)/female<br>Total population: 0.85 male(s)/female (2010 est.) |
| Infant mortality rate | Total: 10.56 deaths/1,000 live births<br>Country comparison to the world: 152<br>Male: 12.08 deaths/1,000 live births<br>Female: 8.94 deaths/1,000 live births (2010 est.) |

*continued*

| Table 16-1 **Select Key Demographic and Economic Indicators,** *continued* | |
|---|---|
| Life expectancy | Total population: 66.03 years<br>Country comparison to the world: 162<br>Male: 59.33 years<br>Female: 73.14 years (2010 est.) |
| Total fertility rate | 1.41 children born/woman (2010 est.)<br>Country comparison to the world: 195 |
| GDP—purchasing power parity | $2.11 trillion (2009 est.)<br>Country comparison to the world: 8 |
| GDP—per capita | $15,100 (2009 est.)<br>Country comparison to the world: 72 |
| GDP—composition by sector | Agriculture: 4.7%<br>Industry: 34.8%<br>Services: 60.5% (2009 est.) |
| Agriculture—products | Grain, sugar beets, sunflower seed, vegetables, fruits, beef, milk |
| Industries | Complete range of mining and extractive industries producing coal, oil, gas, chemicals, and metals; all forms of machine building from rolling mills to high-performance aircraft and space vehicles; defense industries including radar, missile production, and advanced electronic components, shipbuilding; road and rail transportation equipment; communications equipment; agricultural machinery, tractors, and construction equipment; electric power generating and transmitting equipment; medical and scientific instruments; consumer durables, textiles, foodstuffs, handicrafts |
| Labor force participation | 75.81 million (2009 est.)<br>Country comparison to the world: 7 |
| Unemployment rate | 8.4% (2009 est.)<br>Country comparison to the world: 95 |
| Industrial production growth rate | -11.9% (2009 est.)<br>Country comparison to the world: 149 |
| Distribution of family income (GINI index) | 42.3 (2008)<br>Country comparison to the world: 53 |
| Investment (gross fixed) | 20.2% of GDP (2009 est.)<br>Country comparison to the world: 92 |
| Public debt | 6.9% of GDP (2009 est.)<br>Country comparison to the world: 124 |
| Market value of publicly traded shares | $861.4 billion (December 31, 2009)<br>Country comparison to the world: 7 |
| Current account balance | $48.97 billion (2009 est.)<br>Country comparison to the world: 5 |

*continued*

| Table 16-1 Select Key Demographic and Economic Indicators, *continued* | |
|---|---|
| Debt (external) | $369.2 billion (December 31, 2009 est.)<br>Country comparison to the world: 20 |
| Debt as a % of GDP | —— |
| Exports | $303.4 billion (2009 est.)<br>Country comparison to the world: 13 |
| Exports—commodities | Petroleum and petroleum products, natural gas, wood and wood products, metals, chemicals, and a wide variety of civilian and military manufactures |
| Exports—partners | Netherlands 10.62%, Italy 6.46%, Germany 6.24%, China 5.69%, Turkey 4.3%, Ukraine 4.01% (2009) |
| Imports | $191.8 billion (2009 est.)<br>Country comparison to the world: 19 |
| Imports—commodities | Vehicles, machinery and equipment, plastics, medicines, iron and steel, consumer goods, meat, fruits and nuts, semifinished metal products |
| Imports—partners | Germany 14.39%, China 13.98%, Ukraine 5.48%, Italy 4.84%, United States 4.46%, (2009) |
| Stock of direct foreign investment at | |
| Home | $258.8 billion (December 31, 2009 est.)<br>Country comparison to the world: 19 |
| Abroad | $226.2 billion (December 31, 2009 est.)<br>Country comparison to the world: 16 |

Source: CIA. (2010). *The world factbook.* Retrieved December 16, 2010, from https://www.cia.gov/library/publications/the-world-factbook/

# Introduction

The Russian Federation is the largest state in the world in terms of land mass, located in the eastern part of Europe and the northern part of Asia. The country takes up one ninth of the world's land. In 2008, Russia had 141,780,032 inhabitants, 73% of whom lived in urban areas. There are more than 180 nationalities and more than 100 languages represented in Russia, and 80% of the inhabitants are Russians. The most prominent religion is the Russian Orthodox Church, followed by Islam; however, a large part of the population are atheists, mainly due to the Soviet past (*The World Factbook,* 2010).

According to the constitution, state power is carried out by the president, federal council, and the State Duma. Russia has a federal structure; there are 83 subjects (members) of the federation, defined by administrative-geographical location. There are 14 cities with 1 million or more inhabitants in the country, the largest among them are Moscow (10.5 million) and St. Petersburg (4.6 million).

In 2008, the gross domestic product (GDP) was 41,668 billion rubles, and the level of unemployment was 5.9% (Federal State Statistics Service, n.d.). The economic structure has not undergone any significant changes since 1995; the service sector creates about 60% of the GDP, and industry and agriculture create about 40% of the GDP. The fuel-energy industry is the most important branch of Russian industry; other important branches are pulp and paper, transport, and the metal mining industry.

The three most important periods in the country's political, social, and cultural life are before the October revolution (1917), the Soviet era (between 1917 and the mid-1990s) and the post-Soviet era (since the mid-1990s). Political life is currently in the process of democratization, and presidential government and parliament are in the process of formation. The Russian economy has had many difficulties especially during the last few years, mostly due to volatility in the natural resources sector. The current cultural life is preoccupied with the reconstruction of old Russian traditions, especially religion, and the integration of these in modern life.

## Prevailing Health Issues and Risk Behaviors

From 1990 to 2008, the Russian population decreased by 6 million (from 147,912,992 in 1990 to 141,780,032 in 2008) (World Health Organization, n.d. a). In the Russian Federation from 1940 to 2010, the mortality rate increased from 11.2 per 1,000 to 14.2 per 1,000 (Figure 16-1) and remains significantly higher than in Europe (Figure 16-2). At the same time, the birth rate declined from 13.5 per 1,000 to 10.4 per 1,000 (World Health Organization, n.d. a).

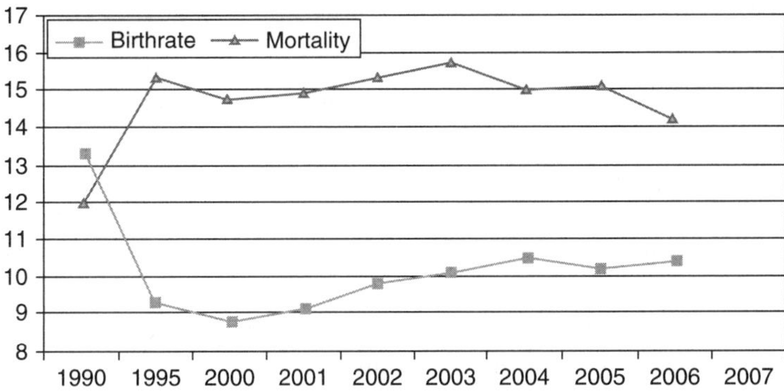


Figure 16-1 Dynamics of the birth rate and mortality (per 1,000) of the Russian population.
Source: http://www.euro.who.int/HFADB

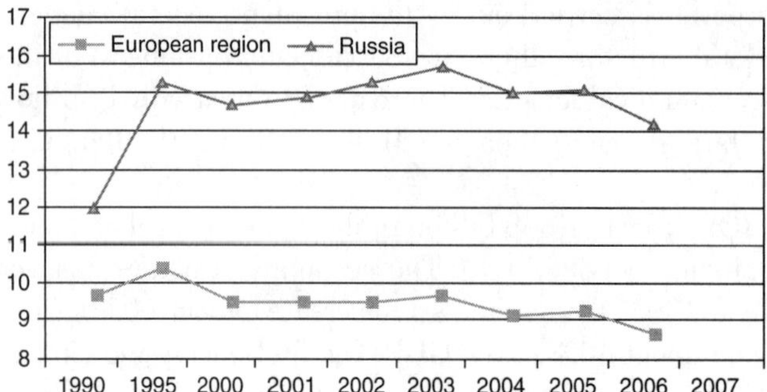


Figure 16-2 Dynamics of the mortality (per 1,000) of the Russian and European population.
Source: http://www.euro.who.int/InformationSources/Data

In 2006, mortality of Russian men 25–64 years of age due to diseases of the circulatory system was 2.5 times higher than European men of the same age (World Health Organization, n.d. b). The high level of mortality of Russians, especially of working age, leads to significant potential years of lost life, losses in gross national product (GNP) and a low life expectancy. As of 2006, Russian men lived 10.8 years fewer than Europeans (Figure 16-3) (Oganov, Komarov, & Maslennikova, 2009). A considerable portion of the premature deaths occur in the working age population.

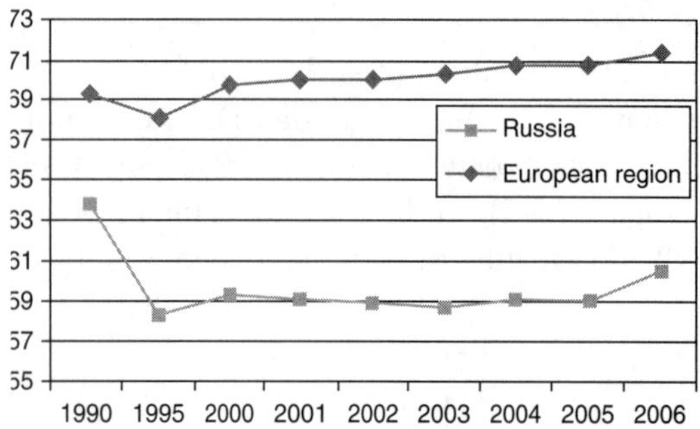


Figure 16-3 Life expectancy at birth, in years of the Russian and European men.
Source: http://www.euro.who.int/HFADB

Noncommunicable diseases (NCDs), cardiovascular diseases, external causes, and cancer account for more then 80% of Russian mortalities. Cardiovascular disease is a leading cause of premature death in men (about half of all cases) as well as in women (two thirds of all cases) (Figures 16-4, 16-5). In men, the second cause of mortality is an external disease, while in women, the second cause is cancer deaths (Oganov & Maslennikova, 2006).

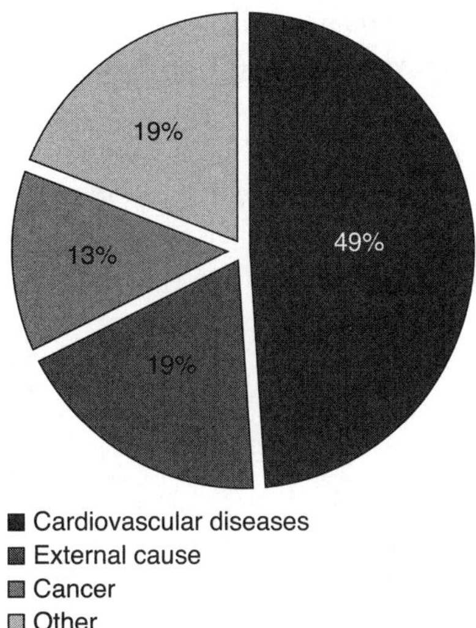


Figure 16-4 Structure of mortality of the Russian men in 2006.
Source: Oganov, Komarov, & Maslennikova, 2009.

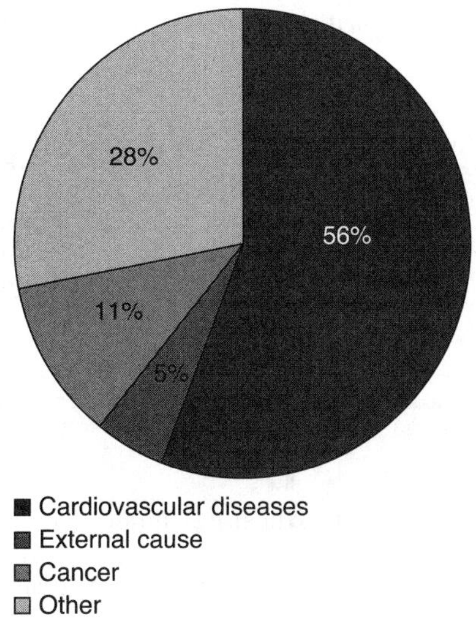


Figure 16-5 Structure of mortality of the Russian women in 2006.
Source: Oganov, Komarov, & Maslennikova, 2009.

## Prevalence of Risk Factors in the Working Age Population

In Russia, the leading causes of death and disability are directly associated with behavioral risk factors. In 2000–2003, under the framework of the Russian Countrywide Integrated Noncommunicable Disease Program (CINDI), six Russian regions conducted behavioral risk factor surveys among 25–64-year-old people on random samples composed of 2,000–3,000 people from each of the six regions. The response rate varied from 60–80% in different regions (Potemkina, 2006).

The criterion for high blood pressure was a systolic blood pressure ≥140 mmHg and/or a diastolic blood pressure ≥ 90 mmHg; or systolic blood pressure <140 mmHg and/or a diastolic blood pressure < 90 mmHg, with a background of treatment with hypotensive preparations during the previous 2 weeks. Regional surveys have shown that up to 45% men and women have an elevated blood pressure (Figures 16-6 and 16-7).

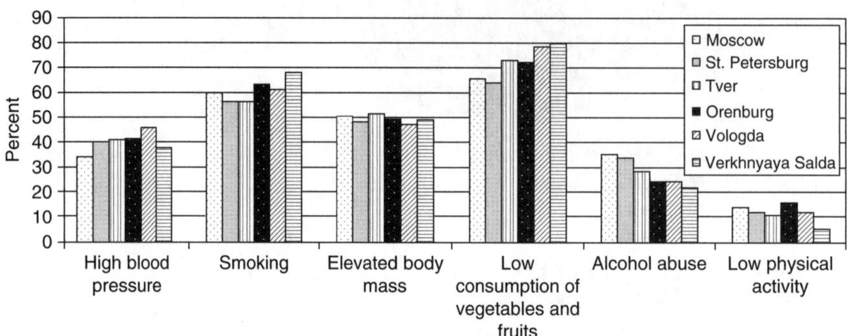


Figure 16-6 Prevalence of risk factors in Russian men ages 25–64 in 2000–2002 (adjusted by age).
Source: CINDI. Behavioral risk factors monitoring in the CINDI-Russia regions, 2000–2002

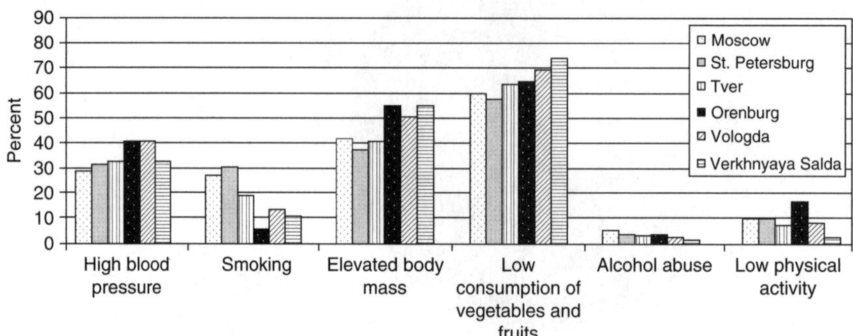


Figure 16-7 Prevalence of risk factors in Russian women ages 25–64 in 2000–2002 (adjusted by age).
Source: CINDI. Behavioral risk factors monitoring in the CINDI-Russia regions, 2000–2002

Persons who had smoked more than 100 cigarettes during their lives and who smoked every day or often were considered to be smokers. Data analysis has shown that up to 68% of men and up to 32% of women are smokers.

Data analysis has also shown that overweight (body mass index ≥ 25) and obesity (body mass index ≥ 30) are highly prevalent in the different geographic and administrative settings in the Russian population; about half of men and two thirds of women are overweight and about one tenth of men and up to one quarter of women are obese.

Across regions, up to 80% of men and women have low consumption of fruits and vegetables. The criterion for a low consumption of vegetables and fruits was accepted as less than 400 grams a day. Regional surveys have also shown that up to 35% men are alcohol abusers. The criterion for excessive consumption of alcohol was accepted as a consumption of more than 20 grams of pure alcohol a day.

In Russia, up to 17% of men and women have a low level of physical activity. Persons with a low level of physical activity included those who said that they mainly sit at work or do not work, walk less than 60 min/day, and do not engage in any kind of exercise in leisure time. Low level of physical activity was also prevalent in the working population; about one third of men and about half of women have mainly sedentary work, and only one fifth to one quarter of respondents engage in leisure time activity at least 30 min/day, 5 days/week or more. Nevertheless, mean walking time varied in the different regions from 70 min/day to 85 min/day in men and from 70 min/day to 90 min/day in women.

## Healthcare System

The current healthcare system was established in the beginning of the 20th century. The main principle of the system is availability and free service. Government health insurance (compulsory insurance) covers all citizens of the country. There is a list of essential health services which the obligatory insurance covers.

Traditionally, planning for the public healthcare budget was based on the number of hospital beds; consequently, the number of beds has been needlessly higher than in other countries, although it declined from 1990 to 2006 (Figure 16-8).

At the same time, public sector expenditures on health as a percentage of gross domestic product (GDP) in Russia stood idle at 5.4% from 2000 to 2010, which is about half of the amount in western European countries (World Health Organization, n.d. a).

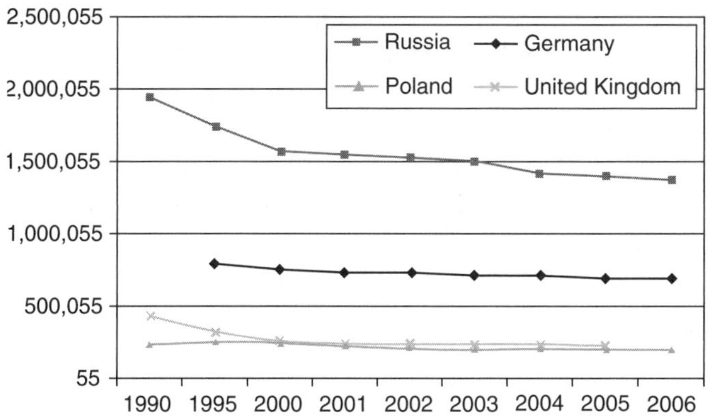


Figure 16-8 Total number of hospital beds per 100,000 population.
Source: http://www.euro.who.int/HFADB

The existing government healthcare system is based on the geographic-territorial principle. Each citizen in Russia has obligatory insurance and could apply for care at the local outpatient clinic, which is typically located close to the place of residence and has a contract with the government insurance company. Primary health care is provided by a district physician, who works at the outpatient clinic. If a patient needs any special medical care (ophthalmology, cardiology, endocrinology, etc.) the district physician refers the patient to a corresponding specialist, who is working at the same outpatient clinic or in a neighboring one. From 1990 to 2010 general practitioners have started working in different regions of Russia, but the system of general practitioners is not widespread.

Since the 1990s, a parallel voluntary insurance system appeared, and private health structures began developing. The system functions on an individual contract basis with health care or through the employer, typically with large commercial operations, which take care of their employees. The Organisation for Economic Co-operation and Development (OECD) characterizes the Russian healthcare system as half-reformed and sees the key challenges in "strengthening primary care provision and reducing the current over-reliance on tertiary care; restructuring the incentives facing healthcare providers; and completing the reform of the system of mandatory medical insurance" (Organisation for Economic Co-operation and Development, 2007).

## Influence of Culture and Mentality

There are 83 regions in Russia and more than 140 million inhabitants with different nationalities, cultures, and religions. In the Soviet era, Russian language was the official language; in addition, local national languages existed in all the Soviet republics. Traditionally, all regional populations speak Russian, and that creates a common cultural bond for the nation. On the other hand, there are a lot of specificities in the national/cultural traditions with regard to health, including behavioral habits, social and physical environments, nutrition, climate differences, and level of urbanization in different regions. For example, the nutritional habits of the populations in the north of Russia differ from those of the southern populations (fruit and vegetable consumption is more prevalent among southern populations; fish and meat consumption is more prevalent among northern populations).

Nevertheless, as it was indicated in the epidemiological studies, the situation from the point of view of the NCD risk factors prevalence is very similar (Figures 16-6 and 16-7) in different regions and comparable with those in other countries. The concept of common NCD risk factors could serve as a basis for the implementation of an integrated approach to health promotion and NCD prevention programs anywhere in the country.

# Drivers of Workplace Health Promotion

There are several economical and humanitarian reasons why workplace health promotion programs are important for business.

## Prosperity of Company and Health of Employees

The prosperity of the company depends on the health of its employees to a great extent. Economical analyses of studies conducted in the business environment have detected that the main impacts of poor employee health for companies are companies' healthcare expenditures and, predominantly, decreases in employees' ability to perform their functions due to poor health. A 2008 economic analysis conducted in a large financial corporation in Russia indicated that financial losses due to worker presenteeism are incomparably bigger than the losses due to absenteeism, and they amount to about 6% of the corporation's annual profits (Potemkina, 2008). From this point of view, it is clear that the strategic direction of preventive programs at the workplace should be not just to minimize healthcare expenditures but also to decrease the risk profile of the working population.

Numerous international programs focusing on decreasing employees' risk factors have shown their effectiveness in improving workers' health indicators as well as economic benefits.

## Prolongation and Retention of Skilled Personnel

The prolongation of the active life of people and retention of skilled personnel at the workplace are important to business.

The aging of the world population and the decrease of the proportion of the working age population creates a gap in future workforces. This gap is especially important to high-technology businesses, which need qualified professionals. The profits of such companies are closely related to well-being and good health of their workers. Competition among large business structures also creates acute demands for qualified personnel. Social workplace programs could be one of the important factors, promoting the employees' health improvement as well as decreasing personnel turnover.

## Reduction in High Risk Factors/Reduction in Costs

Employees with a high-risk profile are very costly to the social services of the company. The prevalence risk factor data obtained from the surveys in 2007 by the random sample of employees of the Russian Financial Corporation URALSIB were matched with the expenses of the corporation for health care in 2006. The results indicated that that those who have a low level of physical activity have double the amount of health expenditures compared to those who have a high level of physical activity. Employees who consume a low level of fruits and vegetables have 32% higher health expenditures compared to those who eat more of these products;

employees with high levels of blood cholesterol have 1.7 times higher health expenditures compared with those who have normal levels (Potemkina, 2008).

### Social Responsibility

Workplace health promotion programs are important for business. However, businesses should also include health promotion services at the workplace in order to assume social responsibility for their employees and to promote health within the country.

## Programs

Workplace health promotion programs have a relatively long history in Russia. In the Soviet era, a healthcare system belonging to the large enterprises existed in parallel to public health care. This system was funded by enterprises and included hospitals, outpatient clinics, and medical units in the enterprises' departments. In general, the system was rather strong in reach, and very often much richer than public health. Presently, only the largest companies (such as GAZPROM) have their own healthcare services; most companies cover the healthcare expenditures of their employees through voluntary medical insurance using public health services or private heath medical institutes.

#### Automotive Industry

The largest enterprise of the Soviet Union's automotive industry obtained impressive results in the beginning of the 1980s (Britov, 1983). Conducting an arterial hypertension control (AH) program through primary and secondary prevention by medical personnel of the enterprise resulted in the reduction of total mortality by 20%, stroke mortality by 70%, and nonfatal myocardial infarction by 22% in 5 years.

#### Heavy Machine-Building Industry, Electrostal-city

Another example of NCD prevention comes from the largest heavy machine-building enterprise at Electrostal-city, located 60 kilometers east of Moscow. The program has been conducted since 1985 among 13,500 employees of the enterprise. The comprehensive approach included integrating different structures in the program, including administrative and financial support from the enterprise authorities, medical personnel also from the enterprise, local mass media, and consultations from researchers in the process planning, implementation, and program evaluation.

Nurses were crucial to the success of the program, heading the work of the medical units in each of the enterprise's departments. The AH control measures emphasized the promotion of a healthy lifestyle among the employees. The nurses were trained to consult on promoting healthy behaviors and treating AH. A random sample of workers had their blood pressures monitored for 5 years. The results showed that the prevalence of AH declined by 2% in men and 4% in women. Another main achievement of the program was an increase in the detectability of AH, which led to improvement of AH control. According to the official data, there was a 26% decrease in the amount of short-term disability due to AH and 28% decrease in the total numbers of days lost due to AH (Solov'eva, 2006).

## URALSIB—Finance and Insurance

A more recent example of health promotion in the workplace occurred at the Russian financial corporation, URALSIB. URALSIB is one of the largest finance and insurance businesses in the Russian Federation. There are more than 20,000 URALSIB employees in different parts of the country. This population differs from those mentioned previously. Most URALSIB employees are office workers with white collar jobs and rather high levels of education. Also, they are rather young; the mean age of the population was 34.8 years for men and 32.6 for women in 2008.

In 2007 and 2008, BRF surveys were conducted among a random sample of employees. The aim of the study was to detect main health problems of the employees and the priorities in the social program development. The standard questionnaire included demographics; education; health status; healthcare accessibility; height and weight; smoking habits; fruit and vegetable consumption; physical activity patterns during working time and leisure time; time spent walking; blood pressure and cholesterol awareness; and seat-belt use data. The surveys were conducted through intranet, e-mail, and telephone interviews. The response rate in 2008 was 81.7%.

Results of the survey have shown that the prevalence of AH was 32% in men and 16% in women, and smoking rates were at 36% and 19%, respectively. Low levels of PA were highly prevalent in the working population; 80% of men and 91% of women have mainly sedentary work, and only 16% and 9% of men and women, respectively, have leisure time activity at least 30 min/day, 5 days/week or more. Mean walking time was about 60 min/day in both genders (30 minutes less compared with the regional CINDI data) (Figure 16-9).

Data analysis of the URALSIB survey has shown that overweight (body mass index ≥ 25) and obesity (body mass index ≥ 30) are highly prevalent in the working population; 56% of men and 31% of women are overweight and 15% of men and 7% of women are obese. Almost 100% of men and women have a low level of fruit and vegetable consumption (fewer than five servings a day) (Figure 16-10). The mean value of fruit and vegetable consumption was less than two servings a day in both genders.

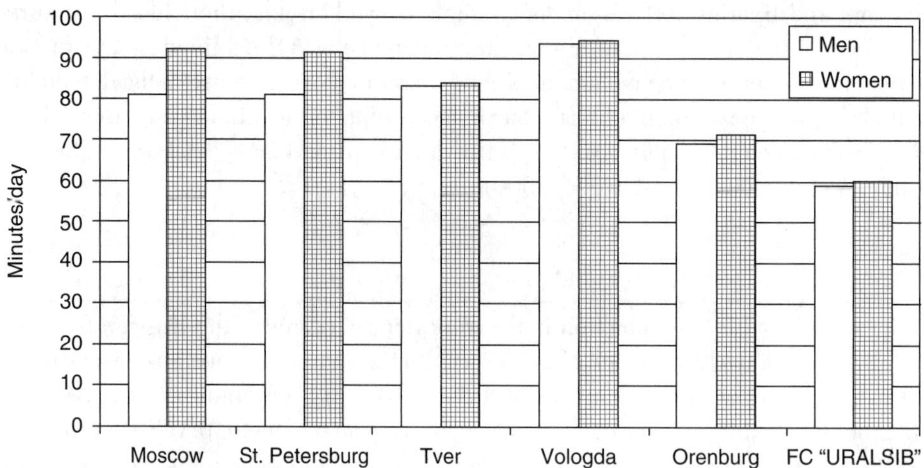


Figure 16-9 Mean walking time of the Russian population in different regions and of the employees of URALSIB.

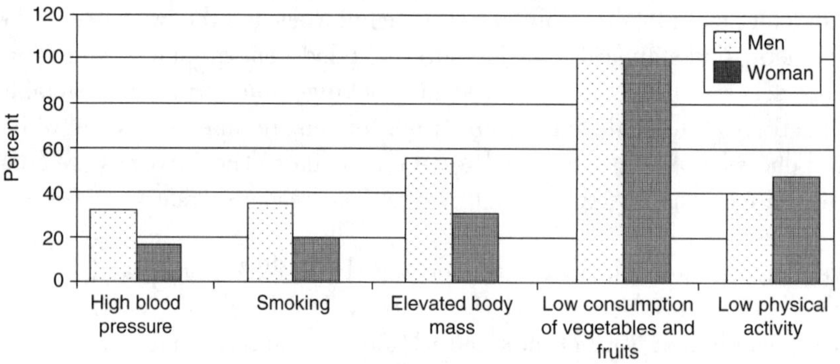


Figure 16-10 Prevalence of risk factors among the employees of URALSIB in 2008.

Data obtained from the surveys were matched with the corporation's healthcare expenses for 2006. The corporation covers employee health expenditures by providing health insurance. It was discovered that those who had a low level of PA had two times higher health expenditures compared with those who had a high level of PA. Employees with a low level of fruit and vegetable consumption had 36% higher health expenditures with 1.7 times higher health expenditures compared with those who had a normal level (Potemkina, 2008).

Survey results were used for the corporation's social policy development as well as for implementing health promotion programs at the workplace. The physical activity promotion, smoking cessation, and healthy nutrition programs for employees were adopted by the corporation in 2008. The motto of the health promotion program was: Healthy choices should be easy.

Different from two previous worksite cases (the motor-car industry and heavy machine-building industry enterprises), the corporation does not have its own health services, and the main goal of the health promotion program is to educate and involve the employees through a variety of activities: intranet, leaflets, posters, campaigns, etc. Many partners were involved in these activities, including the enterprise's administration, social services, and human resources services, the local mass media, the cafeteria located at the enterprise, and other partners. Many posters promoting healthy lifestyles were placed in the working environments, such as in dining rooms, elevators, and offices (Figure 16-11). Leaflets were distributed at the worksites. URALSIB created a special health website for the intranet, and campaigns on increasing PA, smoking cessation, and healthy nutrition were conducted.

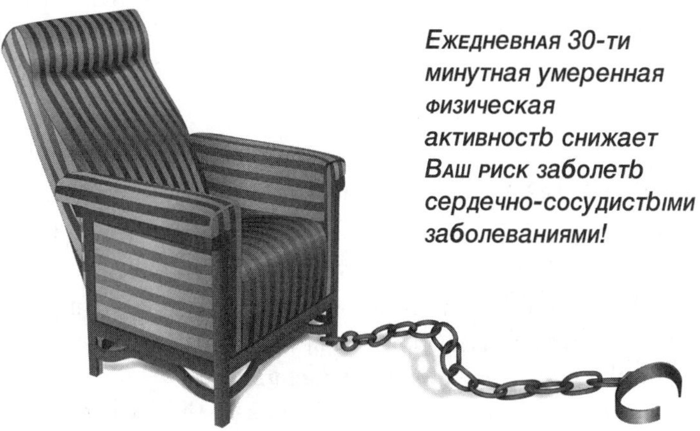
Встанb со своего кресла!
Ежедневная 30-ти
минутная умеренная
физическая
активностb снижает
Ваш риск заболетb
сердечно-сосудистbIми
заболеваниями!

Figure 16-11 Poster advocating additional exercise. "Get off from your armchair! Daily 30 minutes of moderate physical activity decreases your cardiovascular risk."

## Outcomes and Indicators

Several questions appear when evaluating and comparing results at the national and especially at the international level. These include:

- What kind of indicators should one choose?
- How can one detect trends?
- How can one compare results from national and international data?

## What Kind of Indicators Should One Choose?

Experience obtained from Russian worksite programs suggests that two types of indicators could be chosen to evaluate the effectiveness of the programs—economic indicators and health indicators.

Economic indicators include related financial losses, as with presenteeism and direct healthcare expenditures related to the insurance costs covered by employers. Health indicators include data on morbidity with temporary disability (if available) and evaluation of the population's risk profile. Often main causes of morbidity differ between rather young working populations and older populations (for example, women's reproductive health), or the risks are dependent upon professional hazards (for example, sitting at the computer for a long time, leading to ophthalmologic and musculoskeletal diseases). In any case, a needs assessment should be conducted as an initial step in problem identification and priority definition. Nevertheless, NCD risk factors, such as high blood pressure, overweight, low level physical activity, smoking, and others, remain an important focus for all kinds of working populations. Therefore, monitoring these risk factors is essential for the evaluation of workplace disease prevention and health promotion programs.

## How Can One Detect Trends?

It is sometimes difficult to detect significant differences in the prevalence of risk factors at a company because of the short duration of an observation, or because a very high level of employee turnover complicates the dynamics of the risk profile (for example, there is 30% turnover a year at URALSIB). If there is a small number of employees, it's impossible to catch a significant difference in the prevalence of the risk factors.

It seems that in all these cases, monitoring risk factors at the local enterprise is not an acceptable method for the dynamic evaluation of risk factor profile. Workplace health promotion programs should be part of regional/national initiatives, as it is clear that only in these cases can significant changes in risk factors be found.

## How Can One Compare the Results From National and International Data?

Comparability of the results of risk factor prevalence and dynamic evaluation at the international and sometimes at the national level often creates difficulties for investigators. Different languages and cultures make it impossible to use the same questionnaire in different countries, states, or regions. The most difficult issue is to compare evaluations of nutritional habits or physical activity levels. For example, the efforts on creating the international physical activity questionnaire were successful mostly in western European countries, but not in Russia nor in several eastern European countries. These challenges were addressed by creating internationally comparable indicators (for example, body mass index, level of blood pressure or cholesterol level, reaching recommended PA level, or recommended level of fruit and vegetable consumption), which could be defined by questionnaires adapted for various cultures and languages. Another solution is to compare the dynamics of the trends of the indicators.

# Existing Research

The extensive studies on risk factors under the Russian CINDI program and a number of corporate studies in the automobile and heavy machinery industries and the financial service sector were discussed earlier in this chapter. Additional research studies on workplace health promotion do not currently exist in Russia.

# Conclusion

The working environment is very favorable for the organization of intersectoral and comprehensive health promotion programs. There are several reasons why workplace health promotion programs are important for business and the state:

- The prosperity of the company to a great extent depends on the health of its employees. Businesses benefit from the prolongation of active life of people and retaining skilled personnel in the workplace.
- Employees with high risks are very costly for the social services of the company. By improving the risk profile of their employees, companies can save money through decreasing expenditures on health insurance.
- Businesses should be socially responsible.

## Why Should the State Have Business Involved in the Prevention of NCDs?

- The working population is half of all Russians. Every four out of five deaths between the ages of 25–64 in Russia are due to NCD or accidents. NCD prevention and health promotion programs at the workplace could help to decrease premature mortality in the Russian population.
- Preventive programs at the workplace at present will decrease the social expenditures of the state in future.

## What Can Business Do for the Health of the Russian Population?

- Make an impact on the health of the Russian population by encouraging the working population to employ a healthy lifestyle.
- Develop health promotion and disease prevention programs among employees and their families:
  - Healthy nutrition
  - Physical activity
  - Smoking cessation, etc.

- Promote the inclusion of health promotion activities in the work of medical institutions through the commercial insurance system. Currently, large enterprises can choose medical institutions for providing health care for employees covered by the obligatory (voluntary) insurance system. By including preventive services in the features requested from medical insurance, business promotes the development of such services among health providers.
- Contribute to the development of modern NCD prevention programs through international cooperation with the World Bank, the World Health Organization, and the International Labor Organization. The exchange of international experiences in workplace health promotion through the aforementioned organizations could promote modern knowledge in NCD prevention and force action from businesses.

## What Is Necessary for Realization of NCD-Prevention Programs?

- Creation of an intersectoral team to solve health-related problems in the workplace.
- Use of local and international experience in elaboration and realization of disease-prevention and health-promotion programs.
- The legislative support of the state and economic stimulation of social program development among employees.
- The preferential taxation of companies that realize disease-prevention and health promotion programs through the control of an independent expert committee. For example, Moscow regional Duma has adopted the law about preferential taxation of Moscow region (No. 120/2001-03. sub point 2, 3, item 19 from 27 of June 2001). According to this law, companies can transfer up to 2% of their profit tax, which is assigned to the local budget, to public organizations engaged in the population's health enhancement program (www.rosez.ru/law/law0004_007.html).

It is clear that health promotion at the workplace can be beneficial for business as well as for society in general. The success of the process depends a great extent on the interaction between the business sector and society at large.

# Summary

Since 1990s, the Russian population has decreased by 6 million. A considerable portion of premature deaths occur in the working age population. Noncommunicable diseases (NCDs), cardiovascular diseases, external causes, and cancer account for more than 80% of mortality in Russians. All of them are directly associated with the prevalence of a high level of behavioral risk factors (BRF) in the population.

At the same time, the working environment is very favorable for organizing intersectoral comprehensive preventive programs. Experience obtained from the workplace programs in the Soviet Union in the beginning of the 1980s, as well as recent experience, is presented in the chapter. Data on BRF among the working population and economic indicators call for enhanced programming and evaluation of the effectiveness of programs. It is suggested that in several cases, monitoring risk factors at the local enterprise is not an acceptable method for the dynamic evaluation of risk factor profiles, mainly due to employee turnover. Workplace health promotion programs should be part of a regional or national initiative in order to determine significant trends. For reliable evaluation of risk factors, surveys should be conducted at least at the regional level. Workplace health promotion programs should be an essential part of the broader (regional and countrywide) interventions; only in that case can significant changes in the risk factors be monitored and corrected.

Health promotion in the workplace can be beneficial for business and for society in general; the prosperity of a company depends to a great extent on the health of its employees. As the working population represents about half of Russians, NCD prevention and health promotion programs in the workplace could help to decrease premature mortality in the Russian population.

## Review Questions

1. What are the main causes of mortality in Russia? Provide details of each.
2. What is the existing government healthcare system in Russia based upon? How is it funded? Regulated? Managed?
3. What are the economic reasons that workplace health promotion programs are important for Russian businesses?
4. Describe noncommunicable disease prevention efforts that were part of worksite health promotion at Electrostal-city.
5. What type of outcome indicators are important measures for working populations in Russia?

## References

Britov, A. N. (1983). *Detection and method of treatment for hypertension in workers and employees of large industrial enterprise.* Author summary of dissertation for the degree of doctor of medical science, National Research Centre for Cardiology of Russian Federation Moscow.

CIA. (2010). *The World Factbook.* Washington, DC: Central Intelligence Agency, 2009. Retrieved December 2010 from https://www.cia.gov/library/publications/the-world-factbook/index.html

CINDI. (2002). Behavioral risk factors monitoring in the CINDI-Russia regions. Retrieved from http://cindi.gnicpm.ru/monitoring-regiones_2000-2002_eng.htm

Federal State Statistics Service. (n.d.). Homepage. Retrieved November 2009 from http://www.gks.ru/eng/

Oganov, R. G., Komarov, Y. M., & Maslennikova, G. Y. (2009). Demographic problems as a mirror of a nation's health. *Preventive Medicine, 2,* 3–8.

Oganov, R. G., & Maslennikova, G. Y. (2006). Noncommunicable disease in the Russian Federation and the role of risk factors. In *Health promotion and prevention of noncommunicable disease in Russia and Canada: Experience and recommendations* (pp. 3–18). Ottawa, Canada: Public Health Agency of Canada.

Organization for Economic Cooperation and Development. (2007). *Healthcare reform in Russia: Problems and prospects.* Economic Department Working Papers No. 538.

Potemkina, R. A. (2006). Evaluation of health promotion and noncommunicable disease prevention programmes. In *Health promotion and prevention of noncommunicable disease in Russia and Canada: Experience and recommendations* (pp. 80–87). Ottawa, Canada: Public Health Agency of Canada.

Potemkina, R. A. (2008, September). Physical activity and health of the working population: Social costs of poor habits. *1st Annual Conference of HEPA. Europe. Glasgow, Scotland, United Kingdom, 8–9*(87), 174. Retrieved November 2009 from http://www.sparcoll.org.uk

Solov'eva, I. M. (2006). Action against risk factors for noncommunicable disease in the workplace. In *Health promotion and prevention of noncommunicable disease in Russia and Canada: Experience and recommendations* (pp. 65–68). Ottawa, Canada: Public Health Agency of Canada.

World Health Organization. (n.d. a). *European health for all database (HFA-DB).* Retrieved January 2010 from http://www.euro.who.int/HFADB

World Health Organization. (n.d. b). European mortality indicator database (HFA-MDB). *Mortality indicators by 67 causes of death, age, and sex.* Retrieved November 2009 from http://www.euro.who.int/InformationSources/Data

Chapter 17

# Singapore

Neo Seow Ping, Lek Yin Yin, Alan Pui Wee Ming, Low Soo Leng, Annie Ling, and Chew Ling

After reading this chapter you should be able to:

- Identify core strategies that are the focus of workplace health promotion efforts in Singapore
- Describe Singapore's historical evolution of workplace health promotion
- Explain the different approaches employed by corporate health promotion efforts throughout Singapore
- Review the central disease states and health issues driving Singapore's health promotion needs
- Name the components of, and the associated funding sources for, Singapore's healthcare system
- Discuss the impact of culture on Singapore's health status and health promotion efforts

Table 17-1 **Select Key Demographic and Economic Indicators**

| | |
|---|---|
| Nationality | Noun: Singaporean(s)<br>Adjective: Singapore |
| Ethnic groups | Chinese 76.8%, Malay 13.9%, Indian 7.9%, other 1.4% (2000 census) |
| Religion | Buddhist 42.5%, Muslim 14.9%, Taoist 8.5%, Hindu 4%, Catholic 4.8%, other Christian 9.8%, other 0.7%, none 14.8% (2000 census) |
| Language | Mandarin 35%, English 23%, Malay 14.1%, Hokkien 11.4%, Cantonese 5.7%, Teochew 4.9%, Tamil 3.2%, other Chinese dialects 1.8%, other 0.9% (2000 census) |
| Literacy | Definition: age 15 and over can read and write<br>Total population: 92.5%<br>Male: 96.6%<br>Female: 88.6% (2000 census) |

*continued*

| Table 17-1 Select Key Demographic and Economic Indicators, *continued* | |
|---|---|
| Education expenditure | 3.7% of GDP (2001)<br>Country comparison to the world: 123 |
| Government type | Parliamentary republic |
| Environment | Industrial pollution; limited natural fresh water resources; limited land availability presents waste disposal problems; seasonal smoke/haze resulting from forest fires in Indonesia |
| Country mass | Total: 697 sq km<br>Country comparison to the world: 192<br>Land: 687 sq km<br>Water: 10 sq km |
| Population | 5,076,700 (January 2011 est.)<br>Country comparison to the world: 117 |
| Age structure | 0–14 years: 14.4% (male 348,382/female 324,050)<br>15–64 years: 76.7% (male 1,737,972/female 1,833,415)<br>65 years and over: 8.9% (male 184,393/female 229,330)<br>(2010 est.) |
| Median age | Total: 39.6 years<br>Male: 39.1 years<br>Female: 40.0 years (2010 est.) |
| Population growth rate | 0.998% (2010 est.)<br>Country comparison to the world: 128 |
| Birth rate | 0.998% (2010 est.)<br>Country comparison to the world: 216 |
| Death rate | 4.66 deaths/1,000 population (July 2010 est.)<br>Country comparison to the world: 196 |
| Net migration rate | 5.82 migrant(s)/1,000 population (2010 est.)<br>Country comparison to the world: 15 |
| Urbanization | Urban population: 100% of total population (2008)<br>Rate of urbanization: 1.2% annual rate of change (2005–2010 est.) |
| Gender ratio | At birth: 1.08 male(s)/female<br>Under 15 years: 1.08 male(s)/female<br>15–64 years: 0.95 male(s)/female<br>65 years and over: 0.8 male(s)/female<br>Total population: 0.95 male(s)/female (2010 est.) |
| Infant mortality rate | Total: 2.31 deaths/1,000 live births<br>Country comparison to the world: 224<br>Male: 2.51 deaths/1,000 live births<br>Female: 2.09 deaths/1,000 live births (2010 est.) |

*continued*

| Table 17-1 **Select Key Demographic and Economic Indicators,** *continued* | |
|---|---|
| Life expectancy | Total population: 81.98 years<br>Country comparison to the world: 4<br>Male: 79.37 years<br>Female: 84.78 years (2010 est.) |
| Total fertility rate | 1.1 children born/woman 2010 est.)<br>Country comparison to the world: 221 |
| GDP—purchasing power parity | $243.2 billion (2009 est.)<br>Country comparison to the world: 46 |
| GDP—per capita | $52,200 (2009 est.)<br>Country comparison to the world: 8 |
| GDP—composition by sector | Agriculture: 0%<br>Industry: 26.8%<br>Services: 73.2% (2009 est.) |
| Agriculture—products | Orchids, vegetables, poultry, eggs, fish, ornamental fish |
| Industries | Electronics, chemicals, financial services, oil drilling equipment, petroleum refining, rubber processing and rubber products, processed food and beverages, ship repair, offshore platform construction, life sciences, entrepôt trade |
| Labor force participation | 3.03 million (2009 est.)<br>Country comparison to the world: 102 |
| Unemployment rate | 3% (2009 est.)<br>Country comparison to the world: 22 |
| Industrial production growth rate | -1.6% (2009 est.)<br>Country comparison to the world: 83 |
| Distribution of family income (GINI index) | 48.1 (2008)<br>Country comparison to the world: 29 |
| Investment (gross fixed) | 28.9% of GDP (2009 est.)<br>Country comparison to the world: 31 |
| Public debt | 113.1% of GDP (2009 est.)<br>Country comparison to the world: 8 |
| Market value of publicly traded shares | $474.8 billion (December 31, 2009)<br>Country comparison to the world: 22 |
| Current account balance | $25.35 billion (2009 est.)<br>Country comparison to the world: 14 |
| Debt (external) | $19.2 billion (December 31, 2009 est.)<br>Country comparison to the world: 69 |

*continued*

| Table 17-1 Select Key Demographic and Economic Indicators, *continued* | |
|---|---|
| Exports | $274.5 billion (2009 est.)<br>Country comparison to the world: 14 |
| Exports—commodities | Machinery and equipment (including electronics), consumer goods, pharmaceuticals and other chemicals, mineral fuels |
| Export—partners | Hong Kong 11.57%, Malaysia 11.47%, China 9.76%, Indonesia 9.67%, United States 6.57%, South Korea 4.65%, Japan 4.56% (2009 est.) |
| Imports | $240.5 billion (2009 est.)<br>Country comparison to the world: 16 |
| Import—commodities | Machinery and equipment, mineral fuels, chemicals, foodstuffs, consumer goods |
| Import—partners | United States 11.88%, Malaysia 11.617%, China 10.56%, Japan 7.63%, Indonesia 5.8%, South Korea 5.72% Taiwan 5.22% (2009 est.) |
| Stock of direct foreign investment at | |
| Home | $275.2 billion (31 December 2009 est.)<br>country comparison to the world: 17 |
| Abroad | $190.8 billion (31 December 2009 est.)<br>country comparison to the world: 19 |

Source: CIA. (2010). *The world factbook.* Retrieved December 16, 2010 from https://www.cia.gov/library/publications/the-world-factbook/

# Introduction

Singapore is a densely populated island country located in Southeast Asia. One of the smallest countries in the world, it has a land area of 710 square kilometers. Its population of almost 5 million is multiethnic, comprising three main groups: Chinese, Malays, and Indians (Department of Statistics, 2009).

Due to its lack of natural resources, Singapore has to rely largely on its human capital to forge ahead as a First World economy. Hence, the government invests heavily in developing its human capital. Singapore has a high literacy rate of 96%. The Singapore government encourages female participation in the workforce, and the rate of female participation has increased by about 15% over the last 15 years. This has led to the dual roles of women and contributed to declining birth rates in the country. The dramatic fall in the number of births (total fertility rate of 1.28 per female in 2008), coupled with an improvement in life expectancy (average life expectancy at birth of 80.9 years in 2008), is causing Singapore to undergo a rapid transition into an aging society.

From 1999 to 2009, the median age of the Singapore workforce rose from 38 years to 41 years (Ministry of Manpower, 2009). It is expected that the median age for the entire Singaporean population will increase to 49.7 years by 2050; i.e., by 2050, the proportion of older persons aged 65 years and above will reach 38% of Singapore's total population (as compared to 8.3% in 2006) (U.S. Census Bureau, 2006). An aging workforce potentially threatens a nation's productivity, and the increasing burden of chronic diseases will contribute to a rise in healthcare expenditure.

In recent years, Singapore has depended on the influx of foreigners to meet some of its manpower needs. Foreign manpower constitutes both the high and low ends of the working population spectrum. Over 85% (about 580,000) of the foreign workers in Singapore are lower skilled workers. The remaining 13.4% are skilled workers and professionals (Yeoh, 2007).

With Singapore's reliance on human capital, the emergence of lifestyle-related diseases, and the aging population, the Singapore government recognizes the need to invest in the good health of the nation. Therefore, health promotion efforts to encourage healthy behaviors, such as staying smoke free, participating in regular physical activity, having good dietary practices, and going for regular screening for chronic diseases, have remained among the priorities of the Singapore Ministry of Health (MOH) to build an excellent healthcare system. Since Singapore's economy depends heavily on its workforce, a healthy workforce is vital for optimal productivity and performance, thus ensuring a sustained competitive edge that the country has in the global market. Bearing this perspective in mind, workplace health promotion (WHP) becomes an important facet of Singapore's health promotion framework.

## Prevailing Health Issues and Risk Behaviors

The state of health in Singapore is good by international standards, with high life expectancy at birth. This can be attributed to its high standards of living and sanitation, good housing, safe water supply, high levels of education, quality medical services, and active health promotion.

However, like most developed countries, Singapore faces the health challenge of emerging lifestyle-related diseases. Cancer, heart diseases, stroke, and diabetes mellitus are major causes of morbidity and mortality. Lung, colon, rectum, and breast cancers were the top specific causes of cancer burden in 2004 (Ministry of Health, 2004a). Singaporeans have one of the highest diabetes prevalences globally, and young adults contribute a third of the national diabetic case burden.

These lifestyle-related diseases contribute to about 60% of deaths among Singaporeans (Ministry of Health, 2008). These diseases share a common set of risk factors, namely poor dietary habits, physical inactivity, obesity, smoking, hypertension, and high blood cholesterol, all of which are modifiable through living healthier lifestyles.

To define and describe the prevalence and distribution of these risk factors, every 6 years, Singapore's Ministry of Health conducts a population-based National Health Survey (NHS) (Ministry of Health, 1998, 2004b), which comprises both interviews and biometric measurements. This is complemented by an interview-only National Health Surveillance Survey (NHSS) (Ministry of Health 2001, 2007) every 6 years in between each pair of NHSs.

## Dietary Habits

The National Nutrition Survey was conducted in conjunction with the NHS (Health Promotion Board, 2004). It served to provide information on the population's dietary practices, as well as to track changes in the diet of Singaporeans.

The National Nutrition Survey 2004 showed that Singaporeans had improved in some areas. For consumption of fruit and vegetables, 28% reported consuming ≥ 2 servings of fruit per day, as compared to 20.4% in 1998. Similarly, 42.8% reported consuming ≥ 2 servings of vegetables per day, as compared to 14.9% in 1998. Compared to 1998, more Singaporeans reported not adding salt or sauces when eating (63.7% vs. 39.8%) and met recommendations for wholegrain foods (13.3% vs. 8.4%).

However, Singaporeans were also found to consume excessive calories, total fat, saturated fat, and cholesterol, which were above and beyond the recommended intake. For example, 48.2% of adult Singaporeans consumed excess calories while 42.7% consumed excess total fat, as compared to 31.8% and 24.9%, respectively, in 1998. These dietary habits would pose a concern because of the associated risks for hypertension, high blood cholesterol, heart disease, and stroke.

## Physical Activity

Based on NHSS 2007, about 23.6% of Singapore residents exercised regularly during their leisure time. (Regular exercise refers to participation in at least moderate-intensity sports or exercise for at least 20 minutes, for 3 or more days a week.) The often-cited reason for not exercising regularly is the lack of time due to work and family commitments. Therefore, a key challenge here is getting people to take time off to be physically active.

More recently, there have been changes in the international guidelines that recognize that physical activity in domains other than leisure-time exercise could benefit health. These other domains are: (1) performing physical activity at work (paid or unpaid work, including household chores), and (2) walking while commuting to and from places. The domains, including that of leisure activity, could be assessed using the Global Physical Activity Questionnaire developed by the World Health Organization (WHO). With the new guidelines, sufficient total physical activity is considered to be the equivalent accumulation of at least 150 minutes of moderate-intensity activities per week. Accumulation should occur at a minimum of 10 minutes per session.

## Obesity

The NHS has shown that the prevalence of obesity among Singapore residents aged 18–69 years rose from 5.1% in 1992 to 6% in 1998, and to 6.9% in 2004. The measure of obesity is based on the WHO international body mass index (BMI) cut-offs, where an individual with a BMI of ≥ 30 kg/m$^2$ is considered obese. This trend increase, though not significant, is certainly a cause for concern. Furthermore, based on a WHO expert consultation review in 2002, it was recommended that a different set of lower BMI cut-off points be used for Asian populations to determine risks for cardiovascular disease and diabetes mellitus (World Health Organization [WHO] Expert Consultation, 2004). With these new cut-offs for Asians, 16% of Singapore residents had high risk (BMI 27.5 or more) for these diseases in 2004.

## Smoking

NHSS 2007 showed that 13.6% of Singapore residents aged 18–69 years smoked cigarettes daily (Ministry of Health, 2007). The proportion of daily smokers was 6 times higher among males (23.7%) than among females (3.7%). Although Singapore has one of the lowest smoking rates in the world, one worrying trend is the increase in daily smoking among young adults (aged 18–29 years) from 12.3% in 2004 (Ministry of Health, 2004a) to 17.2% in 2007 (Ministry of Health, 2007).

## Diabetes, Hypertension, and High Blood Cholesterol

For NHS, biometric measurements were conducted on the participants. Promising trends had been observed for the prevalence of diabetes mellitus, hypertension, and high blood cholesterol among Singapore residents (18–69 years old) between 1998 and 2004. Prevalence of diabetes mellitus dropped from 9.0% in 1998 to 8.2% in 2004; prevalence of hypertension fell from 21.5% in 1998 to 20.1% in 2004; and that of high total blood cholesterol decreased from 25.4% in 1998 to 18.7% in 2004.

## Health Screening

Health screening is an important strategy for early detection and management of diseases. Singapore has in place national screening programs for diabetes mellitus, hypertension, high blood cholesterol, and for breast and cervical cancers.

NHSS 2007 found that health screening for diabetes mellitus, hypertension, and high blood cholesterol was commonly practiced by Singapore residents aged 40–69 years who had not been told by a doctor that they had these conditions. Among adults without known diabetes mellitus, 72.2% had been screened for the condition within the past 3 years. A proportion of 63.9% without known hypertension had their blood pressure checked in the past year. Of those without known high blood cholesterol, 78.0% had been screened within the past 3 years.

Breast cancer is the leading cancer affecting women in Singapore today. During a five-year period from 2002 to 2006, the incidence of breast cancer in the resident population was 73.6 per 100,000 women per year (National Registry of Diseases Office, 2008). Therefore, the awareness and practice of mammography are important attributes for early detection of breast cancer. In 2007, 83.2% of women aged 50–69 years were aware of mammography, as compared to only 46.7% in 2001. Overall, 61.3% of women aged 50–69 years had gone for a mammography screening at least once, with 40.9% having gone for a mammography screening within the last 2 years in 2007.

Cervical cancer is the sixth most common cancer among women in Singapore. With early detection before it becomes invasive, cervical cancer is almost 100% curable. The Papanicolaou (Pap) smear test has been accepted as an effective screening tool for cervical cancer. The NHSS 2007 showed that 87.4% of women aged 25–69 years were aware of the Pap smear, as compared to 69.3% in 2001. Almost 6 in 10 (59.2%) women aged 25–69 years had gone for a Pap smear within the past 3 years in 2007.

# Healthcare System

Singapore's healthcare philosophy begins with building a healthy population through preventive healthcare programs and promoting a healthy lifestyle. Singapore's healthcare system ensures that basic services are affordable for all, while individual willingness to pay determines the access to higher levels of services. This philosophy promotes individual responsibility towards healthy living and medical expenses.

In terms of healthcare financing, Singapore has a unique hybrid system that combines government subsidies (funded through taxes) with the 3Ms—Medisave, MediShield, and Medifund. Medisave is a compulsory national medical savings scheme, which allows the individual Singaporean to save up for his/her healthcare costs. MediShield is a catastrophic medical insurance scheme initiated by the government to protect individuals against large hospital bills that Medisave may not be sufficient to cover. Medifund is a health endowment fund to help poor and needy Singaporeans pay for their medical expenses.

The safety net provided by government subsidies and Medifund makes sure that no Singaporean is denied access to healthcare services because of the inability to pay. At the same time, to foster discipline in choice of health services and to instill self-responsibility, patients who are able to pay have to co-finance their healthcare costs through Medisave, MediShield, or out-of-pocket payments. This healthcare financing system has secured good healthcare outcomes for the Singapore population. Moreover, these outcomes have been achieved with a consistently small national healthcare expenditure, which is below 4% of its gross domestic product (GDP), although it would be expected to increase with an aging population.

## Influence of Culture and Mentality

Singaporean society is multiethnic and multicultural, comprising 74.5% Chinese, 13.5% Malays, 9% Indians, and 3% of other ethnic origins. Singaporeans speak many different languages. There are four official languages, including Malay, Chinese, Tamil, and English. The majority speaks at least two of them.

Besides the myriad of languages spoken in Singapore, there is also a host of cultural and religious festivals celebrated throughout the year. The strong racial harmony in the country means that such festivities are often celebrated with participation from the various ethnic groups.

With such a wide mix of ethnic and cultural groups, it is inevitable that these different groups would have different health risk behaviors, and so, certain groups are more predisposed to some chronic diseases than others. Therefore, the practice of workplace health promotion must understand the influence of culture on the health needs of individual ethnic groups, and tailor its interventions accordingly.

## Drivers of Workplace Health Promotion

Overall, 65.6% of the resident population aged 15 years and above participated in the labor market (Ministry of Manpower, 2008). As most Singaporeans spend a considerable amount of time at work, the workplace presents an excellent captive setting to promote physical, social, and mental health, early detection of chronic disease, and timely follow-up interventions.

The need for workplace health promotion in Singapore is made more urgent by an aging workforce, which could potentially result in a higher burden of chronic diseases. If chronic diseases are not detected and managed early, there would be a negative impact on national productivity and workplace healthcare expenditure. For the Singapore healthcare financing system to be sustainable with a consistently small national healthcare expenditure, it is imperative that measures be taken to help Singaporeans, in particular those in the workforce, to stay healthy for as long as possible.

Therefore, to this end, the National Workplace Health Promotion Programme (WHPP) underpins the Singapore government's commitment to build a healthy workforce. The Singapore government is the principal driver of workplace health promotion. It works with various stakeholders to improve the health of the workforce. Employers are encouraged to promote workplace health through training, grants, and other incentives.

Currently, the Singapore Health Promotion Board (HPB) champions the National WHPP. The HPB was set up in 2001 with the vision of being the agency to build a nation of healthy and happy people in Singapore. HPB's strategic framework encompasses looking after the health of those in the different phases of the life cycle (i.e., children, adolescents, adults, elderly) through its various health promotion screening and disease management programs. At each life cycle phase, HPB implements programs to address the needs of those in the different stages of health status (the healthy, the at-risk, the unhealthy), as well as those in the different settings of society, of which the workplace is one.

The workplace health movement in Singapore started more than 20 years ago. In the 1980s, promotion of workplace health focused on provision of fitness facilities and health education activities. In 1984, the Ministry of Health set up a Workplace Health Education Unit to promote better health among employees from both the public and private sectors.

In 1999, the first National Tripartite Committee was formed comprising the employer's federation, trade unions, and government to expand and improve the National WHPP. The committee reviewed local and international evidence on workplace health promotion, consulted with experts, and identified issues. In 2000, the *Report of the National Tripartite Committee* was published, and a National Intersectoral Committee comprising employer and employee unions and key government and private agencies was also established to oversee the implementation of recommendations made by the Tripartite Committee.

The recommendations of the Tripartite Committee provided the strategic framework and foundational strategies to jump-start the national WHPP. An integrated, comprehensive, and ecological approach was undertaken to promote workplace health addressing the work environment, organizational policies, and lifestyle change interventions. Key strategies of the national WHPP included building sustainable collaborations with key partners and stakeholders, alignment and integration at the national level, establishment of supportive environments and

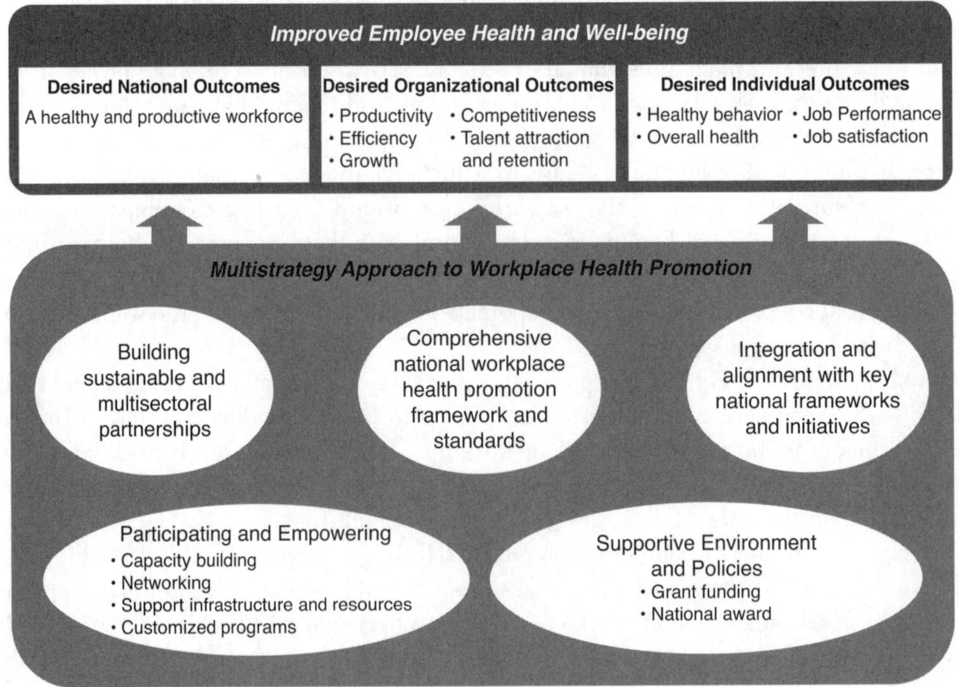


Figure 17-1 An integrated approach to workplace health promotion.

policies through a national award scheme, and empowerment of both employers and employees through building a comprehensive ecosystem of support (Figure 17-1).

The national WHPP continues to review its efforts to build healthy, productive, and vibrant workplaces. A second National Tripartite Committee on Workplace Health (TriCom) was formed in January 2009 to recommend key strategies that will address the challenges of an aging population and an increasing burden of chronic disease. The formation of the second TriCom underscores the importance of strengthening a tripartite partnership among the government, private sector, and public sector in promoting workplace health.

The committee will be releasing its recommended strategies in the final report by the end of 2010. These strategies will serve to guide the national WHPP in its next lap to promote workplace health.

# Programs and Good Practices

## Establishing Strategic Partnerships at a National Level

The WHPP utilizes a broad-based strategy framework involving multiple stakeholders, which include employer and employee unions, private sector companies, key government agencies, and business and trade associations.

## Alignment and Integration at the National Level

### *Establish Standards and Indicators Linked to Business Outcomes*

Workplace health promotion standards and outcome indicators are essential components of total strategy to improve workplace health promotion. They will provide clear direction about the outcomes to be achieved and the best ways to achieve them. A workplace health promotion standards framework was developed to guide organizations in designing and monitoring their programs. These standards were then used to measure and recognize the success of organizations' workplace health programs.

### *Integration With the Productivity Movement*

It is recognized that a healthy workforce is one of the key contributors to business excellence and national productivity. The alignment of workplace health promotion with the nationally recognized business excellence standard, which recognizes organizations' attainment of world-class quality and people development standards, has been critical to acknowledge the close relationship between health and productivity.

### Alignment With Other National Initiatives

To further enhance the alignment of WHP with other national initiatives, the HPB developed a conceptual framework on workplace health in 2003 to enable a whole-of-government approach to more systematically address all work-related factors related to the health and well-being of the employees. It aims to encourage greater integration at a national level and reinforces a whole-of-government approach involving all national workplace health-related initiatives, namely workplace safety and health, work–life harmony, and workplace health promotion.

## Establishing Supportive Environments and Policies

### National Award

A national workplace health award, named HEALTH Award (Helping Employees Achieve Life-Time Health Award) was established in 1999 to give national recognition to companies with commendable WHPPs. The key objectives of the award are as follows:

- To generate awareness of the benefits of an effective workplace health program
- To identify healthy workplaces that will serve as role models for other companies to emulate
- To challenge workplaces to engage in regular assessment and continuous improvement of their health promotion programs

Selection of award recipients is based on a set of criteria that include:

- A comprehensive program with activities to raise awareness, motivate, and empower employees to make informed decisions to improve their health
- A workplace environment that supports and sustains health
- Systematic planning and implementation of the program
- Regular monitoring and evaluation of the program
- Strong management support and committee
- Employee participation
- Sustainability

These criteria are based on the World Health Organization's principles of effective health promotion (WHO Expert Committee, 1998). Based on the above criteria, participating workplaces are awarded platinum, gold, silver, or bronze medals.

The number of award recipients more than doubled from 132 workplaces in 1999 to 358 in 2008. In 2008, out of the 358 award recipients, there were 41 platinum, 120 gold, 72 silver, and 125 bronze winners.

### *Grant Funding*

The Workplace Health Promotion Grant, introduced in 2001, was designed to help companies jump-start and sustain their workplace health programs. Currently, companies can receive up to $10,000 to start and sustain their health program initiatives.

The grant cofunds for health screening, health risk assessment, and health programs on healthy eating, exercise, mental well-being, smoking control, chronic diseases, and other health-related topics. A company is eligible to apply for the grant as a newcomer and again when the company attains an award in a higher Singapore HEALTH Award category (bronze, silver, gold, and platinum). This mechanism works to incentivize companies to work toward continuous improvements in their health promotion programs to progress to the next award category of the Singapore HEALTH Award.

## Empowering Employers and Employees Through a Comprehensive Support Eco-System

### *Capacity Building*

The HPB provides structured training courses on workplace health promotion, seminars, and forums on health topics to equip employers, human resource personnel, workplace health managers, and facilitators with the skills and knowledge to organize effective workplace health promotion programs. An annual National Conference on Workplace Health Promotion invites local and regional expert speakers to share and provide updates on the latest trends and developments in workplace health.

In addition, the HPB also offers consultancy services to companies via phone, email, and face-to-face meetings. With the goal of increasing companies' access to WHP consultancy services and support, the HPB has implemented a structured training course and audit process in order to expand the pool of health promotion service providers. This training course equips health service providers with the skills and knowledge to provide health promotion consultancy and ensure quality in its delivery.

### *Networking and Sharing*

Club HEALTH is a peer support network for companies' health facilitators from the Singapore HEALTH Award companies. Club HEALTH organizes quarterly best practice sharing sessions to facilitate opportunities for members to exchange ideas and share challenges, solutions, and best practices. An online forum is also provided to facilitate exchange of ideas and best practices among health facilitators.

### Resources

Companies have easy access to a tool kit of resources and handy references that includes comprehensive guides on how to plan and implement effective WHP programs, health education materials, and case studies on best practices. The workplace online health portal, Health@Work (www.hpb.gov.sg/healthatwork/), was developed as a one-stop resource platform for workplaces to obtain resources and information in organizing workplace health promotion programs. A quarterly newsletter, the *Workplace Health Digest*, aims to keep companies abreast of the latest developments in workplace health, featuring best practices on workplace health, new initiatives and programs from HPB, and interviews with workplace health experts and facilitators.

### Customized Programs

The HPB has developed and made available to the working population customized workplace programs on a range of healthy lifestyle topics, including mental health education, communicable diseases education, nutrition, smoking control, and physical activity. For example, *Fitness at Work* and *I-run* bring weekly aerobics workout and running sessions, respectively, to the doorsteps of many Singaporeans working in the central business district and major industrial parks.

## Reaching Out to Small and Medium Enterprises

In Singapore, small and medium sized enterprises (SMEs) account for 62% of employment and provide 1.7 million jobs. Reaching out to SMEs is key to improving the healthy lifestyle behaviors and health of the Singapore workforce. Compared to larger enterprises, SMEs face more barriers and challenges in starting and sustaining a workplace health promotion program, such as lack of management support, budget constraints, lack of staff demand, limited experience in planning WHP programs, and constraints in organizing activities during office hours (Health Promotion Board, 2006, 2008). To help SMEs overcome these challenges, the strategies shown in Figure 17-2 were adopted.

### WHP@SMEs' Doorsteps Program

HPB pioneered a collaboration with commercial and industrial building owners and trade associations to bring health programs and health screening to their tenants' doorsteps. This program takes a clustering approach, which includes pooling for critical mass and more efficient use of resources.

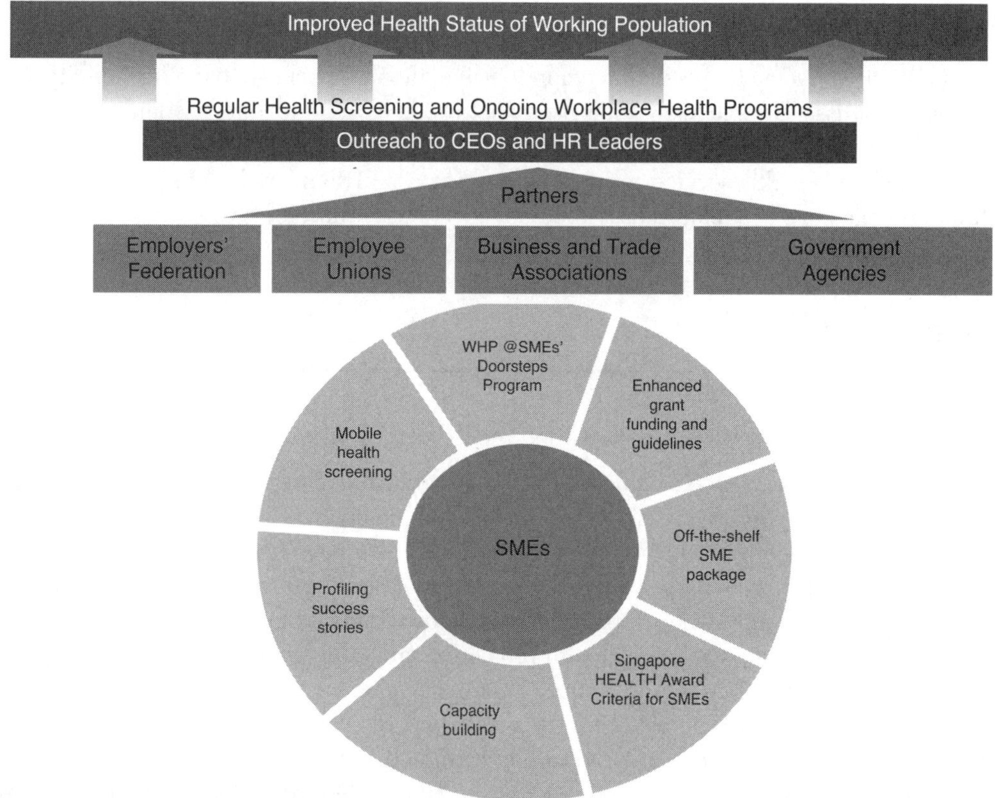


Figure 17-2 Strategies for small and medium enterprises.

### *Screening on Wheels Program*

The Health Screening on Wheels program was introduced to make health screening more accessible to SMEs' employees. A mobile screening bus was deployed to industrial estates to screen SME employees for chronic diseases such as obesity, high blood pressure, high blood cholesterol, and diabetes.

## Enhanced Grant Funding for SMEs

The enhanced SME grant was introduced to meet the needs of SMEs, which may face budget constraints and need an added impetus to jump-start their WHP programs. This grant funds up to 90% for SMEs' WHP programs, capped at $10,000 per application. The grant can be used to fund essential health screening and follow-up programs, health education, and promotion activities such as talks and workshops on various healthy lifestyle areas. The enhanced grant also has funds for off-site health programs, such as health screening at clinics and health talks, workshops, and exercise classes in the community.

## Health Package for SMEs

HEALTHWORKS is an off-the-shelf, comprehensive, flexible package that offers on-site WHP programs to SMEs. The package comprises health screening and interventions on four key areas of healthy lifestyles. To overcome the challenges that most SMEs faced on resource constraint, appointed health service providers coordinate and deliver the programs on-site. In addition, the package is subsidized by the enhanced WHP grant for SMEs.

# Outcomes

## Prevalence of Workplace Health Promotion

The prevalence of workplace health promotion programs in Singapore has demonstrated a steady increase over the years among private sector companies. Prior to the setup of the national WHPP, a 1998 study of private sector organizations revealed that only 33% of companies had a comprehensive workplace health program, covering about a quarter of the workforce. (Note: A comprehensive program was defined as one that addressed organizational policy, environmental facilities, and health promotion and education activities).

Between 2003 and 2006, the prevalence of companies having a workplace health promotion program had risen from 45% to 59%, covering 59% and 76% of workers, respectively, as noted in Figure 17-3. The rise in prevalence can be attributed to the successful implementation of recommendations made by the National Tripartite Committee in 1999; that is, to develop a more comprehensive and integrated approach to workplace health promotion in Singapore.

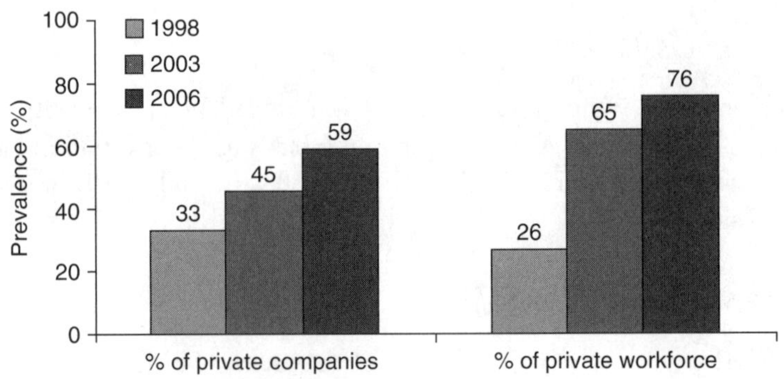


Figure 17-3 Prevalance of workplace health promotion.
Source: National Workplace Health Promotion Survey 1998, 2003, 2006.

## Health Status of the Working Population

The increased prevalence of workplace health promotion programs over the years has resulted in positive improvements to the health status of working adults. The National Health Survey 2004 showed that working adults between the ages of 18 and 69 years had lower prevalence of diabetes, hypertension, high blood cholesterol, and obesity compared to the general population. Between 1998 and 2004, as noted in Table 17-2, the prevalence of working adults exercising regularly increased by 7% while the percentage of working adults who smoke decreased by 2.5% (Ministry of Health, 1998, 2004a).

Table 17-2 **Health Indicators for General Population and Working Population**

| | Working Population (%) | | General Population (%) | |
|---|---|---|---|---|
| | 1998 | 2004 | 1998 | 2004 |
| Diabetes | 6.5 | 6.6 | 9 | 8.2 |
| Hypertension | 19.1 | 18.7 | 27.3 | 20.1 |
| High total cholesterol | 24.7 | 18.6 | 25.4 | 18.7 |
| Exercise | 14.2 | 21.2 | 16.8 | 24.9 |
| Obesity | 5.2 | 6.6 | 6 | 6.9 |
| Smoke | 17.6 | 15.1 | 15 | 12.6 |

Source: Singapore National Health Survey 2004, 2008.

# Existing Research

Since the establishment of the national WHPP in 2001, the Health Promotion Board has conducted the National Workplace Health Promotion Survey once every 3 years to track the prevalence of WHP in Singapore and assess its continual progress. The surveys were conducted in 2003 and 2006. Besides determining the prevalence, the survey also finds out the nature and scope of WHP programs, barriers to the development of WHP, and the perceived costs and benefits of WHP among private companies in Singapore. The findings have provided useful insights to the national WHPP on the progress of WHP and its strategies to create a comprehensive support infrastructure for the workplaces.

The next National Health Promotion Survey was scheduled to be conducted in 2010. With the formation of the new Tripartite Committee in 2009 and the increased focus on SMEs, the 2010 survey included private companies with fewer than 50 employees. The findings will provide insights on the current status of WHP among SMEs in Singapore.

## Conclusion

The National Workplace Health Promotion Program has achieved some measure of success as evidenced by the increase in workplace health prevalence and the improved health status of the working population. Tackling the challenges of an aging workforce and the rising burden of chronic diseases will require a multiyear effort, close intersectoral collaborations, strong committed leadership, and a responsive workforce.

The HPB and the Tripartite Committee continue to review their efforts to build healthy, productive, and vibrant workplaces and will post recommendations based on three key goals (Figure 17-4), namely:

1. Further integration and alignment of workplace health promotion with other relevant national initiatives and frameworks
2. Increasing uptake of WHP among employers, specifically the SMEs and industry sectors
3. Increasing participation in WHP among employees with a focus on creating a greater sense of ownership for health among employees

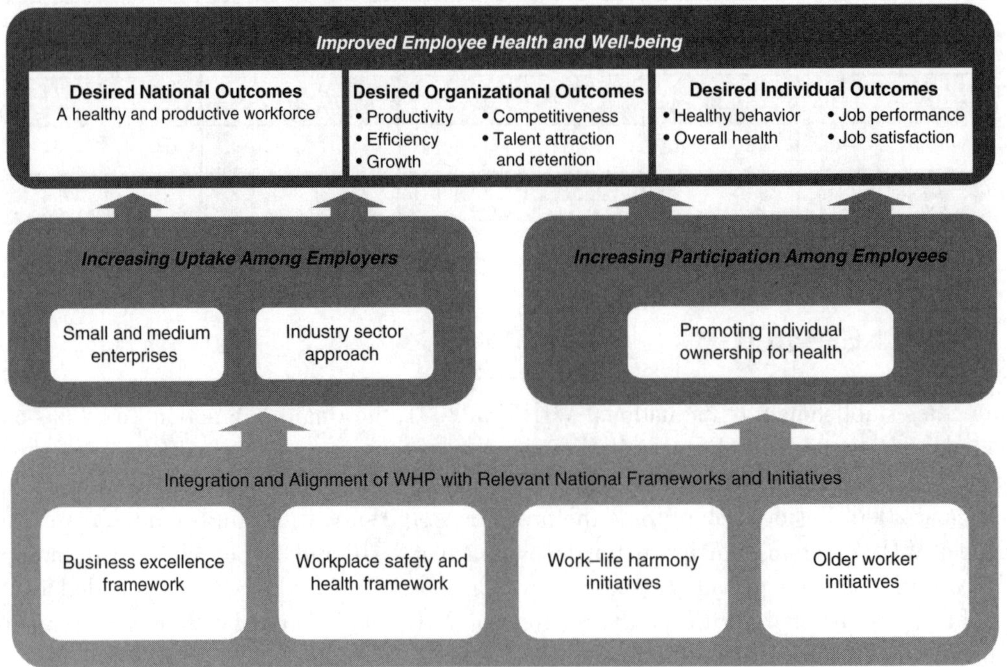


Figure 17-4 Key goals of the national tripartite committee on workplace health.

To shift from the current "wait-for-sickness" mind-set to one that empowers individuals to take ownership for health and employers to appreciate and value the benefits brought about by a healthy and vibrant workforce, the HPB and Tripartite Committee will tap into local and international best practice experiences and recommend a health incentive framework, which will serve to engage corporations and individuals towards greater health and wellness.

## Summary

The Singapore government recognizes that a healthy workforce is the cornerstone for sustainable development. Like most developed countries, Singapore faces challenges such as aging population, dominance of lifestyle diseases, and rising healthcare costs, which indicate a need to proactively manage the health risks facing the workforce.

The National Workplace Health Promotion Program is championed by the Singapore Health Promotion Board (HPB). Multipronged strategies are used to engage organizations to implement a comprehensive and effective workplace health promotion (WHP) program. Strategies include engaging with key stakeholders, such as employers' and employees' unions, private sector companies, key government agencies, and business and trade associations; introducing an integrated conceptual framework on WHP; recognizing the achievement of companies via a national award; providing funding to start and improve WHP programs; and setting up a comprehensive support ecosystem, which includes training, free consultancy, and resources on WHP and introducing customized programs on a range of healthy lifestyle topics.

The efforts over the years have reaped tangible results. The National Workplace Health Promotion Survey showed that prevalence of WHP programs among private sector workplaces has increased from 33% in 1998 to 58.7% in 2006. The National Health Survey 2004 also showed that the health risk status of the working population had improved.

HPB has continued to review its efforts to build healthy, productive, and vibrant workplaces and will put up its recommendations based on three key focus areas, namely, further integration of WHP with relevant national initiatives and frameworks; increasing uptake among SMEs and industry sectors; and increasing participation among employees.

## Review Questions

1. What is the role of human capital in Singapore's corporate health promotion efforts?
2. What is the common set of risk factors that contribute to Singaporean's lifestyle-related diseases?
3. Name the health screening strategies that are in place for early detection and disease management in Singapore.
4. What is unique about the financing of health care in Singapore?

5. Is there an urgent need for workplace health promotion in Singapore? Explain why or why not.
6. List the key strategies of the national WHPP.
7. Describe the objectives and selection criteria of Singapore's HEALTH award.
8. How do workplace health promotion organizations share information about best practices?

## References


Department of Statistics. (2009). *Key annual indicators.* Retrieved from http://www.singstat.gov.sg

Health Promotion Board. (2004). *National nutrition survey.* Singapore: Author.

Health Promotion Board. (2006). *National workplace health prevalence survey.* Singapore: Author.

Health Promotion Board. (2008). HPB-SME focus group discussions (unpublished).

Ministry of Health. (1998). *National health survey.* Singapore: Author.

Ministry of Health. (2001b). *National health surveillance surveys 2001.* Singapore: Author.

Ministry of Health. (2004a). *National Health Survey.* Singapore: Author.

Ministry of Health. (2004b). *Singapore burden of disease study.* Singapore: Author. Ministry of Health.

Ministry of Health. (2007). *National Health Surveillance Surveys 2001, 2007.* Singapore: Author.

Ministry of Health. (2008). *Health facts Singapore: Principal causes of death.* Singapore: Author.

Ministry of Manpower. (2008). *Report on the labour force in Singapore.* Singapore: Author.

Ministry of Manpower. (2009). *Singapore workforce.* Singapore: Author.

National Registry of Diseases Office. (2008). *Singapore Cancer Registry interim report: Trends in cancer incidence in Singapore 2002–2006.* Singapore: HPB.

U.S. Census Bureau. (2006). *Midyear population projection.* Retrieved November 16, 2006, from http://www.census.gov/cgi-bin/ipc/idbagg

WHO Expert Committee. (1998). Health promotion for working populations: Report of a WHO Expert Committee. *WHO Technical Report Series, No. 765.* Geneva, Switzerland: WHO.

WHO Expert Consultation. (2004). Appropriate body-mass index for Asian populations and its implications for policy and intervention strategies. *Lancet, 363*, 157–163.

Yeoh, B. S. A. (2007). *Singapore: Hungry for foreign workers at all skill levels.* Washington, DC: Migration Information Source.

Chapter 18

# South Africa

Tanya Kalas, Wolf Kirsten, Gert Strydom, and Cilas Wilders

After reading this chapter you should be able to:

- Identify core strategies that are the focus of workplace health promotion in South Africa
- Describe the historical evolution of South Africa's workplace health promotion efforts
- Explain the different approaches employed by corporate health promotion throughout South Africa
- Review the central disease states and health issues driving workplace health promotion in South Africa
- Name the components of, and the associated funding sources for, the South African healthcare system
- Discuss the impact of culture on the health status and health promotion efforts within South Africa

Table 18-1 **Select Key Demographic and Economic Indicators**

| | |
|---|---|
| Nationality | Noun: South African(s)<br>Adjective: South African |
| Ethnic groups | Black African 79%, white 9.6%, colored 8.9%, Indian/Asian 2.5% (2001 census) |
| Religion | Zion Christian 11.1%, Pentecostal/Charismatic 8.2%, Catholic 7.1%, Methodist 6.8%, Dutch Reformed 6.7%, Anglican 3.8%, Muslim 1.5%, other Christian 36%, other 2.3%, unspecified 1.4%, none 15.1% (2001 census) |
| Language | IsiZulu 23.8%, IsiXhosa 17.6%, Afrikaans 13.3%, Sepedi 9.4%, English 8.2%, Setswana 8.2%, Sesotho 7.9%, Xitsonga 4.4%, other 7.2% (2001 census) |
| Literacy | Definition: age 15 and over can read and write<br>Total population: 86.4%<br>Male: 87%<br>Female: 85.7% (2003 est.) |

*continued*

| Table 18-1 **Select Key Demographic and Economic Indicators,** *continued* | |
|---|---|
| Education expenditure | 5.4% of GDP (2006)<br>Country comparison to the world: 52 |
| Government type | Republic |
| Environment | Lack of important arterial rivers or lakes requires extensive water conservation and control measures; growth in water usage outpacing supply; pollution of rivers from agricultural runoff and urban discharge; air pollution resulting in acid rain; soil erosion; desertification |
| Country mass | Total: 1,219,090 sq km<br>Country comparison to the world: 25<br>Land: 1,214,470 sq km<br>Water: 4,620 sq km<br>*Note:* includes Prince Edward Islands (Marion Island and Prince Edward Island) |
| Population | 49,052,489<br>Country comparison to the world: 24 |
| Age structure | 0–14 years: 28.9% (male 7,093,328/female 7,061,579)<br>15–64 years: 65.8% (male 16,275,424/female 15,984,181)<br>65 years and over: 5.4% (male 1,075,117/female 1,562,860)<br>(2010 est.) |
| Median age | Total: 24.4 years<br>Male: 24.4 years<br>Female: 25 years (2010 est.) |
| Population growth rate | 0.281% (2010 est.)<br>Country comparison to the world: 174 |
| Birth rate | 19.93 births/1,000 population (2010 est.)<br>Country comparison to the world: 99 |
| Death rate | 16.99 deaths/1,000 population (July 2010 est.)<br>Country comparison to the world: 8 |
| Net migration rate | -0.13 migrant(s)/1,000 population country<br>Comparison to the world: 93<br>*Note:* there is an increasing flow of Zimbabweans into South Africa and Botswana in search of better economic opportunities (2010 est.) |
| Urbanization | Urban population: 61% of total population (2008)<br>Rate of urbanization: 1.4% annual rate of change (2005–2010 est.) |
| Gender ratio | At birth: 1.02 male(s)/female<br>Under 15 years: 1 male(s)/female<br>15–64 years: 1.02 male(s)/female<br>65 years and over: 0.69 male(s)/female<br>Total population: 0.99 male(s)/female (2010 est.) |

*continued*

| Table 18-1 **Select Key Demographic and Economic Indicators,** *continued* | |
|---|---|
| Infant mortality rate | Total: 44.42 deaths/1,000 live births<br>Country comparison to the world: 61<br>Male: 48.66 deaths/1,000 live births<br>Female: 40.1 deaths/1,000 live births (2010 est.) |
| Life expectancy | Total population: 48.98 years<br>Country comparison to the world: 212<br>Male: 49.81 years<br>Female: 48.13 years (2010 est.) |
| Total fertility rate | 2.38 children born/woman (2010 est.)<br>Country comparison to the world: 104 |
| GDP—purchasing power parity | $505.3 billion (2009 est.)<br>Parity country comparison to the world: 26 |
| GDP—per capita | $10,300 (2009 est.)<br>Country comparison to the world: 104 |
| GDP—composition by sector | Agriculture: 3%<br>Sector industry: 31.1%<br>Services: 65.8% (2009 est.) |
| Agriculture—products | Corn, wheat, sugarcane, fruits, vegetables, beef, poultry, mutton, wool, dairy products |
| Industries | Mining (world's largest producer of platinum, gold, chromium), automobile assembly, metalworking, machinery, textiles, iron and steel, chemicals, fertilizer, foodstuffs, commercial ship repair |
| Labor force participation | 17.38 million economically active (2009 est.)<br>Country comparison to the world: 35 |
| Unemployment rate | 24% (2009 est.)<br>Country comparison to the world: 172 |
| Industrial production growth rate | -7.2% (2009 est.)<br>Country comparison to the world: 126 |
| Distribution of family income (GINI index) | 65 (2005)<br>Country comparison to the world: 2 |
| Investment (gross fixed) | 22.4% of GDP (2009 est.)<br>Country comparison to the world: 67 |
| Public debt | 29.5% of GDP (2009 est.)<br>Country comparison to the world: 87 |
| Market value of publicly traded shares | $805.2 billion (December 31, 2008)<br>Comparison to the world: 18 |

*continued*

| Table 18-1 Select Key Demographic and Economic Indicators, *continued* | |
|---|---|
| Current account balance | $-11.53 billion (2009 est.)<br>Country comparison to the world: 177 |
| Debt (external) | $73.84 billion (30 June 2009 est.)<br>Country comparison to the world: 39 |
| Debt as a % of GDP | ——— |
| Exports | $66.64 billion (2009 est.)<br>Country comparison to the world: 38 |
| Exports—commodities | Gold, diamonds, platinum, other metals and minerals, machinery and equipment |
| Exports—partners | China 10.34%, United States 9.19%, Japan 7.59%, Germany 7.01%, United Kingdom 5.54%, Switzerland 4.72% (2009) |
| Imports | $66.02 billion (2009 est.)<br>Country comparison to the world: 36 |
| Imports—commodities | Machinery and equipment, chemicals, petroleum products, scientific instruments, foodstuffs |
| Imports—partners | China 17.21%, Germany 11.24%, United States 7.38%, Saudi Arabia 4.87%, Japan 4.67%, Iran 3.95% (2009) |
| Stock of direct foreign investment at | |
| Home | $73.67 billion (December 31, 2009 est.)<br>country comparison to the world: 42 |
| Abroad | $51.36 billion (December 31, 2009 est.)<br>country comparison to the world: 230 |

Source: CIA. (2010). *The world factbook.* Retrieved December 16, 2010, from https://www.cia.gov/library/publications/the-world-factbook/

# Introduction

South Africa is a country situated at the southern tip of Africa, with a total land area of slightly more than 1.2 million square km and a coastline of more than 2,500 km. It is twice the size of France and three times that of Germany. There are nine provinces in South Africa—each of varying land sizes. The country's three capital cities are Cape Town, the legislative capital; Bloemfontein, the judicial capital; and Pretoria, the administrative and ultimate capital of the country. Johannesburg is the nation's biggest city and serves as its economic hub.

At present, it is estimated that South Africa has a population of over 47.9 million people of different backgrounds, cultures, languages, and beliefs. It is further estimated that South Africa's population mainly consists of Africans, of whom there are approximately 38 million, or 79.6% of the population. The white population represents one of the population's minorities, with 4.3 million (9.1%), followed by the colored population of 4.2 million (8.9%), and lastly the Indian/Asian population of approximately 1.2 million (2.5%).

South Africa has 11 official languages, which are: Afrikaans (spoken by 13.3% of the total population), English (8.2%), Ndedele (1.6%), Xhosa (17.6%), Zulu (23.8%), Sepedi (9.4%), Sesotho (7.9%), Setswana (8.2%), SiSwati (2.7%), Tsihivenda (2.3%), and Xitsonga (4.4%). Ten of these languages are unique to Africa.

Since the 17th century, the basis of the white population has been formed by the Dutch, German, French, Huguenot, and British immigrants. As with other smaller ethnic groups, the main languages spoken by these groups are Afrikaans and English. The colored people are a mixed race and speak mainly Afrikaans. The Asian population is mainly of Indian origin and is situated in Kwazulu Natal.

The population distribution within the nine provinces is:

- Eastern Cape: 6.9 million (14.4%)
- Free State: 2.9 million (6.2%)
- Gauteng: 9.6 million (20.2%)
- KwaZulu-Natal: 10 million (20.9%)
- Limpopo: 5.4 million (11.3%)
- Mpumalanga: 3.5 million (7.4%)
- Northern Cape: 1.1 million (2.3%)
- North West: 3.4 million (7.1%)
- Western Cape: 4.8 million (10.1%)

Unemployment has been a major problem in the country for many years and in 2009 was estimated at 24% (CIA, 2010). The number of unemployed adults is increasing in urban areas because of the inflow of people into the cities, without a significant increase in job opportunities.

Even though South Africa is a well-to-do country in per capita terms, the majority of households either live in poor conditions or are vulnerable to poverty. This discrepancy is due to the enormous inequality of the distribution of income and wealth among the population. While a small part of the population lives in luxury, the rest live in conditions where access to clean water or energy is still insufficient and obtainment of health care and education is uncommon (Table 18-2).

**Table 18-2 Education Levels of the South African Population**

| Education level | Male (%) | Female (%) | Total (%) |
|---|---|---|---|
| No formal education | 9.0 | 12.1 | 10.6 |
| Less than grade 7 | 19.6 | 18.2 | 18.9 |
| Less than matric | 45.6 | 45.8 | 45.7 |
| Matric and above | 25.8 | 23.9 | 24.8 |

Source: Data from *CIA*, 2010

### Politics

South Africa has a bicameral parliament consisting of two chambers: the National Council of Provinces, which is the upper house and comprises 90 members, and the National Assembly, which is the lower house and comprises 400 members.

Members of the lower house are elected by party-list proportional representation, a voting system used during parliamentary elections that emphasizes population-based proportional representation and proportionally elects each half of the members from national and provincial lists. The prime objective of the National Council of Provinces, which consists of 10 members for each of the 9 provinces, is to represent the individual provinces and their particular points of view. Elections for both chambers are held once every 5 years.

## Prevailing Health Issues and Risk Behaviors

The life expectancy of South African citizens at birth is only 53.5 years for males and 57.2 years for females (CIA, 2010). According to a survey of perceived health among South African citizens, 36.1% of the population feel that they have a good health status, and 12% feel that they have a poor health status. Only 51.3% of the population feel that they have excellent health status (Statistics South Africa, 2004).

The biggest threats for optimal health in South Africa are poverty and diseases such as HIV. The great majority of deaths occur as a result of AIDS-related illness. The total prevalence of HIV is estimated to be 10.6% of the population (5.21 million people), with 17% of adults (ages 15–49) being HIV positive (Statistics South Africa, 2009). Approximately 30% of pregnant women were found to be HIV-infected in 2005 (Department of Health, 2006). The scale of the AIDS crisis in South Africa continues to spiral upwards. Although this burden is projected to have a small effect on the economy as a whole, other repercussions will take a major toll on individual households. In addition, South Africa's population will continually be faced with a deteriorating life expectancy, which will have consequences for the entire nation. Even though the majority of the population are of the Christian religion, the practice and the types of sexual behavior that promote the ongoing epidemic have not been prevented.

It appears that people with a higher education level have a better perceived health status than those with no or lower education levels. Also, in comparison with other cultural groups, white people tend to have a better health status than the other cultural groups in the country. Teenagers (ages 13–17) and preteenagers (ages 7–12) were perceived as having better health than younger children (ages 0–6), most likely due to exposure to unfavorable living conditions during the vulnerable years of childhood (Statistics South Africa, 2004). Malnutrition also had an influence on the perceived health status, since 26.5% of children younger than 7 years went hungry in some stage during the last year because of poverty.

The most common factors influencing the perceived health and wellness of families in South Africa include the following: death of a loved one, serious injury, loss of regular job, theft, fire, destruction of property, bankruptcy, failure of business, cut-off from remittance, divorce, abandonment, and termination of government grants (Statistics South Africa, 2004).

Poverty has an influence on health in various ways. According to Statistics South Africa, 18.6% of citizens living in an overcrowded household feel that they have very poor general health. Poor sanitation facilities also influence perceived health, since 14.5% of citizens without working sanitation facilities have a poor perception of their general health status.

South Africa forms a part of the human trafficking chain, in which people are exploited in different ways, both domestically and internationally. People, especially women from Africa, are transported to South Africa for mostly sexual exploitation. South Africa also forms a shipment hub for several illicit drugs such as marijuana, heroin, and cocaine. On the other hand, a local market for synthetic drugs is increasing.

A prevailing threat to the South African population is the increasing rate of obesity and overweight among adults. About 29.8% of the male population and 54.9% of the female population are obese or overweight (IASO, 2010). Most people would never think of Africa as having an obesity pandemic; however, since 1990, there has been a drastic increase in the rates of overweight and obesity, which can be attributed partly to the change in patterns of physical activity. As a result of urbanization, the type of work that people do has evolved from physical labor to jobs that are less energy demanding. This has contributed not only to obesity but also to multiple other noncommunicable diseases, such as type 2 diabetes, which increases the risk of heart disease.

As a result, the population of South Africa is faced with a double burden. The government must find new strategies to fight not only poverty and the associated consequences such as malnutrition and starvation, but also the obesity epidemic that brings with it multiple health consequences. If action to reverse these patterns is not taken soon, there will be a tremendous burden on the health-care system.

Tobacco consumption in South Africa has been one of the main health concerns of the government. Each year, 25,000 deaths occur due to diseases associated with tobacco (Human Capital Review, 2010). Although the use of tobacco has decreased over the last decade, it still presents a significant threat to the health of the population, especially to men. About 11% of the female population uses tobacco, while three times as many men (37%) use it (WHO, 2006). The government has implemented numerous national antismoking laws, and cigarette taxes have risen drastically. The efforts are paying off, as trends now show a decrease in tobacco use.

Alcohol is available in an estimated 230,000 liquor outlets in South Africa. South Africans consume over 5 billion liters of alcoholic beverages per year, which amounts to 120 liters per person per year, according to a report by the Medical Research Council. The highest levels of fetal alcohol syndrome in the world have been recorded in the cape region: 65.2–74.2 per 1,000 children in the first grade population (Viljoen et al., 2005) have been diagnosed with fetal alcohol syndrome. As a point of comparison, this is 33–148 times greater than fetal alcohol syndrome estimates in the United States.

## Healthcare System

The healthcare system in South Africa consists mainly of a large public sector that provides health care to 80% of the population; however, it is drastically underfunded and suffers shortages of doctors and nurses. As a result of increasing urbanization, the public healthcare system also faces the challenge of attracting and retaining health professionals in areas that are underserved and in dire need of health professionals. The private sector provides health care to the remaining 20%, comprising the predominantly white middle- and upper-income earners. The latter have the luxury of access to technologically advanced, high-quality health services that are unfortunately inaccessible to the rest of the population.

Over the past 30 years, expenditures for health care in the private sector have grown to consume a much larger proportion of total national expenditures on health. In GDP terms, private healthcare expenditures in South Africa are much higher than in most other countries with comparable economic development, and much more similar to high-income countries such as the United Kingdom. The private sector contribution to health care, which caters to a small minority of the population, is 5.2% as a share of GDP. The public sector, on the other hand, contributes a much smaller amount, with a share of 3.5% of GDP, yet it covers the majority of the population (McIntyre & Thiede, 2007).

Even though the overall percentage of GDP that is spent on health is fairly high, health status indicators in South Africa are much worse than those of other countries with an upper-middle income status. Therefore, the primary challenge facing the health sector is not the shortage of resources, but rather the need to use the already existing resources in a more efficient manner.

The South African Constitution sets forth that every individual has the basic right to achieve optimal health. The government has the main responsibility to establish the conditions necessary for this to occur. Unfortunately, this right is not equally enjoyed by all—though some may dispute this—as most resources and quality care services are only provided to those who can afford private health insurance, a situation that leads to racial inequalities.

The costs for private insurance vary from R1,000 (€96) to R2,000 (€192) per month. Premiums can also be higher for the elderly and for comprehensive coverage (that is, insurance that covers 100% of all healthcare costs). There are also many companies and organizations that offer discounted rates for their employees and members, and some employers cover half of employee health insurance costs.

Universal access to health care was implemented by the government in 1994, and this program is currently the primary source of health care for the majority of the population. This service is offered free to all citizens, but it does not cover all health-related costs. Most individuals who wish to be more extensively covered need to have additional coverage or pay out of pocket.

The Department of Health is mainly responsible for providing health services to 80% of the population. However, due to high unemployment rates and high levels of poverty, the department bears the burden of funding most healthcare expenses. This places a great deal of pressure on the department, and as a result of underfunding, the quality and availability of services suffer.

Quality-related problems in health care, such as the inefficient use of resources, poor delivery systems, or inadequate diagnosis and treatment, have been identified in both the public and the private sectors (National Department of Health, 2007). These limitations and drawbacks put the health and lives of patients at risk, further increase healthcare costs, and hinder productivity and efficacy. As a way of addressing these shortcomings, the National Policy on Quality in Health Care has set key goals to improve the quality of care in both the public and private sectors. It is recognized that the goal of a quality healthcare system can be achieved only through a national commitment and an effort to assess, improve, and maintain quality health care for the population. As a first step, it is important to measure and assess the gaps that exist between standards and the practices in place, and to find solutions to eliminate the existing gaps.

There are several projects in place to promote health in order to improve the overall quality of life of South Africans. The South African food-based dietary guidelines have been developed to achieve and promote practical, affordable, sustainable, and culturally sensitive food intake and physical activity in an attempt to help South Africans choose a healthy and adequate diet (Gibney & Vorster, 2001). Like the food-based dietary guidelines, the Be Active guidelines also focus on identifying and tackling obstacles to physical activity within the population. Sparling, Owen, and Lambert (2000) propose that an ecological perspective should be adopted in order to develop appropriate interventions. Here, the aim is to understand the interaction between individual characteristics and environmental factors, as both have an influence on one another.

# Influence of Culture and Mentality

There is no single culture in South Africa, due to the diversity of the population. Food, music, and dance feature heavily in daily life, and a variety of different ethnic cultures can be found within the same region. South African cuisine incorporates numerous meat-based dishes, reflected in the very popular traditional social barbeque gatherings known as *braais*. Binge drinking is ingrained in South African society at all levels, not only among the uneducated. This can be partially attributed to the "dop system" that existed prior to 1980, wherein laborers on many farms were paid partly with alcohol. Although the system is now banned, many farm workers and rural South Africans continue to binge drink after payday, spending their wages on locally available cheap wine that is often sold by the liter at mobile bars (*shebeens*).

The burden of obesity has a tremendous negative effect on the health of the South African population. However, because of cultural views on physical attractiveness, not much concern is given to the consequences of obesity. This is especially the case among black women, who view themselves as more attractive the more they weigh. Another cultural tradition is for a woman to gain weight before her family delivers her to her future husband. This is done because overweight and obesity represent a sign of affluence and family wealth.

A further influence on obesity prevalence is related to mentality. Ever since HIV/AIDS became prevalent, South Africans have been trying endlessly to show that they are not affected. According to Professor Philip James, chairman of the International Obesity Task Force, people intentionally try to become overweight as a sign of being healthy, as the virus is also known as the "slim disease."

In the past, the culture and lifestyle of South Africans have always provided for an active way of living. Physical labor was a predominant aspect of the working culture, and due to lack of transportation, walking was a large part of daily life. However, with urbanization also came along a tremendous change in the lifestyles of many South Africans. Sedentary work and jobs demanding less energy have replaced work involving physical labor. Public transportation has taken the place of physical movement. These factors contribute a great deal to the increasing rate of obesity.

The topic of HIV/AIDS is taboo, which discourages people with the virus from reaching out to others and seeking help. Thabo Mbeki, the former president of South Africa, as well as the former minister of health, Manto Tshabalala-Msimang, have long asserted that the many deaths in the country are attributable to malnutrition and poverty and have refused to acknowledge that AIDS is linked with and is the primary cause of those deaths. Because HIV/AIDS is not openly talked about, many people have misconceptions about it. As a result, millions of people are left in the dark, not knowing how to help themselves or how to prevent infecting others. In spite of numerous, highly visible awareness campaigns, adequate knowledge about the spread and infection of HIV and AIDS is lacking. A major concern is the lack of knowledge regarding how to prevent sexual transmission of HIV. According to a 2008 survey, more than half of all individuals, both men and women, were unaware of both the preventive effect of condoms and the reduction in HIV risk resulting from a decrease in number of sexual partners (Human Sciences Research Council, 2008). The survey further concluded that accurate knowledge and awareness have significantly diminished in recent years.

## Drivers of Workplace Health Promotion

There are multiple key drivers of workplace health promotion (WHP). Mainly private corporations see the benefits of investing in employees, which in return improves the company's morale and productivity. However, the government also plays a large role in setting guidelines and laws for the well-being of employees. The African smoke-free legislation has prohibited smoking in public places, and because worksites are considered public places, the national framework applies to work settings as well.

The government has an inherent interest in WHP, as it is one of the best ways of reaching out to the majority of people and empowering them to change their lifestyles for the better. However, there are still very few effective legislative guidelines that promote workers' health. Instead, large companies are the key drivers of such initiatives. For some multinational companies, it is the company image that drives the program, and for others, it is overall employee productivity and business profitability.

The Global Survey on Health Promotion and Workplace Wellness identified strategic corporate objectives for WHP programs. The key reasons for implementing wellness programs in South Africa were to increase productivity and to decrease absenteeism. The major health risk was identified to be stress, followed by the negative impact of HIV/AIDS on the workforce (Buck Consultants, 2009). Further analysis showed that 30% of surveyed companies in South Africa had already implemented a WHP program and 42% had partially implemented a program. Only 4% indicated that they had no intention of implementing a WHP program. This implies that the benefits of having a wellness strategy is well understood by the surveyed employers.

The biokineticist profession (see description below under "Programs and Good Practices") has been a proponent for WHP since the mid-1990s. This has led to a growing number of biokineticists, both individuals and provider companies. Many other organizations also work in cooperation with trade unions to improve the health and safety of workers.

## Programs and Good Practices

Health promotion at the workplace is still in the early stages in South Africa, but it has undergone considerable growth in recent years and shows promise. Currently, one of the leading causes of employees' ill health, absenteeism, and lack of productivity is HIV/AIDS; therefore, managing it has become a core business practice. In the past, infected employees were either subject to discrimination or left on their own to deal with the ensuing health challenges. Nowadays, fighting the epidemic of HIV/AIDS is slowly becoming an integrated part of business strategy. As HIV/AIDS has become a focus of attention in many larger organizations, there are now many companies with good practice workplace health programs that place an emphasis on this epidemic. These models of good practices set an example of how the HIV/AIDS epidemic can be defeated. By providing employees with necessary resources and educating them on the topic of HIV/AIDS, and by setting corporate guidelines that discourage discrimination, the morale and productivity of workers can be improved drastically. It has been noted that employees who are HIV positive have a low morale and tend to be less productive because they do not see the benefit of contributing to future economic growth. As a result, the business suffers, weakening the already vulnerable workforce.

Fortunately, employers are recognizing the need for workplace health promotion in this area and have programs in place to help employees deal with the burdens. The programs exist mainly within larger multinational organizations and focus on increasing morale, productivity, and overall health. The two examples described here are Johnson & Johnson and Daimler.

## Johnson & Johnson

Johnson & Johnson has taken on social responsibility in South Africa and is committed to improving the overall well-being of its employees. The company has implemented multiple programs at its worksites that help create healthy and safe working environments, help promote mental well-being, and strengthen its workforce and the business. In 2005, Johnson & Johnson implemented a global workplace policy on HIV/AIDS that provides employees with support and access to treatment (Johnson & Johnson, 2010). Nondiscrimination and confidentiality protection for HIV-infected employees and their dependents is incorporated in the policy. All Johnson & Johnson employees and their dependents can receive voluntary testing and counseling, and the policy also focuses on educating employees and implementing awareness programs.

As further evidence of its commitment to improving workers' well-being, Johnson & Johnson has kept close track of HIV prevalence at its sites in South Africa to make employees aware of their status and to evaluate the success of the program. In 2003, there was a 93% participation rate, and the results showed an HIV prevalence rate of 4.5% among the employee population in East London and the Eastern Cape Province. The participation rate increased to 97% in 2007, when results showed a decrease in the HIV prevalence rate, to 4.2%. Currently 80% of Johnson & Johnson employees at these two sites are aware of their HIV status. The results reflect the success of the program, and the findings provide valuable statistical data for further development and improvement of the already excellent program.

## Daimler

Daimler, a multinational automotive engineering company, has set its focus on improving workers' health by implementing good practice programs at its worksites. Since the early 1990s, Daimler has made HIV/AIDS a priority on its agenda and has developed best practices to support its employees. In 2000, the company implemented a workplace program at its South African locations, which was geared not only toward all of the employees at the site, but to their families as well. In 2005, Daimler implemented a global HIV/AIDS policy as a way of providing guidelines on effectively combating HIV/AIDS and promoting antidiscrimination practices in the workplace. The MBSA (Mercedes-Benz South Africa) HIV/AIDS workplace program

- Provides access to voluntary testing and counseling if necessary, and invests in prevention strategies and support systems for workers and their dependents. Employees' right to privacy is given primary consideration and may not be violated.
- Takes corporate social responsibility very seriously.
- Aims to manage and overcome challenges of development, financing, and human resources brought on by the impact of HIV and AIDS, not only within business operations but in local communities as well.

### *Additional HIV/AIDS Programs*

Through the Siyakhana Project (Panter, 2008), the comprehensive approach to managing HIV and AIDS in the workplace has extended to a range of small and medium-sized business partners in the Eastern Cape Province of South Africa.

In addition, there are multiple national and international organizations, such as the Solidarity Center, that work in partnership with the National Union of Metal Workers of South Africa to help companies deal with the HIV/AIDS problem within their organizations and provide support, education, and resources for their employees (Solidarity Center, 2008). The objective is to educate as many individuals as possible and to provide free counseling and treatment options for them. Many manufacturing companies, such as Johnson Matthey Catalysts in South Africa, which has nearly 600 employees working at its factory, have agreed to host these training and education sessions, and to give employees a chance to be tested for HIV and receive a subsequent counseling session (AFL-CIO, 2010). These types of practices are a great start for employees to take control of their health and change their behavior accordingly. The collaboration among nonprofit organizations, unions, and private businesses to improve workers' health is a great step in creating a healthy workforce.

## Biokinetics and Corporate South African National Games and Leisure Activities

The biokinetics profession in South Africa has played a major role in spreading the health promotion message to the corporate sector. The practice of biokineticism is meant to improve a person's physical status and his or her quality of life. It provides individual evaluation of a person's overall physical and emotional well-being and prescribes preventative and therapeutic exercises accordingly.

In 1997, the Biokinetics Association of South Africa took on a project as part of a national initiative known as Corporate South African National Games and Leisure Activities, which aimed at improving the lifestyle behaviors of middle and upper management of South African companies. The Biokinetics Association managed the program and aimed to gather research information on the value of sports and physical activity as a means of optimizing quality of life, wellness, and overall well-being. The goal was to provide business executives with individualized assessments and supply them with the means of altering their behavior for the better, so that they might be empowered to take responsibility for their own health and, as a result, contribute to a healthier company profile. Following the 3-year South African National Games and Leisure Activities initiative, which had been funded by the government, the Biokinetics Association continued to provide its services to a variety of South African companies. Biokineticists are registered as health professionals with the Health Professions Council of South Africa, which gives them a vehicle to speak to other medical partners, health insurers, and companies. Many corporate health promotion programs are using the Biokinetics Association's network of practitioners.

## Discovery Vitality

Discovery is a financial services institution that provides services throughout the world. In South Africa, it operates the country's largest health insurance program, under the name Discovery Health (Discovery Vitality, 2009). One of the company's science-based wellness programs, which is based on providing incentives and rewards for sustaining good health, is its well-known Vitality program. Members are encouraged to make use of the multiple resources and tools provided to them for the purpose of improving the individuals' health. By utilizing these resources, members are rewarded with perks such as discounted rates at selected fitness centers and airlines. Vitality points are also rewarded for numerous healthy activities. Members can have preventative screening tests done and complete online assessments not only to learn about their health status but also to earn Vitality points. The more activities individuals participate in and the more tools they utilize, the more points they earn, and the greater the rewards they attain. The incentive-based program motivates people to improve their health and to lower healthcare costs by doing so.

As a result of workplace health promotion programs implemented in mostly larger organizations, awareness of health risks has become more prominent among workers, and positive behavioral changes continue to result. Although there are some excellent existing programs, the majority of workplaces have not implemented any form of workplace health promotion program, and so there is a real opportunity for health professionals to advance this field. The good practice WHP programs also provide a foundation on which other companies can base their wellness programs.

## Outcomes and Indicators

Most WHP programs are not measured for effectiveness. Although a significant amount of money is invested in these programs, very little attention is given to return on investment. According to the results of the Buck survey, only 16% of the participating organizations that implemented a WHP program report having measured the outcomes. Among that 16%, the biggest impact of the corporate wellness strategy was found to be on company image and employee morale (Buck Consultants, 2009).

## Existing Research

Currently, more than one third (37%) of deaths in South Africa can be attributed to noncommunicable disease. However, by analyzing the health of the employee population and by addressing the main risk factors within the organization, the burden of noncommunicable disease can be reduced significantly.

In 2008 a study on health risk factors among South African employees that negatively impact the rates of noncommunicable disease among the employees was conducted (Kolbe-Alexander et al., 2008). Employees from 18 different South African companies were invited to participate in a health day, where their overall health and risk profiles were assessed. The health risk assessment was based on self-reported health behavior and health status, and clinical measurements of cholesterol, blood pressure, and BMI (body mass index). Participating employees' health insurance medical histories were also made available on a voluntary basis. From the provided data, the health-related age was calculated to determine its deviation from the actual chronological age. It was determined that health-related age was linked to both the number of days away from work and annual healthcare costs. Employees with higher annual medical costs were more likely to be absent from work and to be physically inactive, and they also had an increased number of risk factors. By comparing participating employees with the general South African population, it could be determined that the employees had a higher risk of overweight, smoking, and physical inactivity.

It could be further concluded that the employees, in comparison with the general South African population, were more likely to have poor health and lifestyle habits, which places them at a higher risk of contracting a noncommunicable disease than would normally be expected. The findings of the study provide valuable data on the employees' health and risk profiles, which can aid companies in determining the appropriate interventions for their employee populations and, as a result, decrease the risk of noncommunicable disease.

Although South Africa is increasing the number of health programs not only in the work setting but also in the general population, there is not much research available that demonstrates the effectiveness of the programs. This could be a result of the lack of funding invested in health promotion, but mainly it is because health promotion has entered the health system in South Africa fairly recently, and sufficient knowledge in this field is still lacking.

## Conclusion

South Africa is a country of diverse nationalities and population groups and varying languages. Its recent economic boom has transformed South Africa into an urbanized nation that presents opportunities for development and growth in many fields. However, with the economic development also comes the challenge of keeping up with the population's changing health behaviors and lifestyles. These challenges are enormous considering the HIV/AIDS crisis and rising obesity rates, which as a result will further weaken the workforce and slow down economic growth. Corporations are starting to realize the benefit of a healthy workforce and have begun to implement workplace health promotion programs as a fulfillment of social responsibility and as a business strategy. Unfortunately, measurement and evaluation of these programs have not been made, and as a result, evidence for ROI (return on investment) and the benefits of health promotion programs is lacking. Further research in this area is needed, making it a field in which health promotion professionals can advance.

## Summary

South Africa is a diverse country that has been experiencing economic growth since 1990. However, as a result of urbanization, the population has been exposed to new noncommunicable diseases due to lifestyle and behavior changes. Currently, the two major health challenges facing South Africans are HIV/AIDS and obesity.

The challenge to improving the overall well-being of the majority of the population lies in the lack of financial support for public health promotion programs. Although 8.7% of GDP is spent on overall health expenditures, there is a large gap between public and private funding. The public sector (3.5% of GDP) provides health insurance for 80% of the population, whereas the private sector (5.2% of GDP) provides for the remaining 20%.

The main focus of health promotion has been on HIV/AIDS, and as a result, there are now many good practice programs that focus on HIV/AIDS prevention, education, and empowerment. Most of the progress on health promotion has been made in the worksite setting within large and multinational corporations. However, workplace health promotion is still in the early stages in South Africa, and further research in this field is needed to support a more evidence-based practice.

## Review Questions

1. Aside from HIV, what are the central issues affecting population health in South Africa? Explain.
2. What demographic characteristics affect population health status among South Africans?
3. What are the components of the South African healthcare system and how are they funded? Regulated? Managed?
4. What impact, if any, does the multicultural nature of South Africa have on its health promotion efforts?
5. What are the primary drivers of South Africa's workplace health promotion programs?
6. Describe the differences and similarities between Discovery's and Johnson & Johnson's strategies with regard to their workplace health promotion programs.
7. Explain the impact of current research findings regarding the measurements of success for workplace health promotion programs in South Africa.

## References

American Federation of Labor-Congress of Industrial Organizations (AFL-CIO). (2010). *Combating HIV/AIDS in Africa: Worksite education and testing.* Retrieved February 13, 2010 from http://blog.aflcio.org/2010/02/11/combating-hivaids-in-africa-changing-behavior-with-worksite-education-and-testing/

Buck Consultants. (2009). *Working well: A global survey of health promotion and workplace wellness strategies.* Boston, MA: Buck Consultants.

Central Intelligence Agency (CIA). (2010). *The world factbook.* Retrieved January 16, 2010 from https://www.cia.gov/library/publications/the-world-factbook/geos/sf.html

Department of Health. (2006). Report, national HIV and syphilis antenatal sero-prevalence survey in South Africa 2005. Pretoria, South Africa: Department of Health.

Discovery Vitality. (2009). *You and your famity.* Retrieved January 13, 2010 from http://www.discovery.co.za/portal/loggedout-individual/vitality

Gibney, M., & Vorster, H. (2001). South African food-based dietary guidelines. *The South African Journal of Clinical Nutrition, 14*(3), 1–80.

*Human Capital Review.* (2010, February). Workplace wellness. Retrieved February 4, 2010 from http://www.humancapitalreview.org/content/default.asp?Article_ID=723

Human Sciences Research Council. (2009). *South African national HIV prevalence, incidence, behaviour and communication survey, 2008: A turning tide among teenagers?* Cape Town, South Africa: HSRC Press.

International Association for the Study of Obesity (IASO). (2010). *Global prevalence of adult obesity.* London, England: IASO.

Johnson & Johnson. (2010). *Protecting our people.* Retrieved January 7, 2010 from http://www.jnj.com/connect/caring/employee-health/

Kolbe-Alexander, T., Buckmaster, C., Nossel, C., Dreyer, L., Bull, F., Noakes, T., and Lambert, E. (2008). Chronic disease risk factors, healthy days and medical claims in South African employees presenting for health risk screening. *BMC Public Health, 8*(228). Retrieved from http://www.ncbi.nlm.nih.gov/pmc/articles/PMC2475536/

McIntyre, D., & Thiede, M. (2007). *Health care financing and expenditure.* Cape Town, South Africa: Health Economics Unit.

National Department of Health. (2007). A policy on quality in health care for South Africa. Pretoria, South Africa: National Department of Health.

Panter, C. (2008). The Siyakhana project 2008–2009 (PPP Project E0146): Interim report. East London, South Africa: Mercedes Benz South Africa.

Solidarity Center. (2008). *Promoting worker rights worldwide. 2008 annual report.* Washington, DC: Solidarity Center.

Sparling, P., Owen, N., & Lambert, E. (2000). Promoting physical activity: The new imperative for public health. *Health Education Research, 15*(3), 367–376.

Statistics South Africa. (2004). *Perceived health and other health indicators in South Africa.* Pretoria, South Africa: Statistics South Africa.

Statistics South Africa. (2009). *Mid-year population estimates, 2009.* Pretoria, South Africa: Statistics South Africa.

Viljoen, D. L., Gossage, J. P., Brooke, L., Adnams, C. M., Jones, K. L., Robinson, L. K … May, P. A. (2005). Fetal alcohol syndrome epidemiology in a South African community: A second study of a very high prevalence area. *Journal of Studies on Alcohol, 66*(5), 593–604.

World Health Organization. (2006). *World health statistics 2006.* Retrieved April 15, 2010 from http://apps.who.int/ghodata/

Chapter 19

# Sweden

Jan Winroth and Lars Österblom

After reading this chapter you should be able to:

- Identify core strategies that are the focus of workplace health promotion efforts in Sweden
- Describe the historical evolution of Sweden's workplace health promotion efforts
- Explain the different approaches employed by corporate health promotion throughout Sweden
- Review the central disease states and health issues driving workplace health promotion in Sweden
- Name the components of, and the associated funding sources for, the Swedish healthcare system
- Discuss the impact of culture on the health status and health promotion efforts within Sweden

Table 19-1 **Select Key Demographic and Economic Indicators**

| | |
|---|---|
| Nationality | Noun: Swede(s)<br>Adjective: Swedish |
| Ethnic groups | Indigenous population: Swedes with Finnish and Sami minorities; foreign-born or first-generation immigrants: Finns, Yugoslavs, Danes, Norwegians, Greeks, Turks |
| Religion | Lutheran 87%, other (includes Roman Catholic, Orthodox, Baptist, Muslim, Jewish, and Buddhist) 13% |
| Language | Swedish, small Sami- and Finnish-speaking minorities |
| Literacy | Definition: age 15 and over can read and write<br>Total population: 99%<br>Male: 99%<br>Female: 99% (2003 est.) |
| Education expenditure | 6.7% of GDP (2007)<br>Country comparison to the world: 28 |

*continued*

| Table 19-1 **Select Key Demographic and Economic Indicators,** *continued* | |
|---|---|
| Government type | Constitutional monarchy |
| Environment | Acid rain damage to soils and lakes; pollution of the North Sea and the Baltic Sea |
| Country mass | Total: 450,295 sq km<br>Country comparison to the world: 55<br>Land: 410,335 sq km<br>Water: 39,960 sq km |
| Population | 9,059,651 (July 2010 est.)<br>Country comparison to the world: 88 |
| Age structure | 0–14 years: 15.7% (male 733,597/female 692,194)<br>15–64 years: 65.5% (male 3,003,358/female 2,927,038)<br>65 years and over: 18.8% (male 753,293/female 950,171)<br>(2010 est.) |
| Median age | Total: 41.7 years<br>Male: 40.6 years<br>Female: 42.9 years (2010 est.) |
| Population growth rate | 0.158% (2010 est.)<br>Country comparison to the world: 186 |
| Birth rate | 10.13 births/1,000 population (2010 est.)<br>Country comparison to the world: 194 |
| Death rate | 10.21 deaths/1,000 population (July 2010 est.)<br>Country comparison to the world: 58 |
| Net migration rate | 1.66 migrant(s)/1,000 population (2010 est.)<br>Country comparison to the world: 47 |
| Urbanization | Urban population: 85% of total population (2008)<br>Rate of urbanization: 0.5% annual rate of change (2005–2010 est.) |
| Gender ratio | At birth: 1.06 male(s)/female<br>Under 15 years: 1.06 male(s)/female<br>15–64 years: 1.02 male(s)/female<br>65 years and over: 0.8 male(s)/female<br>Total population: 0.98 male(s)/female (2010 est.) |
| Infant mortality rate | Total: 2.75 deaths/1,000 live births<br>Country comparison to the world: 222<br>Male: 2.91 deaths/1,000 live births<br>Female: 2.58 deaths/1,000 live births (2010 est.) |
| Life expectancy | Total population: 80.86 years<br>Country comparison to the world: 9<br>Male: 78.59 years<br>Female: 83.26 years (2010 est.) |

*continued*

| Table 19-1 **Select Key Demographic and Economic Indicators,** *continued* | |
|---|---|
| Total fertility rate | 1.67 children born/woman (2010 est.)<br>Country comparison to the world: 175 |
| GDP—purchasing power parity | $331.4 billion (2009 est.)<br>Country comparison to the world: 35 |
| GDP—per capita | $36,600 (2009 est.)<br>Country comparison to the world: 30 |
| GDP—composition by sector | Agriculture: 1.6%<br>Industry: 26.7%<br>Services: 71.6% (2009 est.) |
| Agriculture—products | Barley, wheat, sugar beets, meat, milk |
| Industries | Iron and steel, precision equipment (bearings, radio and telephone parts, armaments), wood pulp and paper products, processed foods, motor vehicles |
| Labor force participation | 4.91 million (2009 est.)<br>Country comparison to the world: 75 |
| Unemployment rate | 8.3% (2009 est.)<br>Country comparison to the world: 95 |
| Industrial production growth rate | -9% (2009 est.)<br>Country comparison to the world: 137 |
| Distribution of family income (GINI index) | 23 (2005)<br>Country comparison to the world: 134 |
| Investment (gross fixed) | 17.4% of GDP (2009 est.)<br>Country comparison to the world: 120 |
| Public debt | 35.8% of GDP (2009 est.)<br>Country comparison to the world: 74 |
| Market value of publicly traded shares | $NA (December 31, 2009)<br>Country comparison to the world: 23 |
| Current account balance | $29.5 billion (2009 est.)<br>Country comparison to the world: 12 |
| Debt (external) | $669.1 billion (June 30, 2009 est.)<br>Country comparison to the world: 14 |
| Debt as a % of GDP | ——— |
| Exports | $130.8 billion (2009 est.)<br>Country comparison to the world: 28 |

*continued*

| Table 19-1 **Select Key Demographic and Economic Indicators,** *continued* | |
|---|---|
| Exports—commodities | Machinery 35%, motor vehicles, paper products, pulp and wood, iron and steel products, chemicals |
| Export—partners | Norway 10.61%, Germany 10.2%, United Kingdom 7.45%, Denmark 7.35%, Finland 6.44%, United States 6.36%, France 5.05%, Netherlands 4.67% (2009) |
| Imports | $120.5 billion (2009 est.)<br>Country comparison to the world: 27 |
| Import—commodities | Machinery, petroleum and petroleum products, chemicals, motor vehicles, iron and steel, foodstuffs, clothing |
| Import—partners | Germany 17.9%, Denmark 8.9%, Norway 8.7%, Netherlands 6.17%, United Kingdom 5.56%, Finland 5.14%, France 5.06%, China 4.79% (2009) |
| Stock of direct foreign investment at | |
| Home | $269.2 billion (December 31, 2009 est.)<br>Country comparison to the world: 18 |
| Abroad | $346.9 billion (December 31, 2009 est.)<br>Country comparison to the world: 13 |

Source: CIA. (2010). *The world factbook.* Retrieved December 16, 2010, from https://www.cia.gov/library/publications/the-world-factbook/

# Introduction

Sweden has about 9,300,000 inhabitants in an area of 450,000 square kilometers. Sweden has been a member of the European Union since 1995, yet the currency is Swedish kronor, not euros. The Swedish gross national product in 2009 was 342,400 Swedish kronor per person (U.S. $55,620).

There are many ethnic groups in Sweden. During the 20th century, industrial workers were recruited deliberately from other European countries, and since about 1980, many refugees from countries outside Europe have found their refuge in Sweden.

Sweden is quite secularized. The Church of Sweden is Evangelical Lutheran and coexists with many other denominations. Religion's influence on and importance to working life is almost nonexistent. However, some are of the opinion that Swedes have a Lutheran approach to time and morality, including being on time, respecting deadlines, and being honest and true.

The aging population poses a challenge to Swedish society. Recently, the retirement age increased from 65 years to 67 years, but citizens retained the right to leave work at 65. A so-called working line has been a political doctrine in Sweden regardless of political majority in Parliament. Inhabitants are encouraged to work longer and to be on sick leave as rarely as possible. The proportion of the population aged 65 years and above is 17.2% (for comparison, Germany's is 17.5%, Norway's is 14.8%, and Turkey's is 5.5%) (Central Intelligence Agency, 2009).

Sweden has a high proportion of working women and men; approximately 4.6 million inhabitants participate in the labor market. The public child care service is well developed. Swedish parents of young children have the opportunity to stay home with small children for up to 450 days with compensation from the state. The level of education in Sweden is high. The Swedish people have access to free tax-financed education, beginning with day care centers and preschools, and continuing with the 9-year compulsory school and the voluntary upper secondary school (International Graduate, n.d.).

University and college education in Sweden is also heavily tax financed and is supported by a generous system of study loans and grants. Thus, higher education is accessible to people from all social classes (International Graduate, n.d.).

For many years Sweden has had a large public sector financed by tax systems. This means that the work of a large proportion of the working population is funded by taxes.

The success of the Swedish industry is based on a high level of export. Several large companies are established abroad. Many companies are successful in the international market, but they are also highly influenced by global economic developments.

The nation is affected by the 2009 economic crisis, and forecasts indicate that the unemployment rate, usually about 3–4%, will increase to about 12%. Unemployment is a worrying development and is especially high among young people.

Since the beginning of industrialization in Sweden, a large majority of the workers have become union members. Although about 85% was the norm, since 2005, membership has decreased sharply. Published data shows that only 71% of workers are affiliated with a union (Andersson & Brunk, 2008).

Sweden is adapting to European customs more and more. Trends in Europe generally also become trends in Sweden, and Swedish laws and regulations are gradually adapted to EU legislation.

Swedish legislation on the working environment, health, and safety is well established. The distinct responsibility of the employer with respect to the prevention of illness and rehabilitation of people on sick leave is clear and well known (Björklund, 2008). There are, however, no laws or rules covering workplace health promotion (WHP). WHP has been introduced instead in companies and public sector activities to improve production and productivity and to establish a given company as an employer of choice.

## Prevailing Health Issues and Risk Behaviors

Swedish life expectancy has gradually increased; for women it is 83 years and for men 79 years. The main cause of a longer life is a reduced risk of dying from cardiovascular diseases. Mortality from cancer and injuries has remained basically at the same level since 1990. According to predictions from Statistics Sweden (2006), by the year 2020, the estimated life expectancy will increase to 84.2 years for women and 80.8 years for men.

Other facts of interest pertaining to the health of the Swedish people, from the Swedish National Institute of Public Health (FHI 2008:1), are listed below:

- 71% of men and 66% of women aged 16–84 years stated that they were in good health. Poor health was reported by 6% of men and 8% of women. About 32% of women and 29% of men had a long-term illness with impaired working ability. Severe distress from aches or pains in the locomotive organs was reported by 20% of women and 13% of men, while 22% of women and 15% of men had impaired mobility.
- Severe distress from anxiety, worry, or anguish was most common among women aged 16–29 years. Young women also displayed other signs of mental ill health such as stress, impaired mental well-being, thoughts of suicide, and suicide attempts.
- People with low incomes and those who lacked cash margins or who had been in economic crises suffered considerably more physical and mental ill health than people who had not been in straitened circumstances.

There are signs that both physical and mental aspects of the work environment have improved since the mid-1990s. The work environment survey carried out by Statistics Sweden and the Swedish Work Environment Authority (2006) shows that the proportion of employees in the healthcare sector who reported that they had too much to do has decreased. Within the elderly care sector, figures indicate that the need for heavy lifting every day has declined. Since 2001, an increasing number of workers have reported that they believed they would manage to keep on working until retirement age. There are also contradictory tendencies: for example, symptoms such as tired body after work have increased among both white collar and blue collar workers. In the 2006 survey on work-caused inconveniences; Statistics Sweden reported that nearly one out of four employees in Sweden indicated during the previous 12 months that they had had some kind of physical, stress-related, or psychiatric disorder that they could attribute to work. The proportions of both physical and stress-related mental disorders increased between 1997 and 2003 but has subsequently declined. In the 2006 survey, however, the changes were relatively small compared to figures in 2005.

The following observations on Swedish society are noteworthy:

- The increase in overweight and obesity has ceased, but both are still at very high levels.
- There is continued positive development regarding smoking behaviors. Women are quitting smoking, but at a slower pace than men.

At a company/organizational level, these observations are noted:

- New forms of employment are being established, which means that individuals will have a weaker connection to their workplace.
- A report from the Swedish Trade Union Confederation (2007) points out that women have a poorer work environment than men. For example, three out of four women in the public sector and the private service sector are not able to take a so-called chat break during work hours.

On an individual level these observations are noted from the National Public Health Survey 2008.

## Tobacco Habits

The proportion of females who smoke daily decreased by 5% between 2004 and 2008. It is now 14%. Among men, the decrease during the same period was 3%, to a rate of 11%.

## Alcohol Habits

Sweden has a restrictive alcohol policy; wine and liquor are sold exclusively by a state-owned company. Sixteen percent of men have risky drinking habits. Men with risky drinking habits are more commonly drunk more than 1 or 2 times per month than are women. Women are more likely than men to abstain from alcohol entirely.

## Weight, Overweight, and Obesity

The proportion of men with normal weight (a body mass index of 18.6–24.0) is 45%, and the proportion of women is 58%. In 2008, obesity (a BMI greater than 30) was found in 12% of men and 11% of women.

## Physical Activity

About two thirds of the population consider themselves to be engaging in some type of physical activity for at least 30 minutes a day. A slight decline was noted for men from 2004 to 2008.

Sweden is facing some major challenges in the workplace, including:

- Stressful situations at work, which lead to sleep disorders and other unhealthy phenomena, among other things
- An increasingly aging workforce with different needs and requirements

## Healthcare System

For many years, Sweden has had comprehensive public primary health care, run by county councils. All citizens have access to it, and the fee for a consultation with a doctor or nurse is minimal.

The Swedish government seeks to make it compulsory for the county councils to introduce a care choice system in primary health care. This system would grant the patient the right to choose between a private or public healthcare center, with the funds for health and medical care to follow the patient's choice.

Since the mid-1900s, the number of doctors and nurses in Sweden has increased fivefold. In 1980, Sweden had 18,000 doctors below 65 years of age, 25% of whom were female. In 2005, Sweden had 29,400 doctors below 65 years of age, 43% of whom were women (Västra Götalandsregionen, 2009).

Occupational health and safety services in Sweden were initially based on agreements between parties in the labor market, and such services have covered a relatively large proportion of the labor market, primarily for prevention and treatment of work-related complaints. New data indicate that the proportion of employees who have access to occupational health and safety services has decreased, possibly in part because employers have not seen the direct result of their efforts.

Sweden has a well-developed social security system that covers all citizens and guarantees a minimum income during sick leave. The social insurance is administered by the Swedish Social Insurance Agency and financed through a combination of employer and employee contributions and through taxes. Social insurance expenditures have increased over time, but the severe recession of the early 1990s prompted a number of changes in rules, curbing the increases in expenditures until 1997. Between 1998 and 2003, expenditures rose sharply due to widespread sickness-related absence and the increasing costs of old-age pensions.

In 2008, the public expense for financial security in cases of sickness and disability (including sickness cash benefits, rehabilitation compensation, and sickness/activity compensation) was about 4% of the nation's GDP.

The majority of Swedish employees are also covered by an unemployment fund that guarantees an income during unemployment. In most industries and trades, there is also a structured system of collectively agreed-upon insurances covering loss of income in case of sickness or injury caused by work. Recently, several private insurance companies have launched new services, such as medical insurance, that may be obtained by individuals but which are also offered by employers to key employees.

Some conclusions from a report (SKL, 2008) comparing Sweden with 17 other countries are as follows:

- Sweden manages the most healthcare needs (the highest percentage of elderly people).
- Sweden has good medical outcomes and impacts (for example, the lowest infant mortality rate and a low mortality from cancer).

- Sweden offers good access to care (based on the number of operations per 100,000 inhabitants, such as cataract, hip, and coronary surgery).
- Sweden has moderate costs (based on the cost per inhabitant per year and as a percentage of GNP).
- Sweden offers good preventive care, including vaccinations of children.

The cost of Swedish health care is about U.S. $3,000 per person, as of 2005 (compared with roughly U.S. $2,000 in Portugal and U.S. $6,500 in the United States).

## Influence of Culture and Mentality

Sweden has a relatively small population considering its geographic size. There are extensive areas of land and sea available for an active outdoor life, and for many Swedes, outdoor activities are a natural part of everyday life. Many Swedish families have a summer house or a cottage, in addition to their regular housing. There are particularly attractive areas along the coasts, with a great number of islands and mountainous areas in the north. All working women and men are entitled to at least 5 weeks of vacation each year.

During the 1970s, Sweden developed a kind of workplace democracy that has evolved ever since. Participation agreements are in place, and safety representatives have the legal right to stop dangerous work. A law of employment security regulates how a person can be dismissed from work. Democratic influences have also affected the leadership and management of businesses and public activities. One author (Isaksson, 2007) points out that the Swedish management style is knowledge-based and team-oriented and that it encourages delegation and fosters self-governed employees. Organizational solutions such as decentralization, delegation of responsibilities and duties, independent employees, and teams and groups are common elements in the workplaces. Swedish managers often describe the characteristics of Swedish leadership traditions in terms of confidence, self-governed employees, and time-consuming processes of decision making (Gullers, 2007).

## Drivers of Workplace Health Promotion

When we discuss the concept of workplace health promotion (WHP), we emphasize (1) the organizational approach, (2) the setting approach, and (3) the health promotion approach. In Sweden, there is no fixed meaning of WHP; it is rather a mixture of approaches and angles. Sweden has a long-standing tradition of focusing on occupational health and safety. Lifestyle and living habits (in Swedish, *friskvård*) has played a prominent role in corporations and organizations since the mid-1980s. In recent years, human resource issues have been linked to health more often, and in certain organizations, issues of work activities and health have also been linked. As a basis for further discussion, we present a working model (Figure 19-1) in order to facilitate an understanding of how we choose to discuss WHP (Winroth & Rydqvist, 2008).

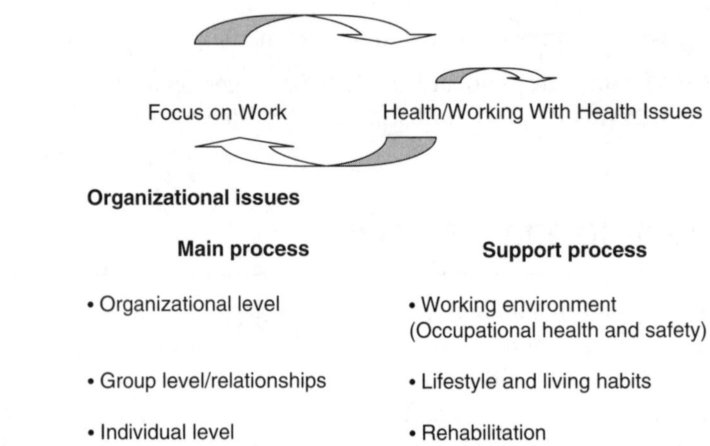


Figure 19-1 A working model for workplace health promotion, basic version.

When we henceforth discuss WHP from a Swedish perspective, it will encompass a mix of the various parts in the model in Figure 19-1.

Corporations and organizations such as municipalities and county administrations have contributed to the development and furthering of these issues. Initially, these activities were mostly considered to be social activities for the staff, with the added benefit of contributing to the quality and efficiency of the work in a positive way. Today, more businesses and organizations tend to see the connections among work, profit, and health, and regard WHP as an issue strongly linked to the organizational approach and to HR issues (Johanson, Ahonen, & Roslender, 2007).

Consultants are also important actors when WHP is put into practice. They often develop their own concepts, which they then sell to businesses and organizations. This means that they choose to emphasize a specific aspect of what we classify as WHP, including leadership development, team development, or different instruments and tools that support health-related goals. The consultants' driving forces are not only having an idea they believe in, but also their interest in securing assignments and earning an income.

Additional actors with an interest in WHP, and who in different ways contribute to its development, are insurance companies and providers of education. One insurance company that has taken a special interest in working life and health is AFA, a company owned by Sweden's labor market parties, which has utilized a program called Suntliv.nu ("Healthy life now"), discussed in detail below in the "Programs" section.

From the perspective of the authorities and the government, the issue is limited to making laws and regulations concerning occupational safety and health that focus on protection and safety (such as the OSH Act 1977:1160, last revision 2009; and Systematic Work Environment Management, AFS 2001:01). Some research on working life and health from a broader perspective is funded with support from the government, such as the Swedish Council for Working Life and Social Research. Prior to 2007, a government research center called the National Institute for Working Life conducted its own research on working life, but it was shut down by the present government. Its researchers now work at various Swedish universities.

## Programs and Good Practices

An example of a comprehensive and thoroughly worked-out program is the previously mentioned, Suntliv.nu (http://www.suntliv.nu), based on well-known research and extensive databases. The program was developed and tested by four large companies and the Karolinska Institutet, which was responsible for the research issues and the evaluation of this 2-year pilot project. The concept of the program is based on the following structure and plan:

<u>Establishing phase (in collaboration with consultants from AFA)</u>

- Gather information
- Establish and define structures
- Conduct management seminars

<u>Continuation phase (with continued support from AFA consultants)</u>

- Questionnaire and visit to the workplace
- In-depth analyses
- Feedback seminars
- Measures and support

<u>Independent phase</u>

- Continuing work
- Evaluation

A 2003 Swedish Work Environment Authority review of the methods and concepts used within occupational health care to assess psychosocial ill health found 29 different methods. Several of them also concern organizational aspects; these include SLOT, which is based on systems theory and a biopsychosocial perspective, and SMC's Profiler, which is composed of six different profiles that can be combined in various ways. The concept of HealthSCORE (http://www.halsopromotiongruppen.se) should also be mentioned in this context, as it is a tool focused on the health-promotive perspective, which sheds light on both the individual and group level as well as the organizational and management level.

Various forms of situation analyses are a part of many concepts, often as questionnaires but also in the form of interviews, focus groups, and different kinds of measurements and tests. A very established method for arriving at an individual's health status is the Health Profile Assessment, a scientifically based method that has been used in Sweden for more than 30 years (Andersson, 1987; Andersson & Malmgren, 1976; Malmgren, 1987). An example of a questionnaire used to attain a picture of the present situation concerning self-reported physical and psychological health is Short Form 36 (http://www.hrql.se). When it comes to broader questionnaires regarding work activity, staff, and working environment, every large organization uses various standardized instruments for situation analyses and follow-ups. An example of a tool used for business and management control is the balanced scorecard (Kaplan & Norton, 1996).

## Health-Promotive Workplaces (Social Insurance in Östergötland, Eastern Sweden)

This program's starting point was the idea that health-promotive workplaces are created through the education of leaders and managers on various levels and health inspirers who can support the managers in their respective workplaces. Approximately 30 first-line managers participated in a leader development program of 12 days spread over 1 year. In a parallel process, the management group received supervision and education based on the same material given to the operative managers. Approximately 50 health inspirers, who were educated in 2 rounds, participated in a process-focused university course offering 7.5 higher education credits.

The leadership program was structured in three phases. Phase one was a starting phase, in which a common platform was created and a common goal for the course was formulated. The intention was to make the participants a part of the process, something that is a core idea in health promotion work. The focus of the course content was their own work and its conditions, and also the development of strategic foresight and an analysis of the structural conditions. Phase two was focused on building knowledge and providing participants with tools to enable them as leaders to work toward a health-promotive workplace. The content involved how work-related issues and health are linked, which factors influence health, and what it means to promote health and prevent ill health in practice, as well as improvement work at various levels. The role of the leader was also a central part of the education, as the program involved leading both activities and people and also helping them achieve results.

The purpose of the third phase was to put the health-promotive way of thinking into practice. This phase focused on how best to create conditions for a health-promotive workplace on an organizational level, for example with support processes in place for the leaders. Another section was aimed at developing one's own leadership. To initiate action, the participants were given various tasks in order to establish a health-promotive workplace. The course for the health inspirers featured certain elements concerning health, health promotion, and improvement work that were also to be found in the leadership course. This was done deliberately to create a common language. However, one difference was that since the health inspirers' course was a university course with credits, the requirements were greater, including the reading of course materials and the completion of various types of exams. So what was the result? In order to obtain a comprehensive picture of the process, a researcher was engaged who followed the process and documented the results in three reports (Thomsson, 2004, 2005, and 2007). The researcher concluded her last report with some advice for other workplaces aspiring to be health-promotive. According to Thomsson (2007) some suggestions are:

- Work on developing leadership
- Make sure the management wants the workplace to be health promotive
- Provide all coworkers with basic knowledge of health promotion
- Have health inspirers who collaborate and support each other
- Let managers and health inspirers receive continuous supervision, preferably both together and separately
- Make sure there are funds available
- Supply nutrition and energy for perseverance
- Be concrete

## Scania—Focus on the Healthy; Let's Fight Ill Health by Focusing on Good Health

Scania is one of the world's leading manufacturers of trucks and buses for heavy transport applications, and of industrial and marine engines. Scania operates in about 100 countries and has nearly 35,000 employees. Its research and development activities are concentrated in Sweden, and production takes place in Europe and South America. In Sweden there are 12,000 employees, of whom 2,400 are women. The average age of the workers is 39 years. The absentee rate decreased from 8% to below 4% during the period 1998–2009.

Listed below are some historical dates from the OHS service in Scania:

1950s: The first occupational physician was employed

1990s: The OHS service was outsourced

2000s: The OHS service was brought back into the Scania parent company, but with a new strategic role

2002: Scania provided primary health care for all employees

2006: Scania provided primary health care for employees' family members

2008: Scania signed an agreement with the Stockholm county council that led to tax-financed support for OHS activities.

The multifunctional team that operates within the OHS service consists of:

- Health scientists
- Ergonomists
- Safety engineers
- Psychologists
- Occupational nurses
- Occupational physicians
- Health economists

They all work from the perspective of meeting their customers' demands. Scania has created strong values regarding customers, quality, and employees. The OHS service has based its principles and methods upon those values, and its results are regularly measured. These are illustrated in Figures 19-2 and 19-3.

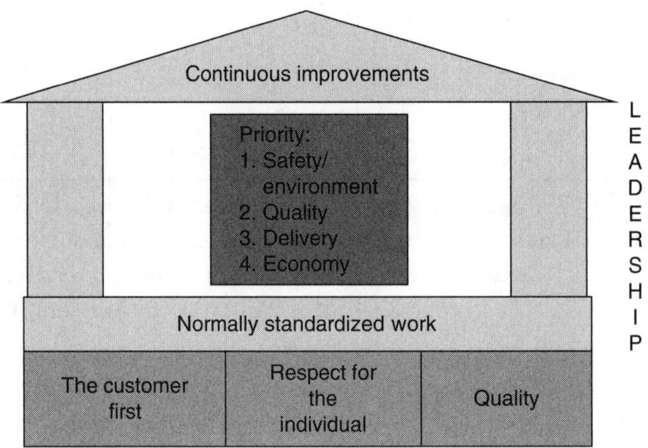


Figure 19-2 The Scania house.

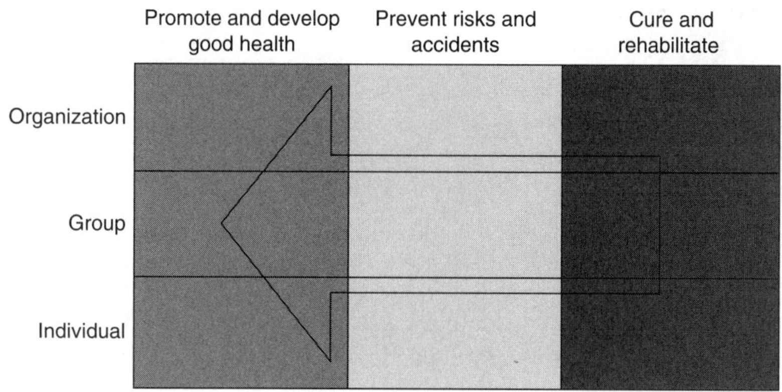


Figure 19-3 Scania's health principles.

The company's health principles are:

- All employees are responsible for their own health
- Working together toward good health

The methods are:

- Systematic health work
- Systematic work-environmental work

The following results are continuously measured:

- Degree of healthy presence (a counterpart to absenteeism)
- Degree of long-term healthy presence
- Accidents at work
- Near-accidents
- Personnel turnover
- Inquiries to the employees

The degree of healthy presence is regularly measured and plotted for each department so that the OHS service can act properly. The result can also be compared with other figures such as "reclamation per vehicle," as shown in Figure 19-4.

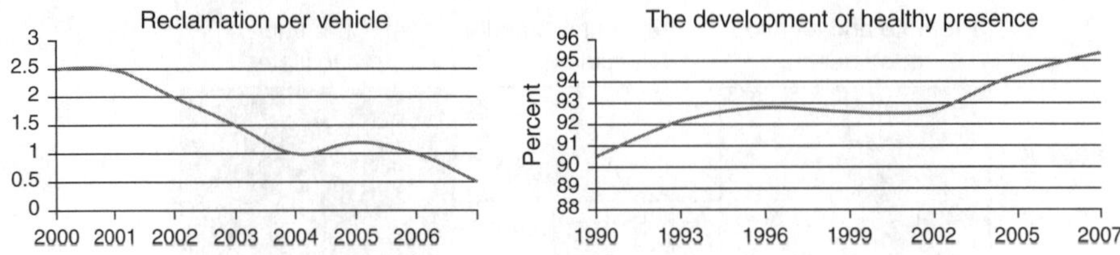


Figure 19-4 Reclamation per vehicle. The development of healthy presence.

Scania also measures improvements in productivity, and the management often refers to the degree of healthy presence. Of course this development has a great impact on the company's economy, as illustrated in Figure 19-5.

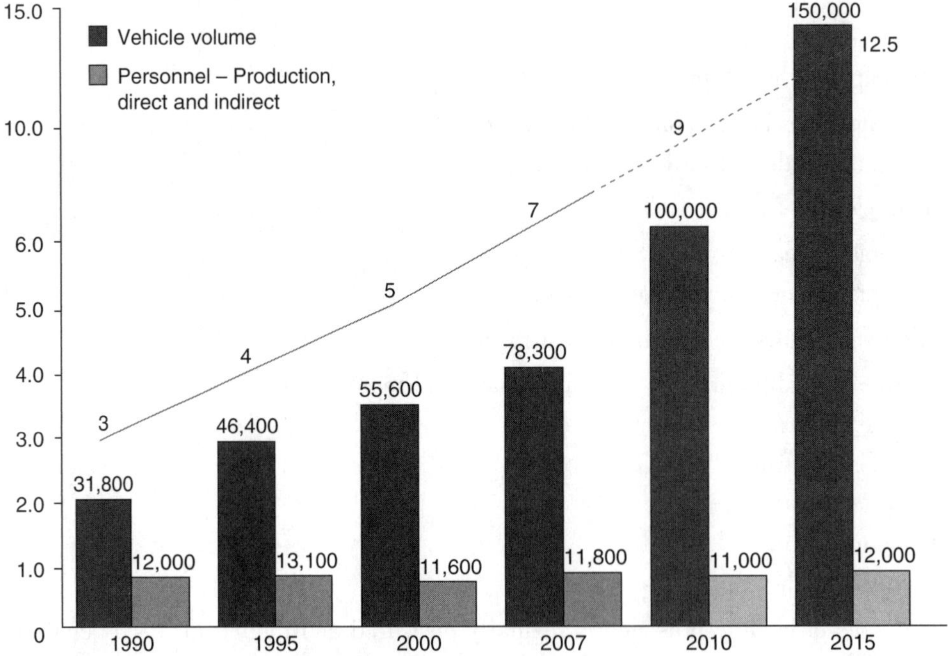


Figure 19-5 Productivity improvements.
**The ascending line signifies the amount of vehicles per person employed per year.**

Among the WHP activities that take place at Scania, the Health School for employees is important. The Health School is meant for employees at risk for absenteeism due to pain, stress-related problems, and other symptoms. Employees are contacted and encouraged to participate. Those returning from a longer period of absence due to illness may also benefit from the Health School. Every school consists of a 1-year program comprising 6 weeks of half-day programs, during which the employees are trained in health issues through lectures, physical training, and individual participation including work analyses. Follow-ups are conducted every 3rd month.

Scania's WHP activities also place a special focus on healthy leadership, with programs for managers and prospective managers.

The primary driving forces at Scania can be summarized as:

- Strong common values
- Fully integrated and multicompetent OHS service
- OHS service's being regarded as a strategic partner
- Long tradition and sustainability (S. Persson & C. Albiin, OHS Scania, personal communication)

# Outcomes and Indicators

Those who commit to and carry out any kind of change or development work are also interested in the results. Depending on the resources and skills available, results can be measured through a variety of methods from simple follow-ups to sophisticated evaluations to advanced research. In Example 1 in the "Programs and Good Practices" section, relatively large resources were applied to the evaluation. Apart from the researcher contracted to describe and evaluate the process, an additional researcher was contracted to design a questionnaire as a further means of assessing results and patterns. Since education was a central strategy in this program, the goal was to increase the level of knowledge and consciousness relating to the creation of a health-promotive workplace. But as mentioned earlier, obtaining a more tangible result requires further efforts. Results from education can be seen as impact goals that can be related to other goals in the following way, as illustrated in Figure 19-6.

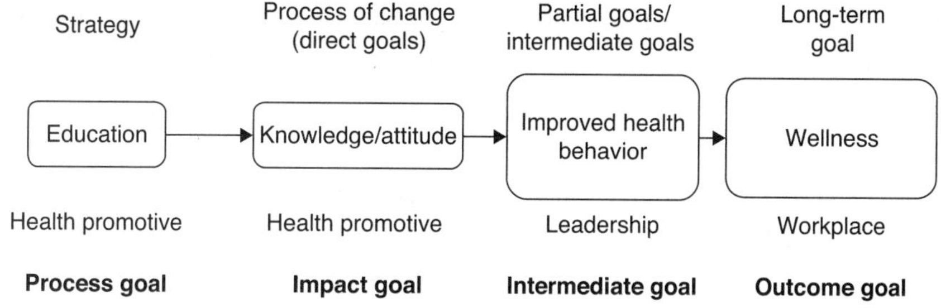


Figure 19-6 Different forms of goals.

Understanding that it is possible to see results in several stages is a central part of the more extensive WHP programs. Nutbeam and Bauman (2006) note the following effects linked to short-term and long-term results: raised awareness and participation, short-term program impact, social and behavioral outcomes, and health status and disease changes.

If we consider the aforementioned in the context of indicators and results, we can say that education and behavior are indicators, while new knowledge, changed attitudes, and changed behavior are results.

If we look at outcomes and indicators in a more general way, it may look like the following:

Outcomes

- Motivated and committed employees
- Job satisfaction
- Low degree of absenteeism and high degree of long-term health
- Increased productivity

Indicators

- Reward system
- Education, training, and development
- Lifestyles program/behavior
- Absenteeism and presenteeism

Time is an important dimension when looking for effects, and a more holistic program is problematic when evaluating cause and effect. One way to work with more holistic programs is to differentiate among process evaluation, impact evaluation, and outcome evaluation (Green & Kreuter, 1999), and through these distinctions capture the various forms of results generated by the program.

## Existing Research

As WHP is interdisciplinary and complex, understanding the state of current research demands certain parameters. The fundamental questions on which this chapter focuses are:

- What variables and factors in the workplace contribute to perseverance, quality, efficiency, and health?
- What are the links among work, working environment, leadership, and health?
- What factors constitute healthy factors in one's working life and in the workplace?

Among the key words and phrases are work ability, sustainability, positive health, leadership and health, work-integrated learning, setting, management, occupational health, lifestyle, and sense of coherence.

Our literature search generated 3 doctoral theses, 8 research reports, and 11 articles of great relevance to issues concerning WHP, according to Figure 19-6. The following is a selection of the results.

The level of work ability and factors that influence this are an important part of WHP-oriented work. Lindberg (2006) found out that determinants linked to excellent work ability were leisure exercise, satisfaction with working hours, good working positions, role clarity at work, low psychological demands, and positive feedback from the manager. He also learned that clear objectives and appreciation from the immediate manager are important health factors in a workplace.

Arnesson (2006) states that an essential characteristic of WHP is "full participation, comprising processes of empowerment, social support and learning" (p. 18). She also notes that a systemic procedure and an ecological approach in the intervention method facilitate WHP interventions. A shift to focusing on the organization as an arena for health promotion is also an essential characteristic of future interventions aiming to promote the health of employees at a worksite.

Important factors concerning health promotion leadership are:

- Showing consideration toward subordinates
- Initiating structure when needed, especially in stressful situations
- Allowing subordinates to control their work environment, giving access to empowerment structures, and affording opportunities for participation, autonomy, and control
- Inspiring employees to see a higher meaning in their work
- Providing intellectual stimulation
- Being charismatic (Nyberg, Bernin, & Theorell, 2005, p. 31)

These factors are in line with what Dellve, Skagert, and Vilhelmsson (2007) have determined, and they further state that "multi-focused WHP interventions had the largest effect on work attendance."

The following are certain recurrent variables in research that are crucial for perseverance and health:

- A balance between demands and resources
- Approachable managers who state the targets for an assignment, are supportive when things are difficult, and provide feedback on performed work
- Social support from managers and coworkers
- Time for recovery and development
- Employees' possessing resources such as competence, strength, and a feeling of being able to have an influence on their own workplace

This pattern also emerges if we put together a compilation of "healthy factors in working life" (Abrahamsson et al., 2003), as illustrated in Figure 19-7.

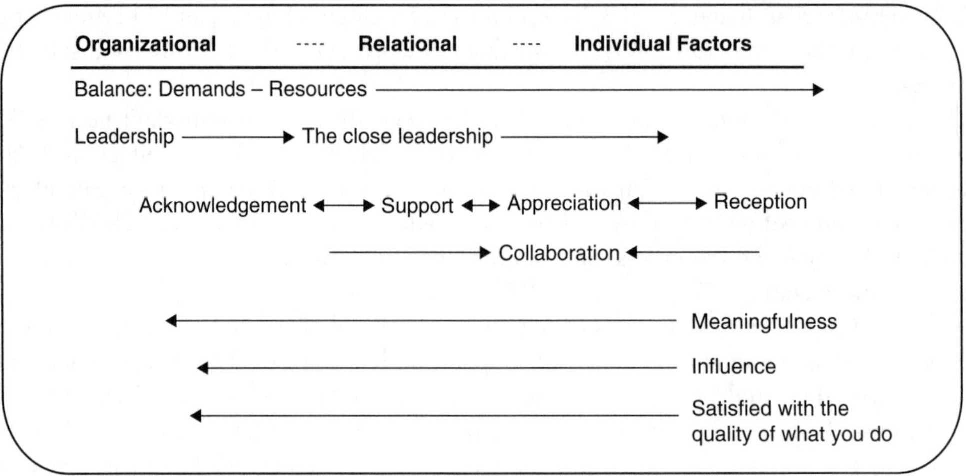


Figure 19-7 Healthy factors in working life.

The basic structure is founded on the three system levels—organizational, group, and individual—and how these influence one another. The arrows indicate that organizational factors also influence the social aspects and the individual coworkers, that the social variables to a large extent involve interaction and interplay, and that the individual factors reflect how we act toward one another and how we perform our tasks.

# Conclusion

Workplace health promotion involves a process that enables organizations, groups, and individuals to increase their control over factors influencing health, thereby improving it. We are of the opinion that the term "workplace" indicates that it is primarily an organizational issue, which is why management and steering systems must be involved. Further, it involves systems thinking and a setting approach in which both the central and local levels of an organization are included, and where enabling is central (for example, through policies and resources) and acting is local, with concrete programs in the actual workplace. When emphasizing the promotive idea even further, participation becomes a central aspect and also a salutogenic starting point for thought and action (Antonovsky, 1979; Antonovsky, 1987).

WHP is far from a unanimously supported concept in Sweden. It concerns issues regarding work activities, working environment, and health that are handled by many actors and professions with somewhat different perspectives on the issue. The following structure is of guidance regarding various focus on these issues. WHP as:

Work activity and organizational issue

- Management and steering, strategic issue, health account

Human resource issue

- Focus on personnel issues, reports of staffing accounts

Work environment issue

- Focus on safety and protection, systematic work-environment work, Occupational Health Service

Fitness work issue

- Focus on an individual and group level, lifestyle and living habits

Every part is important, but in this chapter we have attempted to highlight the links among work, work environment, and health and to demonstrate how to think and work in order to maintain or improve health in an organization, a workplace, or an individual according to the presented model. To be able to pursue long-term work for health in an organization, certain things are essential: an idea and clear goals; professionals who have the authority to move the issue forward; and, finally, resources. Further, to the largest extent possible the design of the program needs to be worked out in collaboration with those concerned. We therefore do not consider standardized programs to be the best solution, as the prerequisites of organizations and workplaces vary greatly along with the culture and the people involved. There are, on the other hand, good reasons for having a clear structure for the work, and also for utilizing existing knowledge about what contributes to increased health at different systems levels (see earlier research).

Traditionally, work focusing on work environment issues has dominated the arena in, for example, Sweden, because of the existing laws and regulations. Fitness work developed strongly during the 1980s and 1990s. There also has been a tendency in recent years toward linking health issues to human resource work to a larger extent. Subsequently, more businesses have raised health issues to an organizational level, for example by inserting them into leadership courses, when they realize the increased financial value that can be gained from systematic health work (Johanson, Ahonen, & Roslender, 2007; Malmqvist, Vinberg, & Larsson, 2007). Health work focusing on the organization can be based on other concepts, but these are nevertheless strongly related to the main ideas of WHP, such as work ability or total quality management (Johanson, Ahonen, & Roslender, 2007).

## Summary

Sweden has about 9,300,000 inhabitants. The Swedish life expectancy is 83 years for women and 79 years for men. Sweden has a well-developed social security system covering all citizens; for many years Sweden has had a large public sector financed by tax systems. This means that the work of a large proportion of the working population is funded by taxes. Sweden has a well-established legislation on working environment and health and safety.

In Sweden, there is no fixed meaning of workplace health promotion (WHP); rather, it is a mixture of approaches and angles. Sweden has a long-standing tradition of work regarding occupational health and safety. Individual-based fitness work has played a prominent part in corporations and organizations since the mid-1980s. In recent years, human resource issues have been linked to health more often, and in certain organizations, issues of work activities and health have also been linked.

Corporations and organizations such as municipalities and county administrations have contributed to the development and furthering of WHP. From experiences and from existing research, we can find some driving forces for WHP, including:

- Interested people/key people: managers and leaders, coworkers, professional support processes.
- Meetings that encourage dialogue and participation, strategic efforts that enable further action—where education is the main strategy.
- Meaningfulness: transforming an idea worth fighting for into goals that are evaluated.
- Health issues' being a part of the ordinary management and steering system.

## Review Questions

1. Long life expectancy in Sweden is credited to what elements of population health?
2. How is the Swedish healthcare system funded and managed?
3. What approaches are emphasized in Swedish workplace health promotion?
4. Describe the structure and plan of the Suntliv workplace health promotion program.
5. Explain the difference between outcomes and indicators within Swedish workplace health promotion programs.
6. Name the recurrent variables in Swedish research that have proven to be effective guides for workplace health promotion efforts.
7. Identify how Sweden links work, work environment, health, and how to think and work to improve individual health status.

# References


Abrahamsson, K., Bradley, G., Brytting, T., Eriksson, T., Forslin, J., Miller, M., … Trollestad, C. (2003). *Friskfaktorer i arbetslivet.* Stockholm, Sweden: Prevent.

AFA Insurance. Stockholm, Sweden. Retrieved from http://www.afaforsakring.se

AFA Insurance. Stockholm, Sweden. Retrieved from http://www.suntliv.nu

Anderson, G., & Malmgren, S. (1976). *På jakt efter hälsoprofilen.* C- och D- Uppsats i sociologi. Universitetet i Linköping.

Andersson, G. (1987). *The importance of exercise for sick level and perceived health.* (Linköping University medical dissertation No. 245).

Andersson, P., & Brunk, T. (2008, September 7). *Trade unions take action to counter membership decline.* Retrieved August 2009, from http://www.eurofound.europa.eu/eiro/2008/06/articles/se0806029i.htm

Antonovsky, A. (1979). *Health, stress, and coping.* London, England: Jossey-Bass Publishers.

Antonovsky, A. (1987). *Unraveling the mystery of health: How people manage stress and stay well.* London, England: Jossey-Bass Publishers.

Arbetsmiljölagen. (1977:1160). Senaste revideringen gjord 2009.

Arbetsmiljöverket. (2003). *Metoder för att uppmärksamma och bedöma psykosocial ohälsa—en inventering inom företagshälsovården.*

Arnesson, H. (2006). *Empowerment and health promotion in working life.* Doktorsvhandling Linköpings universitet (National Center for Work and Rehabilitation, medical disseration).

Björklund, E. (2008). *Constituting the healthy employee? Governing gendered subjects in workplace health promotion Pedagogiska institutionen.* (2010). Umeå Universitet, Nr. 90.

Central Intelligence Agency (CIA). *The world factbook.* Retrieved December 2010, from https://www.cia.gov/library/publications/the-world-factbook

Dellve, L., Skagert, K., & Vilhelmsson, R. (2007). *Leadership in workplace health promotion projects: 1- and 2-year effects on long-term work attendance. European Journal of Public Health, 17*(5), 471–476.

Engqvist, C., & Werkö, L. *Sverige har inte för få läkare.* Region Västra Götaland, Sweden.

Green, L. W., & Kreuter, M. W. (1999). *Health promotion planning: An educational and ecological approach* (3rd ed.). Mountain View, CA: Mayfield Publishing Company.

Gullers, M., (2007). *Is the Swedish management competitive?* (VINNOVA Report VR 2007:13). Stockholm, Sweden.

*Hälsa på arbetsplatsen.* (2002). Policydokument. Vänersborgs kommun.

*International Graduate*. (n.d.) Graduate study in Sweden. Retrieved August 2009 from http://www.internationalgraduate.net/sweden.htm

International Labour Organization. (2009). OSH Act 1977:1160. Last revision.

International Occupational Safety and Health Information Centre. (2003.) *Law modifying the Working Environment Act*. Retrieved from http://www.ilo.org/dyn/cisdoc/cisdoc_legosh.view_record?p_mfn=101556&p_ctry=swe&p_lang=E

Isaksson, P. (2007.) *Leading companies in a global age*. (VINNOVA Report VR 2007:14). Stockholm, Sweden.

Johanson, U., Ahonen, G., & Roslender, R. (2007). *Work health and management control*. Stockholm, Sweden: Thomson Fakta AB.

Kaplan, R. S., & Norton, D. P. (1996, January–February). Using the balanced scorecard as a strategic management system. *Harvard Business Review*, 75–85.

Lindberg, P. (2006). *The work ability continuum: Epidemiological studies of factors promoting sustainable work ability*. Doktorsavhandling KI.

Malmgren, S. (1987). *A health information campaign and health profile assessment as revalatory communication*. (Linköping University Medical Dissertation No. 246).

Malmqvist, C., Vinberg, S., & Larsson, J. (2007). *Att styra med hälsa–från statistik till strategi*. Metodicum.

Nutbeam, D., & Bauman, A. (2006). *Evaluation in a nutshell: A practical guide to the evaluation of health promotion programs*. Sydney, Australia: McGraw-Hill Australia.

Nyberg, A., Bernin, P., & Theorell, T. (2005). *The impact of leadership on the health of subordinates*. SALTSA—Joint Programme for Working Life Research in Europe. The National Institute for Working Life and the swedish trade unions in cooperation.

SKL. (2008). *Swedish health care in an international comparison*. Swedish Association of Local Authorities and Regions.

Swedish Trade Union Confederation. (2007). Reports. Retrieved from http://www.lo.se/home/lo/home.nsf/unidView/3A9B4822B896CF7C1256E4B00435784

Swedish Work Environment Authority and Statistics Sweden (2006). *Annual report*. http://www.av.se/inenglish/

Systematiskt arbetsmiljöarbete. AFS 2001:1 och AFS 2003:4. (Systematic Work Environment Management). Retrieved from http://www.av.se.

Thomsson, H. (2004). *En hälsofrämjande arbetsplats. Försäkringskassan i Östergötland startar en förändringsprocess*. Försäkringskassan.

Thomsson, H. (2005). *Ett utvecklande ledarskap vid en hälsofrämjande arbetsplats—erfarenheter från en pågående process hos Försäkringskassan i Östergötland*. Försäkringskassan.

Thomsson, H. (2007). *Att vara och förbli en hälsofrämjande arbetsplats—erfarenheter från Försäkringskassan i Östergötland*. Försäkringskassan.

Västra Götalands regionen. (2009). Homepage. Retrieved from http://www.vgregion.se/en/Vastra-Gotalandsregionen/Home/

Wadman, C., Boström, G., & Karlsson, A-S. (2008) *Health on equal terms? Results from the 2006 Swedish National Public Health Survey.* FHI 2008:1.

Winroth, J. (2007). *Hälsostrategiskt förändringsarbete i Vänersborgs kommun 2001–2006.* FoU-rapport.

Winroth, J., & Rydqvist, L-G. (2008). *Hälsa & Hälsopromotion. Med fokus på individ- grupp- och organisationsnivå.* SISU Idrottsböcker. Retrieved from http://www.halsopromotiongruppen.se

Chapter 20

# United Kingdom

Peter R. Mills and Katy Cherry

After reading this chapter you should be able to:

- Identify core strategies that are the focus of workplace health promotion efforts in the United Kingdom
- Describe the historical evolution of workplace health promotion in the United Kingdom
- Explain the different approaches employed by corporate health promotion efforts throughout the United Kingdom
- Review the central disease states and health issues driving the United Kingdom's health promotion needs
- Name the components of, and the associated funding sources for, the U.K. healthcare system
- Discuss the impact of U.K. culture on health status and health promotion efforts

Table 20-1 **Select Key Demographic and Economic Indicators**

| | |
|---|---|
| Nationality | Noun: Briton(s), British (collective)<br>Adjective: British |
| Ethnic groups | White (of which English 83.6%, Scottish 8.6%, Welsh 4.9%, Northern Irish 2.9%) 92.1%, black 2%, Indian 1.8%, Pakistani 1.3%, mixed 1.2%, other 1.6% (2001 census) |
| Religion | Christian (Anglican, Roman Catholic, Presbyterian, Methodist) 71.6%, Muslim 2.7%, Hindu 1%, other 1.6%, unspecified or none 23.1% (2001 census) |
| Language | English, Welsh (about 26% of the population of Wales), Scottish form of Gaelic (about 60,000 in Scotland) |
| Literacy | Definition: age 15 and over has completed 5 or more years of schooling<br>Total population: 99%<br>Male: 99%<br>Female: 99% (2003 est.) |

*continued*

| Table 20-1 **Select Key Demographic and Economic Indicators,** *continued* | |
|---|---|
| Education expenditure | 5.6% of GDP (2007)<br>Country comparison to the world: 43 |
| Government type | Constitutional monarchy and commonwealth realm |
| Environment | Continues to reduce greenhouse gas emissions (has met Kyoto Protocol target of a 12.5% reduction from 1990 levels and intends to meet the legally binding target and move toward a domestic goal of a 20% cut in emissions by 2010); by 2005 the government reduced the amount of industrial and commercial waste disposed of in landfill sites to 85% of 1998 levels and recycled or composted at least 25% of household waste, increasing to 33% by 2015 |
| Country mass | Total: 243,610 sq km<br>Country comparison to the world: 79<br>Land: 241,930 sq km<br>Water: 1,680 sq km<br>*Note:* includes Rockall and Shetland Islands |
| Population | 61,113,205 (July 2010 est.)<br>Country comparison to the world: 22 |
| Age structure | 0–14 years: 16.7% (male 5,233,756/female 4,986,131)<br>15–64 years: 67.1% (male 20,774,192/female 20,246,519)<br>65 years and over: 16.2% (male 4,259,654/female 5,612,953) (2010 est.) |
| Median age | Total: 39.8 years<br>Male: 38.6 years<br>Female: 40.9 years (2010 est.) |
| Population growth rate | 0.279% (2010 est.)<br>Country comparison to the world: 176 |
| Birth rate | 10.65 births/1,000 population (2010 est.)<br>Country comparison to the world: 182 |
| Death rate | 10.02 deaths/1,000 population (July 2010 est.)<br>Country comparison to the world: 63 |
| Net migration rate | 2.16 migrant(s)/1,000 population (2010 est.)<br>Country comparison to the world: 40 |
| Urbanization | Urban population: 90% of total population (2008)<br>Rate of urbanization: 0.5% annual rate of change (2005–2010 est.) |
| Gender ratio | At birth: 1.05 male(s)/female<br>Under 15 years: 1.05 male(s)/female<br>15–64 years: 1.03 male(s)/female<br>65 years and over: 0.76 male(s)/female<br>Total population: 0.98 male(s)/female (2010 est.) |

*continued*

| Table 20-1 **Select Key Demographic and Economic Indicators,** *continued* | |
|---|---|
| Infant mortality rate | Total: 4.85 deaths/1,000 live births<br>Country comparison to the world: 194<br>Male: 5.4 deaths/1,000 live births<br>Female: 4.28 deaths/1,000 live births (2010 est.) |
| Life expectancy | Total population: 79.01 years<br>Country comparison to the world: 36<br>Male: 76.52 years<br>Female: 81.63 years (2010 est.) |
| Total fertility rate | 1.66 children born/woman (2010 est.)<br>Country comparison to the world: 177 |
| GDP—purchasing power parity | $2.128 trillion (2009 est.)<br>Parity country comparison to the world: 7 |
| GDP—per capita | $34,800 (2009 est.)<br>Country comparison to the world: 35 |
| GDP—composition by sector | Agriculture: 1.2%<br>Industry: 23.8%<br>Services: 75% (2009 est.) |
| Agriculture—products | Cereals, oilseed, potatoes, vegetables, cattle, sheep, poultry, fish |
| Industries | Machine tools, electric power equipment, automation equipment, railroad equipment, shipbuilding, aircraft, motor vehicles and parts, electronics and communications equipment, metals, chemicals, coal, petroleum, paper and paper products, food processing, textiles, clothing, other consumer goods |
| Labor force participation | 31.37 million (2009 est.)<br>Country comparison to the world: 18 |
| Unemployment rate | 7.6% (2009 est.)<br>Country comparison to the world: 75 |
| Industrial production growth rate | -9.4% (2009 est.)<br>Growth rate country comparison to the world: 143 |
| Distribution of family income (GINI index) | 34 (2005)<br>Income (GINI index) country comparison to the world: 92 |
| Investment (gross fixed) | 15% of GDP (2009 est.)<br>Country comparison to the world: 138 |
| Public debt | 68.1% of GDP (2009 est.)<br>Country comparison to the world: 22 |
| Market value of publicly traded shares | NA (December 31, 2009)<br>Country comparison to the world: 5 |

*continued*

| Table 20-1 Select Key Demographic and Economic Indicators, *continued* | |
|---|---|
| Current account balance | $-32.68 billion (2009 est.)<br>Country comparison to the world: 184 |
| Debt (external) | $9.088 trillion (June 30, 2009 est.)<br>Country comparison to the world: 2 |
| Debt as a % of GDP | ——— |
| Exports | $357.3 billion (2009 est.)<br>Country comparison to the world: 10 |
| Exports—commodities | Manufactured goods, fuels, chemicals, food, beverages, tobacco |
| Export—partners | United States 14.71%, Germany 11.06%, France 8%, Netherlands 7.79%, Ireland 6.89%, Belgium 4.65%, Spain 4% (2009) |
| Imports | $486 billion (2009 est.)<br>Country comparison to the world: 7 |
| Import—commodities | Manufactured goods, machinery, fuels; foodstuffs |
| Import—partners | Germany 12.87%, United States 9.74%, China 8.88%, Netherlands 6.94%, France 6.64%, Belgium 4.86%, Norway 4.84%, Ireland 4.01%, Italy 3.99% (2009) |
| Stock of direct foreign investment at | |
| Home | $1.032 trillion (December 31, 2009 est.)<br>Country comparison to the world: 3 |
| Abroad | $1.586 trillion (December 31, 2009 est.)<br>Country comparison to the world: 3 |

Source: CIA. (2010). *The world factbook*. Retrieved December 16, 2010, from https://www.cia.gov/library/publications/the-world-factbook/

# Introduction

Although often referred to in political and economic discussion as a single entity, the United Kingdom of Great Britain and Northern Ireland is actually the union of four separate countries: Great Britain, which consists of England, Scotland, and Wales; plus Northern Ireland. Although the separate member countries do have some autonomous powers, the majority of judicial and economic regulation occurs from the U.K. parliament located in London, England.

The shape, culture, and economy of U.K. society has changed greatly over the last half century, which in turn has impacted the prevailing health issues and the delivery of health care. In 2008, the combined population of the United Kingdom was 61.4 million, with over a quarter populating the capital, London, and the southeast of England (Office for National Statistics, 2005; Office for National Statistics, 2009d). Approximately 85% of the population of the United Kingdom lives in England, with another 8% living in Scotland, and the remainder spread between Wales and Northern Ireland. Although to some 61.4 million may not sound like a large population, it is when you consider that the area of the United Kingdom is only 245,000 square kilometers, a little over half the size of California.

The population of the United Kingdom continues to gradually increase in size, with this figure projected to rise to over 71.6 million by 2033 (Office for National Statistics, 2009b), the majority of which is attributed directly or indirectly to migration. However, 2008 was the first year to see natural change overtaking net migration as the main contributor to population growth in almost 10 years (Office for National Statistics, 2009b). The last national census estimated the size of the United Kingdom's ethnic population to be 7.9%, or 4.6 million people (Office for National Statistics, 2003). Indians account for the largest ethnic group, followed by Pakistanis, individuals of mixed ethnic backgrounds, and black Caribbeans. Most minority ethnic populations live in urban areas, and 45% live within the London region (Office for National Statistics, 2003).

In line with global trends in the developed world, the United Kingdom's population is aging, due in part to medical and other advances causing people to live longer, but also due to people having fewer children. This shift in the population has seen the number of people of pensionable age exceed the number of children under 16 for the first time, with the fastest increase over the past couple of decades seen in the number of people aged 85 and over (Office for National Statistics, 2009e). Overall, life expectancy is at an all-time high of 77 years for men and 81 years for women, an immense increase from 45 and 49 years, respectively, recorded in 1901 (Office for National Statistics, 2009a). However, this increase has not been matched by healthy life expectancy gains (the number of years of good health over a person's lifetime), estimated at 68.0 years for men and 70.3 years for women in 2004 (Health Improvement Analytical Team, 2007). Indeed, it appears that although life expectancy is gradually increasing, many of these extra years are spent in suboptimal health (Office for National Statistics, 2008).

U.K. gross domestic product (GDP) is approximately U.S. $2.65 trillion, and it is the fifth largest country economy in the world (World Bank, 2009). Three quarters of the U.K. GDP is delivered by the service sector, with less than a quarter from industry and manufacturing. The global economic downturn of the final years of the 1st decade of the 21st century has not been kind to the U.K. economy. The GDP is contracting and is estimated to be 5% lower in 2009 compared to the previous year. In addition, national debt is approaching 60% of economic output, all signs that the United Kingdom will struggle to maintain its position as a G8 nation in the years to come.

The most recent figures put the U.K. unemployment rate at 7.8%, which shows an increase but remains below the European Union average of 9.2% (Human Resource Management, 2009). The employment rate of working age individuals is 72.5%.

## Prevailing Health Issues and Risk Behaviors

Since the 1920s, the most common cause of death in the United Kingdom has been circulatory disease (encompassing heart disease and stroke), which currently accounts for 33.7% of deaths in England (National Health Service [NHS] Choices, 2009b). Rates have been steadily decreasing over the last 50 years and were estimated at 312 per 100,000 males and 194 per 100,000 females in 2002 (Office for National Statistics, 2004). Following circulatory disease is cancer, accounting for 23.4% of all deaths in England, with lung cancer being the most common. This is followed by respiratory diseases, which account for 13.7% of all deaths. Despite declining mortality rates for many of the main killers, a number of largely preventable conditions and health issues continue to increase in prevalence that could have a significant impact upon future rates and healthy life expectancy.

### Obesity

The number of people in England who are above the healthy weight range has seen an unprecedented rise over the past few decades. Over 60% of adults in England and 31% of children are now classified as overweight or obese, with almost a quarter of adults falling into the obese category (Department of Health, 2009). In addition, 41% of women and 33% of men have a waist circumference above the recommended threshold of 88 cm and 102 cm, respectively (Craig & Shelton, 2008). It's predicted that if no action is taken, obesity rates could rise to 60% for men, 50% for women, and 25% for children by 2050 at huge societal cost (Butland et al., 2007).

### Diabetes

As well as contributing to circulatory and cancer deaths directly, obesity greatly increases an individual's risk of developing type 2 diabetes. The prevalence of type 2 diabetes has risen from 2.60 cases per 1,000 patient years in 1996 to 4.31 in 2005, and the percentage of newly diagnosed individuals who are obese has risen from 46% to 56% (Gonzalez, Johansson, Wallander, & Rodriguez, 2009).

### Hypertension and High Cholesterol

Hypertension and high cholesterol also contribute considerably to ill health and mortality in the United Kingdom, giving rise to a number of campaigns to increase awareness of the importance of regular screening for these conditions, which often go undiagnosed for long periods of time. Hypertension is the chief contributor to cardiovascular disease rates in the United Kingdom and is defined as a systolic blood pressure of 140 mmHg or more and/or a diastolic blood pressure of 90 mmHg or more and/or taking antihypertensive drugs. The 2007 Health Survey of England estimated the overall prevalence of hypertension in England at 31% for men and 29% for women (Craig & Shelton, 2008). Treatment rates are improving and an earlier study calculated that achieving adequate blood pressure control for all hypertensive individuals in England could prevent 21,400 deaths from stroke and 41,400 ischemic heart disease deaths annually (He & MacGregor, 2003).

The U.K. government recommends a total cholesterol level of below 5 mmol/L (193 mg/dl) —a level achieved by 43% of men and 39% of women in England as of 2006 (Craig & Mindell, 2008). The overall average of 5.3 mmol/L (205 mg/dl) for men and 5.4 mmol/L (209 mg/dl) for women makes the country's total cholesterol concentration one of the highest in the world.

The main lifestyle factors contributing directly to mortality and healthy life expectancy, or indirectly by their influence on the contributory conditions discussed, are closely interlinked with social and cultural factors in society, and as a result, form the chief focus of preventative health strategies.

## Inactivity

With the decline in industry and an increasing shift towards technology-based work environments and leisure activities, physical inactivity and barriers to more active lifestyles present a major challenge to society. It is now widely recognized that active lifestyles can help to prevent premature death, halve the risk of developing many chronic conditions, and increase quality of life in later life (Craig & Shelton, 2008). The yearly estimated cost of inactivity to the government is £8.2 billion (U.S. $13.3 billion) in England alone, which includes costs related to sickness absence and treating attributable diseases (National Institute for Health and Clinical Excellence, 2009a). Using data from the World Health Report 2002 to assign mortality to specific risk factors, the NHS Atlas of Risk cites physical inactivity as causing 6% of all deaths (NHS Choices, 2009b).

Although there has been an increase in overall levels of recreational activity since 2000, people tend to do less as part of their daily routine (Department of Health, 2004), and there is still much work to be done, with 60% of men and 72% of women failing to meet the recommended levels (NHS Information Centre, 2009a). Common perceived barriers to being more active include work commitments and a lack of time, although over two thirds of individuals would like to do more (Health Improvement Analytical Team, 2007; NHS Information Centre, 2009a). At a higher level, cultural and societal values and the conduciveness of a person's environment to his or her activity behavior all play a part (National Obesity Observatory, 2009). Although initiatives are on the increase, there clearly remains a widespread lack of knowledge of the national physical activity guidelines, with fewer than 1 in 10 persons being able to state the current minimum level in 2007 (Health Improvement Analytical Team, 2007).

## Nutrition

The main dietary issues contributing to the ill health of the nation are low fruit and vegetable intake, and high salt and saturated fat intakes. These issues are apparent in society as a whole but are consistently more prevalent among lower socioeconomic groups, who are also more likely to eat more sugar and processed meats and less whole-grain bread (Nelson, Erens, Bates, Church, & Boshier, 2007). It is estimated that dietary improvements could save the health service £6 billion (U.S. $9.7 billion) a year by reducing costs associated with conditions such as circulatory disease, diabetes, and cancer (Allender, Peto, Scarborough, Boxer, & Rayner, 2006).

Fruit and vegetable intakes are rising slightly but fall well short of the recommended five a day in the United Kingdom, with only 13% of men and 15% of women meeting the target (Hoare et al., 2004). On average, people eat fewer than three portions a day (Hoare et al., 2004). It tends to be those from higher income households who achieve the recommended intake, with people in the top income quintile consuming 15% more fruit and vegetables than those in the lowest (Allender et al., 2006).

Trends are similarly poor for daily salt intake recommendations, with 15% of men and 31% of women meeting the target of less than 6 g (Hoare et al., 2004). In addition, mean intakes increased from 9 g a day in 1986–1987 to 9.5 g per day in 2000–2001. Overall, average total fat intakes are falling gradually and are close to the recommended 35% of food energy intake for the population. However, saturated fat consumption exceeds the recommendation of 11% of food energy by 2%, forming a chief area for focus to reduce elevated cholesterol levels (Nelson et al., 2007).

Over three quarters of the population believe they would benefit from making dietary improvements. However, predominant perceived barriers, which include lack of time, cost, and lack of confidence in changing eating habits, must be addressed if healthy eating strategies are to succeed (Health Improvement Analytical Team, 2007).

## Alcohol

Excessive alcohol consumption has become increasingly ingrained in U.K. society in recent years, and as a result, alcohol-related diseases are rising. Intakes have doubled since the 1970s and associated treatment costs are spiraling, estimated at £7.3 billion (U.S. $11.8 billion) for crime and public disorder, £6.4 billion (U.S. $10.4 billion) for workplace costs, and £1.7 billion (U.S. $ 2.8 billion) for healthcare costs (Academy of Medical Sciences, 2004). In 2007, the General Household Survey reported that 37% of adults drank over the recommended daily limits (2–3 units for women and 3–4 units for men) and were tending to drink more in the home (Office for National Statistics, 2009c). Although awareness is increasing, with around 90% of the population having some knowledge of alcohol units, few know the exact unit recommendations for their gender (Craig & Shelton, 2008).

## Smoking

In 2007, the year a nationwide smoking ban was introduced in all enclosed public spaces, smoking prevalence fell to the lowest recorded level of 21% of the adult population—a substantial decline from 39% recorded in 1980 (NHS Information Centre, 2009b). The falling rate appears to be predominantly due to increasing numbers of people who have never smoked or only smoked occasionally. Despite this reduction in rates, the cost of treating smoking-related conditions accounts for around 5.5% of total healthcare costs in the United Kingdom, and the habit is a major contributor to health inequalities in the United Kingdom (Craig & Shelton, 2008; NHS Information Centre, 2009b).

## Mental Health

In the U.K. workplace, stress consistently features as one of the main causes of absenteeism. The total cost of mental ill health in England is calculated to be as high as £77 billion (U.S. $125 billion), a third of which can be ascribed to economic losses as a result of the impact on a person's work ability (Sainsbury Centre for Mental Health, 2003). At any given time, it is estimated that between 1 in 3 and 1 in 6 persons in the United Kingdom will suffer from some form of mental health problem, the most prevalent being anxiety and depression (Health, Work, and Well-being, 2009; Office for National Statistics, 2006). The average national sickness absence level runs at about 7 days a year per employee, and it is estimated that approximately 40% of these days are due to mental health issues. The Sainsbury Centre for Mental Health estimates that 70 million working days a year are lost to mental illness at a cost of £8.3 billion (U.S. $13.5 billion), with 1 in 7 of these days being directly due to work-related issues (Sainsbury Centre for Mental Health, 2007). In addition, it is thought that the cost of presenteeism (lost productive time at work owing to ill health) could be as high as 1.5 times that of sick leave.

# Healthcare System

After World War II, massive health reform in the United Kingdom ensued, and in 1948 the National Health Service (NHS) was born. Prior to this development, health care in the United Kingdom was largely for the wealthy, and thus, the chief aims of the new service were to provide immediate care to all, free at the point of delivery, by financing services from a central taxation system that was contributed to according to individual means. From this point onward, there have been periodic reforms by successive governments and the NHS has grown to be the largest publicly funded health service in the world, employing over 1.7 million people. In 2008–2009, the NHS budget exceeded £100 billion (U.S. $162 billion), 60% of which was allocated to employee pay (NHS Choices, 2009a).

Using a broadly similar approach, the health services of England, Scotland, Wales, and Northern Ireland are managed separately but from a centrally allocated budget. The health departments for each country devote a portion of the service to strategy, policy, and management, and the rest to primary (frontline) and secondary care service provision. In England, 152 local primary care trusts (PCTs) manage the frontline care for their area, with each PCT usually covering approximately 200,000 residents. PCTs provide general practitioner (family physician) services and some dental, some pharmacy, some optometry, and community care services to the populations they serve. In addition, PCTs commission secondary care from NHS hospitals, and sometimes private providers of secondary care services. Accountable to 10 local strategic health authorities, they command over three quarters of the total NHS budget.

Secondary care services are delivered by a number of hospitals, or groups of hospitals, commonly referred to as NHS trusts (see Figure 20-1). These trusts often have service-level agreements with their local PCTs and are almost exclusively devoted to delivering care to the resident population of one or two PCTs.

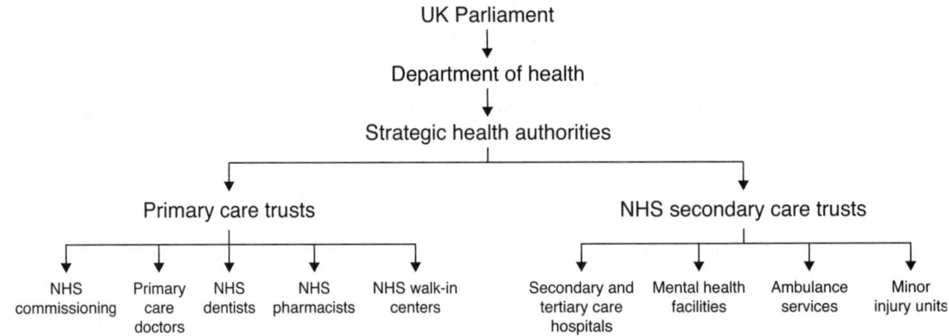


Figure 20-1 Organizational structure of the National Health Service.

Given that every U.K. resident has free access to comprehensive health care from the NHS and has no option to opt out of tax contribution to the service, the factors influencing the decision to purchase private medical insurance (PMI) are an important area for consideration and often relate directly to perceived or actual shortcomings of the NHS. The key driving forces behind purchasing a private medical package of some form include the guarantee of fast access to treatment, a preferable care environment, and greater choice around appointment times, doctors, and provider facilities compared with the NHS (Foubister, Thomson, Mossialos, & McGuire, 2006).

The PMI sector provides many of the same services delivered by the NHS, but these are supplementary rather than comprehensive. Most PMI policies cover the costs for treating acute illnesses as well as elective surgical procedures and associated services, such as accommodation or outpatient visits where necessary. PMI does not usually cover primary care physician visits or ongoing treatment of existing or chronic conditions (Foubister et al., 2006; King & Mossialos, 2005). Since the 1970s, the number of people with PMI has more than tripled from 2.1 million in 1971 to almost 6.9 million in 2000 (Office for National Statistics, 2002). Since 1997, the proportion of the U.K. population covered by PMI has barely changed and consistently remains around the 12% mark; however, during this time the number of people paying individually for PMI has declined, with a concurrent rise in the proportion of employer-paid policies. The PMI market in the United Kingdom is worth approximately £3 billion (U.S. $4.9 billion), a figure dwarfed by the £100 billion (U.S. $162 billion) total annual governmental expenditure on the NHS (Datamonitor, 2008).

Over the last 10 years, PMI has become the *de facto* employee benefit offered to those in senior positions within private corporations. Indeed, in a number of industries, PMI is considered the entry-level benefit required to attract appropriate staff. An analysis of the British Household Panel Survey 1997–2000 identified the main factors contributing to both individual and employer-paid PMI polices in the working population are income, age, gender, and political preference (King & Mossialos, 2005).

With an increasing understanding of how a healthy workforce can not only impact healthcare costs and utilization, but also improve the productivity and performance of employees, both the private and public providers of health care in the United Kingdom have invested more time and resources over the last few years to develop effective workplace health promotion strategies. The chief drivers for U.K. employers (be they private or public sector) are broadly twofold: (1) reducing costs incurred from absenteeism, voluntary staff turnover, and presenteeism; and (2) reducing costs related to treating health conditions and diseases relating to poor lifestyle choices.

## Influence of Culture and Mentality

As general acceptance of disease prevention and health promotion increases within society, there is a necessity for better understanding of the factors that influence lifestyle choices and health behaviors of the U.K. population. Recognizing the complex interaction of sociocultural, environmental, and psychological factors and developing strategies that are sensitive to these issues will be instrumental in their ultimate success. In addition, an understanding of how certain behaviors tend to coexist, and for what reasons, is also an important consideration for a cost-effective, multipurpose strategy.

It is worth noting that the concept of free health care at the point of access has become engrained within the belief systems of the majority of the U.K. population. Generally speaking, people are disinclined to pay directly for healthcare services. It is likely that any sustainable measures that are implemented to promote health and decrease the burden of disease within society will have to be at least partially sponsored by the central government.

At the forefront of the U.K. government's public health strategy is overcoming inequalities and creating environments that are conducive to healthy behaviors. Improvements in life expectancy within the U.K. population as a whole mask some stark variations. In certain areas, and among certain groups (often ethnic minorities), life expectancy can be up to 10 years less.

The workplace is gaining greater acceptance as a venue for health promotion and is ideally suited to reduce some of these observed inequalities. First and foremost, it enables large numbers of individuals to be reached with targeted programs in an environment that has been shown to have a direct influence on health and well-being. In addition, elements of the workforce ethic, such as ambition, organization, and competition, can often help to promote behavioral change.

Although research has repeatedly shown us that work is an important driver for good health and mental well-being, work in the 21st century in the United Kingdom (like many other countries) is characterized by ever-fast-paced lifestyles despite increasing automation in all aspects of our lives. Many workers experience long working hours, despite the European Working Time Directive; long commutes to urban centers of commerce; and a high cost of living. Couple these factors with increasing consumerism and an increasingly secular and fragmented society, and it is not altogether surprising to see why lifestyle choices become compromised.

When it comes to dietary choices, individuals will all too frequently opt for processed, fast, or takeout options for ease, rather than preparing food at home. In other cases, particularly in poorer, urban areas, a lack of affordable healthy options and an abundance of fast food outlets often leave little choice. In a similar fashion, a lack of affordable, accessible, and safe facilities, as well as limited leisure time, can impede more active lifestyles in some population groups.

Recent years have seen a concerted effort by government and policy makers to reverse the trends of the last few decades. New residential schemes are being created with a better understanding of how the built environment can impact health, and existing urban areas are being renovated and enhanced. The huge 2012 London Olympics project has at its heart the intent of regeneration and sustainability for the people of the United Kingdom. The mayor of London has actively encouraged cycling in the capital with greater investment being made in cycle routes and dedicated traffic-free areas. In parallel with these environmental changes, there has been a notable shift in attitude from many large retailers. The last few years have seen an increase in healthy options being offered in supermarkets, together with a voluntary code of greater transparency in food labeling. The challenge the United Kingdom has is making sure that these initiatives are accessible to all of society and not just those who can afford them.

In light of such cultural and socioeconomic influences on health behavior, developing health promotion programs in partnership with the target population is a key element to their success. Whether this be employers working in partnership with their employees or local health service providers within their communities, the tailoring of interventions at the population and individual level is imperative for sustainability.

## Drivers of Workplace Health Promotion

Like many countries, the provision of workplace health promotion initiatives in the United Kingdom have been, until relatively recently, patchy and fragmented. The main reason for this is the perceived lack of clear need by employers to improve healthcare costs, due to the universal, tax-funded healthcare system. However, the last decade has seen a steady increase in awareness and understanding among employers, the NHS, and private medical insurers of the business and societal benefits that can be achieved through preventing disease and enhancing health status. U.K.-centered research has highlighted the clear relationship between health and worker productivity and how improving individuals' health status can positively impact their productivity and performance and potentially provide an employer with a competitive advantage (Mills, Kessler, Cooper, & Sullivan, 2007).

Industry in the United Kingdom, in concert with many other developed nations, is increasingly focused upon service provision. The more traditional manufacturing sector, which now only contributes less than one quarter of U.K. GDP, is either being off-shored, heavily automated, or ceasing to exist entirely. This gradual but continued shift in industrial focus has meant that employers are in competition with each other for the brightest, most innovative, and productive individuals, which in turn has awoken them to the need to maintain their workforce as their most important asset.

Another driver of the increasing adoption of the workplace health promotion in the United Kingdom is the influence of large global employers. Many of these organizations are either headquartered, or at least have a large presence in, the United States and they have been increasingly aware of the need to provide health management and promotion services to all of their employee base, not just those working in America. Organizations like GlaxoSmithKline, Unilever, and BP have led the way in rolling out global health strategies that provide all of their employees with access to geographically and culturally relevant initiatives.

The emergence of vendors that solely supply workplace health solutions has occurred in tandem with the greater acceptance of workplace health promotion as a sound business strategy over the last decade. Organizations such as VieLife, Road to Health, and Working Health have established themselves during this time to provide specifically the health promotion services that corporations wish to deliver to their staff. Despite this, these boutique workplace health promotion organizations still have a relatively small slice of the market share, with the more traditional healthcare service providers and insurers, such as Bupa, Nuffield, and Axa, as well as occupational health providers, making up the bulk of the service provision through the specific workplace health promotion services they have added to their product lines.

More recently, the U.K. government has also joined the fray by investing significantly in the NHS Choices website as well as offering the private sector occupational health and health promotion services via its NHS Plus arm. Active governmental involvement in the workplace health promotion arena is promising, and although some vendors naturally feel skeptical of the government's motives, the added emphasis that this brings to the marketplace should theoretically drive greater acceptance by the corporate world. Testament to the U.K. government's increasing understanding of the need to promote health within the working population is the creation of the Health, Work, and Well-being initiative in 2005. Health, Work, and Well-being brought together stakeholders from the Department of Health, the Department for Work and Pensions, and the Health and Safety Executive to provide clear guidance and recommendations on how both public and private sector organizations should approach promoting the health of their employees. Headed by Dame Carol Black, the initial report was the first time that a U.K. governmental body had specifically advocated proactive health promotion initiatives centered around the workplace (Black, 2008). Adding weight to this effort is the recently published independent review of the health and well-being of NHS employees, which has categorically recommended that all NHS organizations provide their staff with health and well-being services centered on prevention, and that these should be incorporated within national and local governance frameworks (Boorman, 2009). Time will only tell whether the NHS follows its own advice, but the hope is that these studies will be the impetus needed to increase the currently very small proportion of the total U.K. healthcare expenditure devoted to prevention.

The last few years have seen a veritable explosion in interest in health and well-being in the media. Both television and the daily newspapers regularly have health programs or sections covering popular health topics such as physical activity, nutrition, and weight management. Although these are usually pitched as quick fixes or easy options and not normally focused upon the workplace, they have undoubtedly increased public awareness of health initiatives and the available options.

Finally, the role of charitable and third-sector organizations in raising awareness and promoting health in the workplace should not be overlooked. Charities such as the British Heart Foundation and Mind have specifically delivered promotional programs that target working age individuals. In addition, Business in the Community, through its Business Action of Health campaign, and the Oxford Health Alliance both spend considerable amounts of their time and resources promoting workplace health and acting as facilitators to encourage member organizations to become more involved in the proactive management of employee health.

## Programs and Good Practices

The U.K. workplace health promotion landscape is still quite fragmented, with many local or regional vendors focusing upon specific topics or specific industries. The reason for this is that the majority of the U.K. labor force work within SMEs (small or medium sized enterprises), with some estimates stating as much as 95% of the working population are employed by organizations that have 100 or fewer individuals. Thus, there is always going to be a need, and also a desire, to contract with local providers. Despite this caveat, there are three main areas that organizations, both large and small, consistently purchase: health assessments and wellness screenings, online/technology-based wellness programs, and on-site workplace programs.

### Health Assessments and Wellness Screening

Health assessments and wellness screenings typically are conducted at a vendor's clinic or facility and entail a thorough physical assessment conducted by a doctor in conjunction with other support staff. They can last from 1 hour to a whole day, depending upon the detail and supplemental investigations. Because such an approach is very labor intensive, and hence relatively costly, organizations typically purchase such assessments for their executives and key personnel only.

## Online/Technology-Based Wellness Programs

Online/technology-based wellness programs have gained in popularity and are seen by organizations as a low-cost way of providing a solution to all of their employees. This cost effectiveness, coupled with the increasingly service-based nature of the majority of occupations in the United Kingdom, makes technology-driven programs appealing.

## On-Site Workplace Programs

This type of program has been the mainstay of workplace health promotion for many years. Despite the relatively high cost per participant compared to that of technology-driven programs, on-site programs are often seen as providing a more tangible intervention within the workplace. Seminars, workshops, lunchtime fitness sessions, and support groups (such as Weight Watchers) are all popular, and delivery is ideally suited to local workplace health promotion practitioners. Some larger organizations, especially those that have significant numbers of high value people on one site, have gone one step further and provide permanent facilities for their staff. These range from the provision of an onsite gymnasium to, in the case of some of the large investment banks like Goldman Sachs and Citibank, a full suite of permanent services including dentist, osteopath, physical therapist, and doctor.

It is noteworthy that, unlike in the United States, telephone-based health promotion programs are not very prevalent in the United Kingdom. However, this approach does seem to be gaining some traction within the marketplace with organizations such as CIGNA, Health Dialog, and Healthways modifying their U.S. products to enter the U.K. health promotion and disease management market.

# Outcomes and Indicators

As the majority of U.K.-based organizations have very little visibility on the direct healthcare costs of their employees, the outcomes of interest are predominantly focused upon reducing absenteeism, improving productivity, and enhancing employee engagement. A spectrum of different employer attitudes exists, ranging from employers who want a tangible return on investment from any programs that are implemented, to those who just want to do the right thing and help their employees live a healthier life. There is, however, a growing awareness that workplace health promotion programs can deliver tangible value, and increasingly employers are demanding from vendors management information that demonstrates not only how their programs have reduced health issues within the employee base, but also how that has had an impact upon costs. It is clear that the market is growing more mature and sophisticated, with a number of purchasers of workplace health promotion solutions striking deals that put some of the vendors' fees at risk dependent upon key outcomes being achieved.

Over the last couple of years, the National Institute for Health and Clinical Excellence, a government-funded but independent assessment authority, has published two reports on specific workplace health interventions. The reports on increasing physical activity and smoking cessation outline the existing scientific evidence for different approaches and make recommendations on how such programs should be implemented in the workplace (National Institute for Health and Clinical Excellence, 2007; National Institute for Health and Clinical Excellence, 2009a, 2009b). This guidance, together with the more general evidence synthesis provided by Health, Work, and Well-being, provides a broad framework for how workplace health interventions should be approached, although it stops short of providing a blueprint for evaluation or outcome assessment. Increasingly employers are becoming aware of how employee engagement can drive business performance and success. It is clear that the health of employees is a critical element in whether they are engaged in their work, and companies such as Right Management and Towers Perrin provide employee engagement consulting services that include annual measures of engagement as well as health status.

Unlike the United States, where the National Committee for Quality Assurance (NCQA) and Utilization Review Accreditation Commission (URAC) provide accreditation and certification schemes for health promotion services, no nationally recognized quality assurance mark exists within the United Kingdom. Both the U.K. Department of Health and some health-related charities have indicated that they would be interested in being involved in the creation of an accreditation body; however, to date there is no real progress on this.

## Existing Research

Much of the evidence for efficacy of different approaches to program delivery still comes from the United States. In some respects this is not altogether surprising, as the direct costs associated with ill health and lifestyle issues are more tangible to U.S. employers because of the healthcare funding system there. Yet, there appears to be general acceptance in the United Kingdom that what works in the United States is also likely to work here in terms of improving health outcomes.

Business in the Community, through its Business Action on Health campaign, has amassed a sizeable repository of U.K.-focused case studies highlighting the impact health promotion programs have had in a wide variety of U.K. organizations (Business in the Community, 2009). Although these studies could not be considered robust scientific evidence of efficacy, in total they provide a compelling argument for investing in workplace health promotion programs and are generally sufficient evidence on which most employers can make informed decisions.

British United Provident Association, the largest private healthcare insurer in the United Kingdom, has recently published a review of the effectiveness of workplace health interventions as part of its broader analysis of health and work and the challenges U.K. industry faces in the decades ahead (Vaughan-Jones & Barham, 2009; Vaughan-Jones & Barham, 2010). The report provides a valuable resource for those interested in delving into the evidence for relative and absolute benefits of a number of common workplace health interventions, including alcohol and drug consumption, stress management, seasonal influenza, back pain, and weight management. Importantly, where evidence is available, the analysis separates out the potential benefits to the employee as well as the employer.

The Work Foundation, a not-for-profit research institute, has also provided valuable insight into the area of workplace health promotion through its work on employment and its impact on society as a whole. Its primary focus has been on determining what aspects of work life—including job design, level of autonomy, and managerial style—constitute good work, as it is clear from the seminal Whitehall studies that good work is an essential component of good health for employees (Constable, Coats, Bevan, & Mahdon, 2009; Ferrie, 2004).

One of the only prospective, controlled studies to look specifically at the impact of a multicomponent workplace health promotion initiative on productivity was conducted by one of the authors (P.M.). The study took place at a number of U.K. worksites of Unilever Plc. The study design ensured that a control population was followed for the 12 months of the study, so as to put any changes observed within the intervention group into context. The results showed that, compared to those in the control arm, the intervention group decreased their absence rates by an average of a third of a day a month, decreased their average number of health risk factors by half, and increased their work productivity by 10%. Return on investment analysis showed a substantial 6.2 to 1 (Mills et al., 2007).

Although there is a significant body of research evidence available to support the value and outcomes from workplace health initiatives, there is clearly still a need for further work on approaches to engage individuals from different demographic groups, as well as the relative impact and cost effectiveness of specific interventions and channels of delivery, on a variety of outcome measures.

## Conclusion

Although the health and lifestyle issues experienced by the working population in the United Kingdom are similar to those from other developed nations, the unique healthcare funding and delivery system in the region frames the value of workplace health promotion differently for employers. Without the direct burden of healthcare delivery costs to contend with, employers traditionally have been less inclined to invest in specific employee health interventions; possible reasons include: (1) a lack of perceived value to the bottom line of the business, (2) a general belief that the health and lifestyle choices of employees is the responsibility of the individual and/or government and not the employer, and (3) employee mobility and the length of time an individual stays with one employer makes investing in health interventions nonviable.

This landscape changed in the early 21st century, and it is undeniable that the prevalence of workplace-based wellness programs and interventions has increased substantially over this time. This shift has been driven by many factors, including the gradual change in industrial focus in the United Kingdom towards a predominantly service- and knowledge-based economy, an aging workforce with a relative skills shortage, and more recently, a need by organizations to garner competitive advantage in an increasingly global trading economy. In addition, the greater understanding and acceptance of the fact that optimizing the health status of employees can generate significant enhancements in productivity and performance in addition to reducing healthcare costs has helped the workplace health promotion industry grow.

However, the United Kingdom still lags behind the United States in terms of the depth and breadth of provision of solutions within the working population. Many organizations in the United Kingdom still consider private medical insurance and gym membership to be the extent of employee health initiatives, and further work is needed in order to convince these employers of the short- and long-term benefits of including employee health management in their overall business strategy (Buck Consultants, 2009).

A large majority of U.K. employees work for SMEs, and the workplace health promotion movement faces the challenge of developing and delivering scalable, low-cost, effective solutions to this geographically dispersed workforce. The increasing penetration of the web has certainly helped in this area; however, many organizations still struggle with low engagement in these kinds of programs. Undoubtedly one size does not fit all, and over the coming decade vendors of workplace health promotion initiatives must find ways to integrate the current approaches (web, telephone, on site, paper-based literature, etc.) while harnessing new technologies to create product lines that deliver outcomes that are greater than the sum of their constituent parts.

The healthcare industry has often been accused of being slow to adopt new technologies; however, there is a burgeoning group of health services innovators using social media, web 2.0 applications, and wearable devices that are likely to become more mainstream in the years ahead. Backed up by credible scientific evidence of efficacy, it is likely that these approaches will start to be seen as therapies in their own right. It doesn't take a huge leap of faith to envision physicians prescribing accelerometer-type devices to their patients to aid with weight loss and fitness as a step prior to more invasive pharmacological or operative interventions. Companies like Philips, MiLife (Imperative Health), and Global Fit are already exploring these avenues. In addition, the creation of communities of individuals with common health-related goals will also drive participation. The use of virtual worlds to create visually immersive learning and participatory environments that transcend geographical boundaries could also become more commonplace in the years to come.

By the time this book is published, it is likely that the United Kingdom's national debt will be approaching £1 trillion, equating to over 60% of GDP (Office for National Statistics, 2009f). It is inevitable that with this level of debt, expenditure on public services, including the NHS, will be reduced or at best not increase. As a consequence, employee benefits such as private medical insurance will take on new value. In addition, innovative ways of encouraging and incentivizing the general population to adopt healthy lifestyles and manage existing chronic diseases optimally will take on a greater imperative. New approaches to healthcare financing that share ownership and responsibility between insurer (be that a private insurer or the NHS) and the individual and tie behaviors to costs and levels of coverage are likely to become more prevalent. Organizations like RedBrick Health in the United States are experimenting with such approaches. If they prove to be efficacious in moderating cost inflation, then there is no reason why we should not see them in the United Kingdom during the second decade of the 21st century.

Workplace health promotion is a growing discipline. We have a greater understanding of how the health of employees can impact business performance as well as overall healthcare delivery costs. The innovative deployment of new technological approaches, together with further research into what works, and for whom, make the area a very exciting one in which to be involved. It is clear that if the United Kingdom is to escape its current economic woes and maintain its position as one of the top 10 economic forces in the world, more emphasis will have to be placed upon optimizing and enhancing the health of the workforce.

## Summary

The U.K. population as a whole is aging, yet in parallel with life expectancy gains, the prevalence of largely lifestyle-related conditions such as obesity and type 2 diabetes continue to rise to unprecedented levels. Every citizen of the United Kingdom is entitled to free, comprehensive health care through a tax-funded health service—the largest of its kind with over 1.7 million employees—which has to some extent slowed the impetus for employers to introduce health management initiatives. However, from 2000 to 2010 there was growing appreciation among public and private sector organizations, including private medical insurers (PMIs), of the link between a healthy workforce and reduced costs, whether it be in terms of reduced healthcare expenditure or costs associated with absenteeism, presenteeism, and turnover. Consequently, increased time and resources are being devoted to developing effective workplace preventive health strategies, chiefly by government bodies, PMIs, specialist vendors and some third-sector organizations, accompanied by an explosion in health related press coverage. The most commonly purchased workplace initiatives include clinic-based health assessments, online management tools, and on-site programs. Positive outcome studies and case reports are beginning to amass in the literature, which, alongside the large body of U.S. research evidence, continue to solidify the business case for U.K. employers to invest. Yet, unlike the United States, given the limited visibility U.K. organizations have on the direct healthcare costs of their employees, outcome measures predominantly relate to health risk factors and workforce performance indicators, giving rise to a growing requirement for a demonstrable impact of these outcomes upon organizational costs.

## Review Questions

1. What are the prevailing health issues in the United Kingdom?
2. How are the individual healthcare systems among the countries of the United Kingdom financed and managed?
3. How does the health coverage/payment culture of the United Kingdom affect public health strategy?
4. List and explain the drivers of the United Kingdom's workplace health promotion programs.
5. Describe two examples of effective workplace health promotion practices in the United Kingdom.
6. Who has produced the majority of scientific evidence regarding the effectiveness of workplace health promotion in the United Kingdom?
7. Name three other studies and/or organizations that have made significant contributions to workplace health promotion outcomes and indicators.

## References


Academy of Medical Sciences. (2004). *Calling time. The nation's drinking as a major health issue.*

Allender, S., Peto, V., Scarborough, P., Boxer, A., & Rayner, M. (2006). *Diet, physical activity, and obesity statistics.* London, England: British Heart Foundation.

Black, C. (2008). *Working for a healthier tomorrow.* London, England: The Stationary Office.

Boorman, S. (2009). *NHS health and wellbeing.* London, England: Department of Health.

Buck Consultants. (2009). *Working well: A global survey of health promotion and workplace wellness strategies.* London, England: Buck Surveys.

Business in the Community (2009). *BITC case studies.* Retrieved from http://bit.ly/BITC_Case_Studies

Butland, B., Jebb, S., Kopelman, P., McPherson, K., Thomas, S., Mardell, J., & Parry, V. (2007). *Tackling obesities: Future choices—Project report.* Retrieved from http://www.foresight.gov.uk/Obesity/17.pdf

Constable, C., Coats, D., Bevan, S., & Mahdon, M. (2009). *Good jobs.* London, England: The Work Foundation.

Craig, R., & Mindell, J. (2008). *Health survey for England 2006. Cardiovascular disease and risk factors.* Newport, South Wales: Office for National Statistics.

Craig, R., & Shelton, N. (2008). *Health survey for England 2007. Healthy lifestyles: knowledge, attitudes, and behaviour.* Newport, South Wales: Office for National Statistics.

Department of Health. (2004). *At least five a week: Evidence on the impact of physical activity and its relationship to health.* London, England: Author.

Department of Health (2009, November 30). *Obesity general information.* London, England: Author

Datamonitor. (2008). *U.K. private medical insurance 2007.* London, England: Author

Ferrie, J. E. (2004). *Work stress and health: The Whitehall II study.* London, England: Public and Commercial Services Union.

Foubister, T., Thomson, S., Mossialos, E., & McGuire, A. (2006). *Private medical insurance in the United Kingdom.* Brussels, Belgium: European Observatory on Health Systems and Policies.

Gonzalez, E. L., Johansson, S., Wallander, M. A., & Rodriguez, L. A. (2009). Trends in the prevalence and incidence of diabetes in the U.K.: 1996–2005. *Journal of Epidemiology and Community Health, 63,* 332–336.

He, F. J., & MacGregor, G. A. (2003). Cost of poor blood pressure control in the U.K.: 62,000 unnecessary deaths per year. *Journal of Human Hypertension, 17,* 455–457.

Health Improvement Analytical Team. (2007). *Health profile for England 2007.* London, England: Author Department of Health.

Health, Work, and Well-being. (2009). *Working our way to better mental health. A framework for action.* London, England: The Stationary Office.

Hoare, J., Henderson, L., Bates, C. J., Prentice, A., Birch, M., Swan, G., … (2004). *The National Diet and Nutrition Survey: Adults aged 19 to 64 years.* Newport, South Wales: Office for National Statistics.

Human Resource Management (2009, November 11). *U.K. unemployment.* Retrieved from http://www.hrmguide.co.uk/jobmarket/unemployment.htm

King, D., & Mossialos, E. (2005). The determinants of private medical insurance prevalence in England, 1997–2000. *Health Services Research, 40,* 195–212.

Mills, P. R., Kessler, R. C., Cooper, J., & Sullivan, S. (2007). Impact of a health promotion program on employee health risks and work productivity. *American Journal of Health Promotion, 22,* 45–53.

National Institute for Health and Clinical Excellence. (2007). *Workplace health promotion: How to help employees to stop smoking.* London, England: Author.

National Institute for Health and Clinical Excellence. (2009a). *Physical activity and the environment.* London, England: Author.

National Institute for Health and Clinical Excellence. (2009b). *Workplace health promotion: How to encourage employees to be physically active.* London, England: Author.

National Obesity Observatory. (2009). *Causes of obesity.* Retrieved from http://www.noo.org.uk/NOO_about_obesity/causes

Nelson, M., Erens, B., Bates, B., Church, S., & Boshier, T. (2007). *Low Income Diet and Nutrition Survey.* London, England: The Stationary Office.

NHS Choices. (2009a, April 12). *About the NHS.* Retrieved from http://www.nhs.uk/NHSEngland/aboutnhs/Pages/About.aspx

NHS Choices. (2009b). *NHS atlas of risk.* Retrieved from http://www.nhs.uk/Tools/Pages/NHSAtlasofrisk.aspx

NHS Information Centre. (2009a). *Statistics on obesity, physical activity. and diet: England, February 2009.* London, England: National Health Service.

NHS Information Centre. (2009b). *Statistics on smoking: England, 2009.* London, England: National Health Service.

Office for National Statistics. (2002, January 31). *People insured by private medical insurance.* Retrieved from http://www.statistics.gov.uk/STATBASE/ssdataset.asp?vlnk=5053&More=Y

Office for National Statistics. (2003, February 13). *Ethnicity: Regional distribution.* Retrieved from http://www.statistics.gov.uk/cci/nugget.asp?id=263

Office for National Statistics. (2003b, February 13). *Population size.* Retrieved from http://www.statistics.gov.uk/CCI/nugget.asp?ID=273

Office for National Statistics. (2004, July 29). *Health: Mortality.* Retrieved from http://www.statistics.gov.uk/cci/nugget.asp?id=919

Office for National Statistics. (2005, October 15). *Where people live.* Retrieved from http://www.statistics.gov.uk/CCI/nugget.asp?ID=1306&Pos=2&ColRank=2&Rank=672

Office for National Statistics. (2006, January 17). *Health: Mental health.* Retrieved from http://www.statistics.gov.uk/CCI/nugget.asp?ID=1333&Pos=2&ColRank=1&Rank=374

Office for National Statistics. (2008, January 10). *Health and care: Health expectancy.* Retrieved from http://www.statistics.gov.uk/cci/nugget.asp?id=934

Office for National Statistics. (2009a, October 21). *Health: Life expectancy.* Retrieved from http://www.statistics.gov.uk/CCI/nugget.asp?ID=168&Pos=1&ColRank=1&Rank=374

Office for National Statistics. (2009b, October 21). *National population projections, 2008-based.* Retrieved from http://www.statistics.gov.uk/pdfdir/pproj1009.pdf

Office for National Statistics. (2009c, January 22). *Over a third of adults exceed regular daily drinking limit.* Retrieved from http://www.statistics.gov.uk/pdfdir/ghs0109.pdf

Office for National Statistics. (2009d, August 27). *Population estimates.* Retrieved from http://www.statistics.gov.uk/pdfdir/pop0809.pdf

Office for National Statistics. (2009e, September 23). *Population: Ageing.* Retrieved from http://www.statistics.gov.uk/CCI/nugget.asp?ID=2157&Pos=2&ColRank=2&Rank=224

Office for National Statistics. (2009f). *Public sector—Budgetary deficit.* Retrieved December 13, 2009, from http://www.statistics.gov.uk/cci/nugget.asp?id=206

Sainsbury Centre for Mental Health. (2003). *The economic and social costs of mental illness.*

Sainsbury Centre for Mental Health. (2007). *Mental health at work: Developing the business case.*

Vaughan-Jones, H., & Barham, L. (2009). *Healthy work: Challenges and opportunities to 2030.* BUPA.

Vaughan-Jones, H., & Barham, L. (2010). *Healthy work: Evidence into action.* BUPA.

World Bank. (2009). *U.K. GDP.* Retrieved from http://datafinder.worldbank.org/gdp-current?cid=GPD_29

Chapter 21

# United States of America

Robert C. Karch

After reading this chapter you should be able to:

- Identify core strategies of workplace health promotion efforts in the United States
- Describe the historical evolution of workplace health promotion efforts in the United States
- Explain the different approaches employed by corporate health promotion programs throughout the United States
- Review the central disease states and health issues driving workplace health promotion in the United States
- Name the components of, and the associated funding sources for, the U.S. healthcare system
- Discuss the impact of culture on the health status and health promotion efforts within the United States

**Table 21-1 Select Key Demographic and Economic Indicators**

| | |
|---|---|
| Nationality | Noun: American(s)<br>Adjective: American |
| Ethnic groups | White 79.96%, black 12.85%, Asian 4.43%, Amerindian and Alaska native 0.97%, native Hawaiian and other Pacific Islander 0.18%, two or more races 1.61% (July 2007 est.) |
| Religion | Protestant 51.3%, Roman Catholic 23.9%, Mormon 1.7%, other Christian 1.6%, Jewish 1.7%, Buddhist 0.7%, Muslim 0.6%, other or unspecified 2.5%, unaffiliated 12.1%, none 4% (2007 est.) |
| Language | English 82.1%, Spanish 10.7%, other Indo-European 3.8%, Asian and Pacific Island 2.7%, other 0.7% (2000 census)<br>*Note:* Hawaiian is an official language in the state of Hawaii |
| Literacy | Definition: age 15 and over can read and write<br>Total population: 99%<br>Male: 99%<br>Female: 99% (2003 est.) |

*continued*

| Table 21-1 **Select Key Demographic and Economic Indicators,** *continued* | |
|---|---|
| Education expenditure | 5.5% of GDP (2007)<br>Country comparison to the world: 46 |
| Government type | Constitution-based federal republic; strong democratic tradition |
| Environment | Air pollution resulting in acid rain in both the United States and Canada; the United States is the largest single emitter of carbon dioxide from the burning of fossil fuels; water pollution from runoff of pesticides and fertilizers; limited natural fresh water resources in much of the western part of the country require careful management; desertification |
| Country mass | Total: 9,826,675 sq km<br>Country comparison to the world: 3<br>Land: 9,161,966 sq km<br>Water: 664,709 sq km<br>*Note:* includes only the 50 states and District of Columbia |
| Population | 307,212,123 (July 2010 est.)<br>Country comparison to the world: 3 |
| Age structure | 0–14 years: 20.2% (male 31,639,127/female 30,305,704)<br>15–64 years: 67% (male 102,665,043/female 103,129,321)<br>65 years and over: 12.8% (male 16,901,232/female 22,571,696)<br>(2010 est.) |
| Median age | Total: 36.8 years<br>Male: 35.5 years<br>Female: 38.1 years (2010 est.) |
| Population growth rate | 0.977% (2010 est.)<br>Country comparison to the world: 130 |
| Birth rate | 13.83 births/1,000 population (2010 est.)<br>Country comparison to the world: 154 |
| Death rate | 8.38 deaths/1,000 population (July 2010 est.)<br>Country comparison to the world: 99 |
| Net migration rate | 4.32 migrant(s)/1,000 population (2010 est.)<br>Country comparison to the world: 26 |
| Urbanization | Urban population: 82% of total population (2008)<br>Rate of urbanization: 1.3% annual rate of change (2005–2010 est.) |
| Gender ratio | At birth: 1.048 male(s)/female<br>Under 15 years: 1.04 male(s)/female<br>15–64 years: 1 male(s)/female<br>65 years and over: 0.75 male(s)/female<br>Total population: 0.97 male(s)/female (2010 est.) |

*continued*

**Table 21-1 Select Key Demographic and Economic Indicators,** *continued*

| | |
|---|---|
| Infant mortality rate | Total: 6.22 deaths/1,000 live births<br>Country comparison to the world: 180<br>Male: 6.9 deaths/1,000 live births<br>Female: 5.51 deaths/1,000 live births (2010 est.) |
| Life expectancy | Total population: 78.11 years<br>Country comparison to the world: 49<br>Male: 75.65 years<br>Female: 80.69 years (2010 est.) |
| Total fertility rate | 2.06 children born/woman (2010 est.)<br>Country comparison to the world: 127 |
| GDP—purchasing power parity | $14.14 trillion (2009 est.)<br>Country comparison to the world: 2 |
| GDP—per capita | $46,000 (2009 est.)<br>Country comparison to the world: 11 |
| GDP—composition by sector | Agriculture: 1.2%<br>Industry: 21.9%<br>Services: 76.9% (2009 est.) |
| Agriculture—products | Wheat, corn, other grains, fruits, vegetables, cotton, beef, pork, poultry, dairy products, fish, forest products |
| Industries | Leading industrial power in the world, highly diversified and technologically advanced; petroleum, steel, motor vehicles, aerospace, telecommunications, chemicals, electronics, food processing, consumer goods, lumber, mining |
| Labor force participation | 154.2 million (includes unemployed) (2009 est.)<br>Country comparison to the world: 4 |
| Unemployment rate | 9.3% (2009 est.)<br>Country comparison to the world: 111 |
| Industrial production growth rate | -5.5% (2009 est.)<br>Country comparison to the world: 114 |
| Distribution of family income (GINI index) | 45 (2007)<br>Country comparison to the world: 42 |
| Investment (gross fixed) | 12.3% of GDP (2009 est.)<br>Country comparison to the world: 145 |
| Public debt | 52.9% of GDP (2009 est.)<br>Country comparison to the world: 47 |
| Market value of publicly traded shares | NA (December 31, 2009)<br>Country comparison to the world: 1 |

*continued*

| Table 21-1 Select Key Demographic and Economic Indicators, *continued* | |
|---|---|
| Current account balance | $-419.9 billion (2009 est.)<br>Country comparison to the world: 190 |
| Debt (external) | $13.45 trillion (December 30, 2009 est.)<br>Country comparison to the world: 1 |
| Debt as a % of GDP | ——— |
| Exports | $1.046 trillion (2009 est.)<br>Country comparison to the world: 4 |
| Exports—commodities | Agricultural products (soybeans, fruit, corn) 9.2%, industrial supplies (organic chemicals) 26.8%, capital goods (transistors, aircraft, motor vehicle parts, computers, telecommunications equipment) 49.0%, consumer goods (automobiles, medicines) 15.0% |
| Export—partners | Canada 19.37%, Mexico 12.21%, China 6.58%, Japan 4.84%, United Kingdom 4.33%, Germany 4.1% (2009) |
| Imports | $1.563 trillion (2009 est.)<br>Country comparison to the world: 2 |
| Import—commodities | Agricultural products 4.9%, industrial supplies 32.9% (crude oil 8.2%), capital goods 30.4% (computers, telecommunications equipment, motor vehicle parts, office machines, electric power machinery), consumer goods 31.8% (automobiles, clothing, medicines, furniture, toys) |
| Import—partners | China 19.3%, Canada 14.24%, Mexico 11.12%, Japan 6.14%, Germany 4.53% (2009) |
| Stock of direct foreign investment at | |
| Home | $2.397 trillion (December 31, 2009 est.)<br>Country comparison to the world: 1 |
| Abroad | $3.316 trillion (December 31, 2009 est.)<br>Country comparison to the world: 1 |

Source: CIA. (2010). *The world factbook*. Retrieved December 16, 2010, from https://www.cia.gov/library/publications/the-world-factbook/

# Introduction

An essential foundation for presenting a comprehensive overview of the founding, development, and current status of workplace health promotion programs in the United States of America clearly begins with and centers on a basic understanding of key demographic facts concerning the U.S. population. As noted in the demographic table (CIA, 2010), the United States is one of the largest, most advanced, and most productive countries in the world. More specifically, with an excess of 307 million people, the United States ranks third (following China and India) in population within the world community and possesses the world's fourth largest workforce (after China, India, and the European Union), comprising approximately 154 million workers. That workforce is dispersed in predominately urban settings among some 24 million firms (U.S. Census Bureau, 2002).

Built on a large and technologically advanced service sector economy that comprises 76.9% of the total U.S. economy, its $14.3 trillion 2009 GDP far exceeds that of all other countries in the world. The U.S. economy is supported by a highly educated citizenry; the literacy rate for both males and females is 99%. A large majority of the population (67%) is within the working age range of 15–64 years, with a mean of 38 years for females and 35.4 years for males (CIA, 2010). By any global comparative standard, the health status of the U.S. population is very good and the available medical services are abundant and very advanced. However, it should also be noted that health care in the United States is among the most expensive in the world, consuming $2.5 trillion annually, which accounted for 17.6% of U.S. GDP in 2009 (U.S. Department of Health and Human Services, n.d.). Further, the linkage between healthcare costs and how those costs are associated with workplace health promotion programs will be a recurring theme throughout this chapter. For unlike in most of the other countries in the world, in the United States, the large majority of working individuals obtain their health benefits (and in many cases, benefits for their dependents) through their employer. About one half of the U.S. population—154 million workers in a population of 307 million—is currently part of the workforce. Given that the cost for that care is shared by both employer and employee, it is in the interest of both parties to create and promote programs and services that enhance the health of all employees and their dependents.

## Prevailing Health Issues and Risk Behaviors

As is the case in most other countries, chronic diseases are the leading cause of death and disability in the United States. Also central to health promotion is the fact that the most frequently observed chronic diseases, such as diabetes, heart disease, cancer, stroke, arthritis, and obesity, are also the most costly and preventable. The CDC list of select chronic disease facts shown in Box 21-1 clearly illustrates this point.

### Box 21-1 Select CDC Chronic Diseases Facts

- About 7 out of 10 deaths among Americans each year are from chronic diseases. Heart disease, cancer, and stroke account for more than 50% of all deaths each year (Kung, Hoyert, Xu, & Murphy, 2008).
- In 2005, 133 million Americans—almost 1 out of every 2 adults—had at least one chronic illness (Wu & Green, 2000).
- Obesity has become a major health concern: 1 in every 3 adults is obese (Ogden, Carroll, McDowell, & Flegal, 2007), and almost 1 in 5 youth between the ages of 6 and 19 is obese (BMI ≥ 95th percentile of the CDC growth chart) (Ogden, Carroll, & Flegal, 2008).
- About one fourth of people with chronic conditions have one or more daily activity limitations (Anderson, 2004).
- Arthritis is the most common cause of disability, with nearly 19 million Americans reporting activity limitations (CDC, 2006).
- Diabetes continues to be the leading cause of kidney failure, nontraumatic lower-extremity amputations, and blindness among adults, aged 20–74 (CDC, 2008c).

Source: Centers for Disease Control and Prevention. (2010) *Chronic diseases are the leading cause of death and disability in the U.S.* Retrieved August 2010 from http://www.cdc.gov/chronicdisease/overview/index.htm

Simply stated, the very large percentage of health issues present in the United States can be directly linked to individual behavior with respect to choices its citizens make in everyday living. The challenge for all health professionals, and in particular workplace health promotion professionals, is to provide timely and effective programs so as to assist program participants in modifying those lifestyle behaviors that have led or might lead to undesirable health. From among the many risky lifestyle behaviors that directly contribute to and are responsible for chronic diseases and premature deaths, the U.S. Centers for Disease Control and Prevention has identified five of the most common.

- Poor nutrition
- Tobacco use
- Excessive alcohol consumption
- Excessive eating (overweight and obesity)
- Inadequate amount of physical activity

Unmistakably, the leading cause of death and disability in the United States is lifestyle-linked chronic diseases, which account for 70% of all deaths. Moreover, for one out of ten Americans, heart disease, cancer, and diabetes also cause major limitations in daily living. The CDC list of lifestyle behavior factors shown provides a logical explanation for the onset and severity of such chronic diseases. Further, the impact of chronic diseases not only negatively affects medical costs and the productivity of current adult workers in the United States but also, given the status of chronic disease risk factors present in the younger U.S. population, will affect the performance of the country's future workers as well.

**Box 21-2 Select CDC Lifestyle Behavior Facts**

- More than one third of all adults do not meet recommendations for aerobic physical activity based on the 2008 Physical Activity Guidelines for Americans, and 23% report no leisure-time physical activity at all in the preceding month (CDC, 2008d).
- In 2007, less than 22% of high school students (CDC, 2008e) and only 24% of adults (CDC, 2008b) reported eating five or more servings of fruits and vegetables per day.
- More than 43 million American adults (approximately 1 in 5) smoke (National Center for Health Statistics, 2007).
- In 2007, 20% of high school students in the United States were current cigarette smokers (CDC, 2008a).
- In addition, about 30% of adult current drinkers report binge drinking (consuming four or more drinks on an occasion for women, five or more drinks on an occasion for men) in the past 30 days (Naimi, Brewer, Miller, Okoro, & Mehrotra, 2007).

Source: Centers for Disease Control and Prevention. (n.d.) *Four Common Causes of Chronic Disease.* Retrieved August 2010 from http://www.cdc.gov/chronicdisease/overview/index.htm

# U.S. Healthcare System

The U.S. healthcare system has been specifically designed to provide high-quality healthcare services for more than 300 million U.S. citizens. It is a unique system, as well as complex with regard to how and where care is delivered, who pays for such services, and how payment is made. Not surprisingly, this system has also become by far the most costly in the world in sheer total dollars ($2.5 trillion annually), expenditures on a per capita basis (approximately $8,000) and as a percent of the nation's GDP (17.3%). The three key factors in any discussion of the delivery of healthcare services in the United States are access to care, the quality of care, and the cost of the care.

## Access to Care

A unique aspect of the U.S. healthcare system is that, in spite of the prevalent impression to the contrary, all citizens of the United States have access to quality health care. By law, namely the Emergency Medical Treatment and Active Labor Act of 1986, hospitals and ambulance services cannot turn away anyone in need of emergency medical care. One needs only to visit the waiting areas of emergency departments of almost any hospital to observe the line of people waiting for such access (almost 120 million visits in one year) (National Center of Health Statistics, 2008). It is also worth noting that, given the highly skilled medical professionals that staff such facilities, the services received there are often excellent, though for various reasons, they are also often very expensive.

## Health Resources and Services Administration Health Center

Individuals seeking health care in the United States also have access to the Community Health Centers made possible by the Health Resources and Services Administration, an agency of the U.S. Department of Health and Human Services (HRSA, n.d.). Such centers provide quality health care to underserved communities whose populations are often disadvantaged and who have limited access to health care. Figure 21-1 illustrates that in 2008, some 74% of the individuals visiting such centers were either uninsured (6,559,659, or 38%) or covered under government-provided Medicaid (6,131,553, or 35.8%).

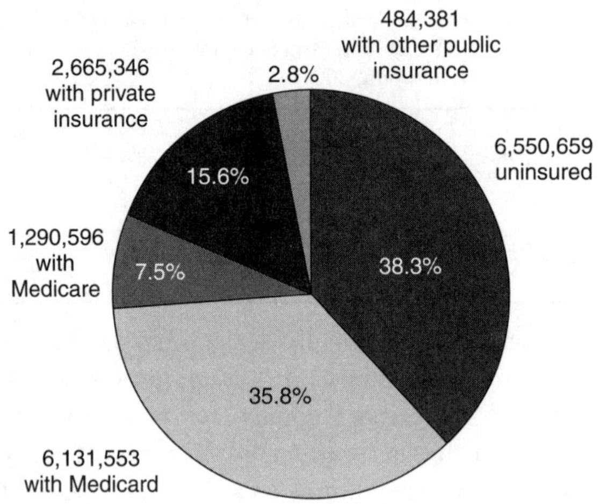


Figure 21-1 Health center patients.
Source: 2008 Uniform Data System. (2008). Health Resources and Services Administration, U.S. Department of Health & Human Services, www.hrsa.gov

## Providers of Healthcare Services

The design of the U.S. healthcare system provides for the delivery of services by numerous medical professionals in multiple settings. A select list and number of medical professionals currently practicing in the United States and the projected 10-year growth trend for those professions is provided in Table 21-2.

Table 21-2 **Medical Professionals and Projections and Trends**

| Professional title | No. in 2008 | Projected No. in 2018 | Growth trend |
|---|---|---|---|
| Physicians | 661,400 | 805,500 | 22% |
| Dentists | 141,900 | 164,000 | 16% |
| Optometrists | 34,800 | 43,200 | 24% |
| Pharmacists | 269,900 | 315,800 | 17% |
| Registered nurses | 2,618,700 | 3,200,200 | 22% |

Source: Bureau of Labor Statistics, U.S. Department of Labor. (2009) *In Occupational outlook handbook* (2010–11 ed.). Physicians and surgeons. Retrieved February 2010 from http://www.bls.gov/oco/ocos074.htm

### *Employer-Sponsored Health Care*

Unlike the residents of most other countries, most individuals in the United States, and in many cases their dependents as well, have access to healthcare services primarily through their place of work. In 2009, some 159 million nonelderly Americans obtained health care through insurance programs provided by an employer. This fact alone might explain why workplace health promotion (WHP) programs have been and remain so important.

Employee-sponsored health insurance is provided through one of the following options: preferred provider organizations, the most popular option, utilized by 60% of employees in 2009; health maintenance organizations, utilized by 20% of employees in 2009; point of service plans, utilized by 10% of employees; high deductible health plans with saving option, utilized by 8% of employees, or a conventional plan, utilized by 1% of employees.

## Scope and Cost of Health Care

Between 1999 and 2009, the annual insurance premium (Table 21-3) for family coverage increased 131% ($5,791 in 1999 to $13,375 in 2009). Employer and employee premium contributions rose from $4,247 to $9,860 and $1,543 to $3,515, respectively (Henry J. Kaiser Family Foundation & the Health Research & Educational Trust, 2009).

Given the fact that, in the United States, most employees obtain their healthcare benefits through their employer and that most employers believe that healthy workers are productive workers, there has developed in most progressive companies a strong health link between workers and employers. Like most companies in other countries in the world, there are many sound reasons why it is desirable for both employees and employers to maximize this interdependence. However, with respect to the United States, the critical issues of the high and ever-increasing cost of medical care as well as a common desire to manage such costs have provided a strong impetus for the establishment of workplace health promotion programs (Table 21-3).

Table 21-3 **Growth and Cost of Health Care**

| | 1970 | 2009 | 2018 |
|---|---|---|---|
| Total cost | $75 billion | $2.5 trillion | $4.3 trillion |
| % of GDP | 7. 2% | 17.6% | 20.3% |
| Per capita | $356 | $8,160 | $13,100 |

Source: Centers for Medicare and Medicaid Services, U.S. Department of Health and Human Services. http://www.cms.hhs.gov

Clearly it is in the interest of both workers, along with their dependents, and employers to maximize opportunities to attain and maintain high levels of individual health. For more than 4 decades in the United States, WHP programs in the corporate setting have played an important role, establishing a unique interrelationship between employees and the healthcare system by offering comprehensive and integrated high-quality health promotion programs. *The Employer Health Benefits Report* (Henry J. Kaiser Family Foundation & the Health Research & Educational Trust, 2009) cited the fact that among all employers who offered health benefits, 58% offered at least one form of a wellness program (93% of the employers with more than 200 employees offered such a program, as did 57% of those with 3–199 employees), which in most cases was provided by an insurance company or outside vendor.

## Influence of Culture and Mentality

The concept of encouraging individuals to embrace and undertake health-enhancing actions, for themselves and for those for whom they are responsible, has been very much a part of the ethos of U.S. society since its founding. The healthcare providers among the early settlers brought with them to the New World their well-established English and/or European traditions and practices with respect to helping their fellow citizens to maintain good health and, when necessary, to treating those who became sick.

There are also a number of distinct cultural traits that have influenced the health status and health-related behaviors of Americans. For one, U.S. society values individualism and ambition, which are responsible for the motivation individuals display in changing health behaviors, such as losing weight or improving fitness, but at the same time those factors could be responsible for an overly ambitious drive to get ahead and thus neglect one's health. The work culture is very prominent in the United States; working hours are among the longest in the world, often leaving people little time for leisure activities. Many people, out of either financial necessity or ambition, work two or three jobs. Interestingly, the term *stress* is not widely used or even accepted in the corporate world and is often understood to be a natural part of the job.

Infrastructure limitations, such as lack of facilities or unsafe conditions, can play a role in making a physically active lifestyle difficult in many cities in the United States. In addition, the nation's multitude of fast food outlets promote quick and mostly unhealthy eating, and food portions have also been an issue of contention with regard to their impact on individual health. However, the United States also has many excellent gyms and athletic facilities, underlining the enormous potential the country has to become healthier.

Since the mid-20th century, the importance of developing positive health behaviors that directly impact lifestyle-linked chronic diseases has been increasingly recognized. The current health promotion mentality in the United States was shaped by a number of documents, acts, and movements. These include:

- **The World Health Organization Constitution (1948):** Emphasized that health is "not merely being the absence of disease but rather…a state of complete physical, mental and social well being …"
- **The U.S. Occupational Safety Act (1970):** Provided a meaningful mandate for focusing on the safety and health of all U.S. workers and provided the impetus for the start of many of the early adopters in workplace health promotion.
- **The 1974 Marc Lalonde report, "A New Perspective on the Health of Canadians":** Affirmed the need to look beyond the traditional healthcare system to improve the general health of the public (Lemco, 1994).
- **The WHO Declaration of Alma Ata in 1978:** Declared that health is a "fundamental human right."
- **The 1979 U.S. Surgeon General's Healthy People Report:** Provided a basic definition of health promotion as being "any combination of health education and related organizational, political and economic intervention designed to facilitate behavioral and environmental adaptation that will improve or protect health."
- **The1980 Promoting Health/Preventing Disease:** Objectives for the Nation 1990: Became the first of what now has become a series of reports that have systematically quantified the nation's progress toward preset health objectives.
- **The WHO Ottawa Charter of 1986:** Defined health promotion and health as "the process of enabling people to increase control over, and to improve, their health. To reach a state of complete physical, mental and social well-being, an individual or group must be able to identify and to realize aspirations, to satisfy needs, and to change or cope with the environment. Health is, therefore, seen as a resource for everyday life, not the objective of living. Health is a positive concept emphasizing social and personal resources, as well as physical capacities. Therefore, health promotion is not just the responsibility of the health sector, but goes beyond healthy life-styles to well-being."
- **The US Healthy People 2000, 2010, and 2020 Objectives:** Increased support for the development of WHP programs in the United States, provided concrete primary goals and specific objectives to help reach those goals, and set a timeframe in which to assess progress.

## Youth Initiatives

As this book is focused on WHP programs, one might wonder why information on the childhood epidemic of overweight and obesity in the United States is relevant. However, one need only a brief pause to realize that in every country in the world, today's youth are tomorrow's workers. It is the present day culture and mentality of the societies in which they live that will determine their future health and, thus, the future of WHP programs.

### Childhood Overweight and Obesity Prevention Initiative

On November 27, 2007, then First Lady, Laura Bush, announced the Department of Health and Human Services launch of the Childhood Overweight and Obesity Prevention Initiative.

> *Our government is working to address one of the greatest dangers to America's young people: childhood overweight and obesity. Nearly one in five school-age children in the United States is overweight and the problem seems to be getting worse. Today, the Department of Health and Human Services is launching a new effort…to coordinate and expand our government's existing childhood-overweight and -obesity prevention programs.* (U.S. Department of Health and Human Services, 2007)

### "The Surgeon General's Vision for a Healthy and Fit Nation"

This document, released in January of 2010, provided a message from U.S. Surgeon General Regina M. Benjamin stressing the magnitude of the epidemic of overweight and obesity present in the United States today. Her call to action included the following six key "vision" areas.

- Individual healthy choices and healthy home environments
- Creating healthy child care settings
- Creating healthy schools
- Creating healthy work sites
- Mobilizing the medical community
- Improving our communities (U.S. Department of Health and Human Services, 2010)

### Let's Move!

On Tuesday February 9, 2010, First Lady Michelle Obama unveiled *Let's Move!*, her plan for a national public awareness campaign focused on the critical state of childhood obesity. The campaign has four parts: helping parents make better food choices, serving healthier food in school vending machines and lunch lines, making healthy food more available and affordable, and encouraging children to exercise more.

*The surge in obesity in this country is nothing short of a public health crisis that is threatening our children, our families, and our future. In fact, the health consequences are so severe that medical experts have warned that our children could be on track to live shorter lives than their parents.* (White House Press, Office of the First Lady, 2010)

# Drivers of Workplace Health Promotion

While the scope and reach of workplace health promotion programs in the United States have dramatically changed since 1970, there remains a core philosophy that is the central tenet of all high-quality programs—the belief that a healthy employee has a greater potential to become and remain a highly productive contributor to a company's success than does an employee in poor health. Thus, one very important factor driving WHP programs has been to make and keep employees healthy, and, when possible, to do the same for their dependents as well. Moreover, and not unique to the United States, it is and will remain very difficult for a corporation to compete successfully in the global marketplace with unhealthy employees.

Four additional key factors that have not only provided the impetus for the initial development of workplace health promotion programs but have also continued to drive progressive development of current WHP programs are as follows:

- Controlling/managing the cost of health care
- Increasing productivity and managing presenteeism
- Recruiting and retaining high-quality employees
- Managing a multinational workforce

## Cost Control and Return on Investment

As discussed previously, the cost of medical services has been increasing at an alarming rate, and in the United States the majority of the 154.5 million people that make up the U.S. workforce obtain their healthcare benefits through insurance programs offered by or through their employer. Therefore, one of the fundamental incentives for corporations to invest in WHP programs is the belief that healthy employees will use fewer healthcare services than the nonhealthy employees. However, when attempts were made to monetize the marginal physiological changes that occurred in healthy employees enrolled in programs that primarily attracted healthy employees, it became almost impossible to build a business case founded on a positive return on investment (ROI). Thus, it became readily apparent that if one of the key purposes of offering WHP programs was the desire to control healthcare costs, a corporation needed to attract a large portion of its employees and their dependents, particularly those who had the most apparent and potentially most costly health risks.

It is worth noting that for some of the earliest employee worksite health promotion programs in the United States, the word *employee* meant only senior level executives. Eventually such programs and facilities were expanded and opened to other employees who had an interest in participating. However, many of those "other employees" already embraced a healthy lifestyle and found it very convenient to participate in such programs at their workplace. The irony of this development was the fact that the already healthy (and also perhaps most productive and happiest) executives, along with similar employees were remaining healthy, happy, and productive. Again, while keeping already healthy people healthy was not an undesirable outcome, it did make it very difficult for proponents of such programs to make a ROI business case that would satisfy a critical key driver—reducing the cost of health care.

This issue became even more critical as detailed reviews of healthcare expenditures revealed the fact that most healthcare expenditures were concentrated on a small subset of the total population. More specifically, it was found that the unhealthiest 10% of a workforce incurred as much as 63% of the total healthcare costs, with 1% of that population consuming 21% of all such costs. It is also worth noting that that the healthiest 50% of the population consumed only 3% of healthcare spending (Henry J. Kaiser Family Foundation, 2009). Thus, a sound ROI case could be made for quality WHP programs that were inclusive of the total workforce as well as dependents and that identified, stabilized, or, better yet, reduced or eliminated employees' risk factors.

## Productivity and Presenteeism

Another significant foundation of U.S. WHP programs over the past several decades is the belief that such programs will have a positive impact on productivity, initially at the individual worker level, and then collectively at the corporate level. Intuitively, it is reasonable to conclude that if employees are healthy, work for a corporation that cares about their health and the health of their dependents, and perform their work in a health-supportive setting, that they would be absent from work less frequently and would be more productive while at work. Many studies were undertaken in the decades of the 1980s and 1990s in an attempt to provide definitive documentation and support for this intuitive belief. (Several such studies and their findings are presented in the "Outcomes and Indicators" section of this chapter.) While some of those studies were of high quality and have been of substantial value in advancing WHP programs in the United States, because of unique differences between programs and a lack of standardization with respect to the research methodologies used across such studies, the collective power of some of the early research has been somewhat compromised. However, from 2000 to 2010, using meta-analysis, numerous researchers have documented positive outcomes for WHP programs that are very consistent with the early intuitive thinking concerning healthy workers.

### Presenteeism

A somewhat newer phenomenon that has become an incentive for U.S. WHP programs is presenteeism. Often considered to be the complement of absenteeism, it has become the term used to describe the loss in productivity resulting in workers' coming to work when they are sick or distracted in some kind of disabling way. This reduced level of presence can be attributable to any one (or more) of a number of illnesses, such as employees' health status, their mental attitude, their lack of desire to work, or even what is occurring in their lives outside the workplace, that distract workers from their focus and effort in the workplace. Further, and as presented in Table 21-4, the broad classifications for illnesses provided by the Society for Human Resource Management (2009) as to why employees are absent from work also provide some insight into personal factors that contribute to presenteeism in the workplace.

| Table 21-4 **Why Employees Are Absent From Work** |
|---|
| 1. Personal illnesses account for 35% |
| 2. Family issues make up 21% |
| 3. Personal needs combine for 18% |
| 4. An entitlement mentality accounts for 14% |
| 5. Stress makes up the final 12% |

Source: Cost of presenteeism surpasses absenteeism. (2007, January 26). *Newswire Today*. Retrieved from http://www.newswiretoday.com/news/13213TS

According to a report by Cigna (Cigna, 2008), each employee averaged 6.9 days of presenteeism during a 6-month period. Whatever the cause or causes, the financial effects of presenteeism on U.S. corporations are serious and increasing; the estimated annual cost associated with presenteeism in U.S. companies is $180 billion, surpassing the annual cost of $118 billion attributed to absenteeism (Weaver, 2006).

## Corporate Image and Retention of Employees

The third factor that has played a very important role in the ongoing development of WHP programs in the United States is the positive cultural value that results from quality programs. More specifically, when a corporation has a definite and visible program dedicated to the health of its employees (and at many corporations, even their dependents), such a commitment greatly enhances both the retention of current employees and the appeal of the company for desirable prospective personnel. Further, quality WHP programs have helped to enhance the external image of publicly traded corporations, which has proven to be rewarding for those companies as well as for their shareholders. Thus, it is more than just a coincidence that when the magazine *Fortune* asked business people to vote for the companies they admired most, nearly all of the top fifty companies named (including Apple, Johnson & Johnson, General Electric, Coca-Cola, IBM, Goldman Sachs, PepsiCo, Starbucks, Caterpillar, AT&T, Intel, UPS, American Express, Nike, and Exxon Mobil) were ones that have made a very substantial commitment to such programs (*World's Most Admired Companies,* 2009).

## Multinational Companies and Workforce

One last driver that only recently has become a focus of multinational companies has to do with the complexity of managing the health needs of a geographically diverse work force. Today many companies have manufacturing and/or marketing and sales activities operating in multiple countries and, with that, employees and in many cases their dependents living and working in settings outside the United States. Progressive companies such as Johnson & Johnson, Caterpillar, and Dow Chemical, after making culturally appropriate adjustments to their U.S.-based workplace health promotion programs, have extended high-quality WHP programs to their respective international operations. For in almost all cases, the same factors that are central to U.S.-based WHP programs are also very important to multinational operations as well.

# Programs (Nature and Examples)

Over the past several decades, most of the focus of U.S.-based WHP programs has mirrored societal trends. Even in its early stages, workplace health promotion focused on promoting the health of individuals. As previously stated, the Ottawa Charter defines health promotion as "the process of enabling people to increase control over, and to improve, their health" (World Health Organization, 1986). Consistent with that definition, most health promotion programs offered in corporate settings in the United States have focused on placing a strong emphasis on informing individuals as to their current health status and then empowering them to assume primary responsibility for its maintenance. Stated differently, the operational empowerment philosophy for many programs has been, "You must do it yourself, but you do not need to do it alone!" And, not surprisingly, most WHP programming conducted in the United States requires an individual to assume primary responsibility for positive health outcomes and comprises activities that are directly linked to lifestyle behaviors. Thus, there are six programming areas that are almost always a part of the core elements found in quality WHP programs:

1. Weight management
2. Stress reduction
3. Smoking cessation
4. Cardiovascular conditioning
5. Flexibility
6. Strength and endurance training

## Policy Development

Beyond designing and delivering specific workplace programming, many leaders of U.S.-based programs are also heavily involved in the development of sound health-enhancing policies that support and are consistent with the overall health philosophy and objectives of their corporations. For many health promotion professionals, this extension of responsibilities has not only been meaningful in increasing their visibility and importance to the corporation, but has also proven to be very helpful in facilitating the integration of many other aspects of a workplace setting, such as employee assistance, safety, and food services.

# Good Practices

While there are thousands of quality WHP programs operating in the United States, the following overview of two particularly well-designed and professionally delivered programs, at the United States Postal Service Headquarters and L.L. Bean, are provided as examples.

## United States Postal Service, Washington, D.C.

### *United States Postal Service Overview*

The United States Postal Service (USPS), an independent government agency headquartered in Washington, D.C., provides domestic and international postal services and, with its almost 700,000 employees, is the second-largest employer in the United States (surpassed only by Wal-Mart). Few corporations have a richer history of service to the citizens of the United States than the USPS. And while all Americans depend on the services of the personnel of the USPS, few fully understand the scope and complexity of everything that the organization does and how well it does it. Those interested in learning more about the scope of USPS history and operations should consult the USPS website at http://www.usps.com/ and for a deeper understanding of USPS business and efficiency, a 2010 article published in *The Washington Post* by John E. Potter, "Five myths about the U.S. Postal Service," provides a very timely and insightful view of the USPS as a competitive business.

### *United States Postal Service Headquarters Workplace Health Promotion Program*

Since 1995, American University's National Center for Health and Fitness has been under contract to provide a comprehensive health promotion program for the employees at the USPS Headquarters located in Washington, DC.

The philosophical basis and operational focus of the USPS program is very similar to those of other health promotion programs and activities conducted by the National Center for Health and Fitness for numerous other federal and private-sector organizations, in that the USPS program has been designed around the wellness model (presented in Figure 21-2) that has been the foundation of the National Center for Health and Fitness as well as of American University's Master's of Science Program in Health Promotion Management since 1980. A key feature of the model is that it places primary responsibility for health on the individual, who must strive for the development and maintenance of the six dimensions of health within their societal structure of norms, values, rules, and ethics.

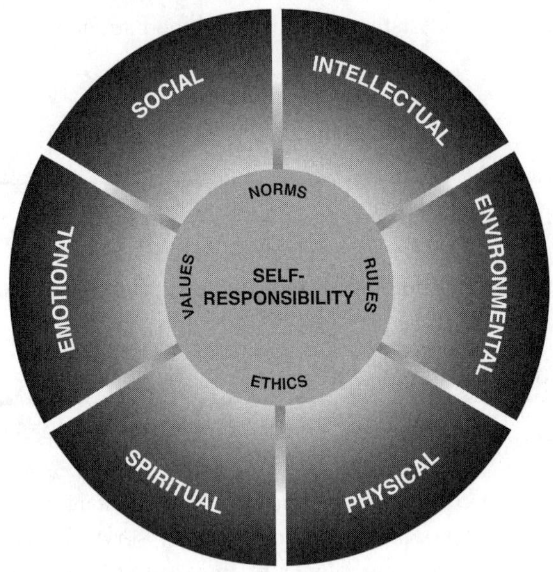


To obtain optimal wellness, individuals must assume responsibility for the continual development and maintenance of the physical, spiritual, emotional, social, intellectual, and environmental components of their health, consistent with the culture in which they reside.

Figure 21-2 American University's National Center for Health and Fitness optimal wellness model.

Source: Karch, R. (1980) *Optimal wellness model*, copyright. All rights reserved. American University's National Center for Health & Fitness.

The specific goals of the USPS Workplace Health Promotion program are designed to improve the quality of life for the several thousand USPS Headquarters employees and where possible, their families as well. Further, all programming has been specifically designed to respond to the known needs and interests of the headquarters employees and then tailored to attract employees to specific programs so as to assist them in developing and then maintaining positive long-term behavioral changes. The clear intent has always been to provide a welcoming and supportive environment and a positive health culture for those who want to improve and manage their health.

Under the supervision of the executive director of the National Center for Health and Fitness, who is also the principal investigator for the project, the USPS headquarters project is staffed by a program director and three full-time and many part-time employees. The principal investigator and program director also work very closely with senior leadership of the USPS to regularly review and, if necessary, adjust program elements to maximize desired outcomes. In addition, extensive data are tracked to monitor participation, outcomes, and costs. The following is a brief list of some of the programs and activities offered at the USPS headquarters:

- Group exercise classes
- Personal training sessions
- Nutrition education programs (healthy eating)
- Weight management (safe and healthy approaches to weight loss)
- Health/risk factor screenings (annual health fair)
- The USPS Postal Stampede (a major annual running and fun event)
- Disease prevention lectures (special speakers on select topics)
- Member recognition programs (awards programs for achieving goals)
- Fitness education classes (small-group topical information sessions)
- Lunch 'n' Learn (timely information sessions on specific health topics)
- Keep Track of Your Holiday (exercise and nutrition)
- USPS Employee Assistance Program
- *Health and Fitness Forum* newsletter featuring timely and informative health topics as well as a list of upcoming events

## L.L. Bean, Inc.

A second program that serves as an excellent example of a quality U.S. workplace health promotion program is L.L. Bean, Inc.'s Healthy Bean Program.

### *Health, Safety, and Wellness Focus*

L.L. Bean has been offering its employees comprehensive on-site wellness programs since 1982. The founding rationale for the Healthy Bean program, one consistent with the company's outdoors heritage, was that there was a direct relationship between the company's desire for its employees to enjoy the outdoors (while using L.L. Bean products) and the need for employees to be healthy and physically fit to do so.

In 1985, the Healthy Bean WHP program was housed in one room; today it has more than a dozen on-site fitness facilities that offer a wide array of classes in physical activity, health promotion, and risk-factor reduction. In addition, L.L. Bean became an early adopter of antismoking policies in 1993 when it mandated a smoke-free workplace, which reduced the employee smoking rate to 8% from a 1986 rate of 24%. L.L. Bean estimates the annual savings from that one healthy policy change alone at $500,000 to $750,000.

The Healthy Bean program was also expanded in 2006 to include safe and healthy living as an additional core value, and in 2007, the company's Healthy Lifestyles Program provided an opportunity for spouses to participate as well. That program now enjoys an 86% participation rate.

Commensurate with its focus on wellness, L.L. Bean also places a very high emphasis on the safety of its employees. The company has achieved national recognition for its occupational health programs as part of the prestigious Voluntary Protection Program from the U.S. Occupational Safety and Health Administration, and for its 57% reduction in employee injuries since 2004.

An obvious testament to the philosophy and culture of L.L. Bean and its WHP program is the company's extremely low (6%) voluntary turnover rate. The words of the company's chief operating officer, Bob Peixotto, provide a clear and factual explanation for such employee commitment: "If you go to work and your life is made better by it, what more strong sense of loyalty can you have (Peixotto, n.d.)?"

It was the early vision of the L.L. Bean corporate leadership, the continued development and expansion of its programmatic offerings, the documented positive health outcomes of its employees, and the vision and support of the current management that have made the Healthy Bean program an excellent example of a high-quality U.S. WHP program. It comes as no surprise that the L.L. Bean Healthy Bean program was a 2009 recipient of the prestigious C. Everett Koop National Health Award.

## Outcomes and Indicators

With the exception of U.S. WHP programs that place a high degree of importance on controlling the medical costs of employees, most programs, independent of country, strive for the same programmatic outcomes and monitor similar indicators of such outcomes. More specifically, most successful health promotion programs are developed with a clear set of predetermined objectives, have well-designed interventions, and utilize an appropriate evaluation methodology. The obvious intent of such an approach is to obtain the desired outcome in the most cost-effective and programmatically efficient way. To that end, most program managers closely monitor the outcomes of the interventions conducted in many of the programmatic areas shown in Table 21-5.

**Table 21-5 Programmatic Areas and Subareas and Desired Outcomes and Indicators**

| Programmatic areas and subareas | Desired outcomes and indicators |
|---|---|
| Health screens | |
| Blood pressure | Identify high risk, reduce, and stabilize |
| Body composition | Assess and establish desirable healthy weight |
| Cholesterol | Assess and establish program and control |
| Blood chemistry | Assess and provide appropriate program |
| Lifestyle behavioral change programs | |
| Stress management | Identify, reduce, and manage |
| Physical activity | Increase if necessary and maintain |
| Weight management | Attain/maintain healthy weight |
| Smoking | Stop or reduce |
| Substance abuse | Increase awareness and educate |
| Educational awareness programs | |
| Work/family balance | Awareness and time management |
| Healthy nutrition | Awareness and education |
| Healthy back programs | Awareness and education |
| Work performance variables | |
| Productivity | Increase and maintain |
| Absenteeism | Decrease |
| Presenteeism | Reduce |
| Employee morale | Increase and maintain |
| Turnover | Reduce and maintain |
| Train/retraining | Reduce turnover and costs |
| ROI | Positive return |

Several prominent researchers, such as Goetzel, Shechter, Ozminkowski, Marmet, and Tabrizi (2007) and O'Donnell (2001), have conducted extensive reviews of the published literature concerning WHP programs, and have concluded that there appear to be a number of common elements or recurring features of those programs that have yielded the best outcomes. In addition, two prominent initiatives in the field of WHP in the United States, the Well Workplace process of the Wellness Councils of America (WELCOA) and the C. Everett Koop National Health Awards, have identified specific criteria for good practice in WHP programs. Common key elements include:

- Organizational commitment and executive management support
- The integration of programs with central corporate operations
- Creating a supportive environment
- Ability to attract and retain participants
- Effective screening, triage, and collection of data
- Operational planning and evidence-based interventions featuring a wide variety of offerings
- Program accessibility and incentives to motivate employees to participate
- Applying appropriate evaluation methodologies
- Ongoing program evaluation
- Communicating successful outcomes to participants and program supporters

For a list of the C. Everett Koop National Health Award winners and a brief description of each winning program, go to http://www.sph.emory.edu/healthproject/koop/index.html. More information on the Well Workplace Awards Program can be found at http://www.welcoa.org/.

## Existing Research

The research literature available on WHP programs in general, and within the United States in particular, is extensive, wide ranging, and of varying quality. Several systematic reviews have looked across many of the more respected studies and have provided succinct conclusions as to the evidence in support of comprehensive workplace health promotion programs. One of the most thorough and current of such reviews is "The Health and Cost Benefits of Work Site Health-Promotion Programs," conducted by Goetzel and Ozminkowski in 2008 and published in the *Annual Review of Public Health.* The following are several select research findings from that review.

### Extent of Program Offerings

"While a 1999 survey reported that 90% of all worksites offered WHP, a 2004 study found that only 6.9% of such programs offered all 5 elements considered to be key components of a comprehensive program" (Linnan et al., 2008).

## Use of Health Risk Appraisals

The use of a health risk appraisal is necessary but is insufficient for successful outcomes if not combined with targeted interventions (Task Force on Community Preventative Services, 2007). The use of a health risk appraisal was shown to be the cornerstone of successful programs for programs designed for retirees (Ozminkowski et al., 2006).

## Importance of Participation Rates

An essential element in all risk-reduction focused WHP programs is employee participation (Serxner, Anderson, & Gold, 2004). Easy access to program interventions offered for risk factor reduction is critical for program success (Erfurt & Foote, 1990; Pelletier, 1999).

## Use of Tailored Messages to Facilitate Behavior Change

"Individuals receiving tailored feedback on their risk profile were 18% more likely to change at least one risk factor" (Kreuter & Strecher, 1996). "Individuals receiving written tailored feedback that was directly linked to their readiness for change demonstrated a 13% increase in physical activity compared to the 1% change for those receiving generic messages" (Peterson & Aldana, 1999).

## Risk Factor Reduction and Behavior Change

"Employees with seven risk factors (tobacco use, hypertension, hypercholesterolemia, overweight/obesity, high blood glucose, high stress, and lack of physical activity) cost employers 228% more in medical costs than an employee not having any such risk factors" (Goetzel et al., 1998).

"There is consistent evidence of a relationship between obesity, stress, multiple risk factors, and subsequent healthcare expenditures as well as subsequent worker absenteeism" (Aldana, 2001).

"There is 'indicative to acceptable' evidence supporting the effectiveness of multi-component WSHP programs in achieving long-term behavior change and risk reduction" (Heaney, & Goetzel, 1998).

"Strong evidence of WSHP program effectiveness has been found with respect to reducing tobacco use among participants, dietary fat consumption as measured by self-report, high blood pressure, total serum cholesterol levels, the number of days absent from work because of illness or disability, and improvements in other general measures of worker productivity" (Task Force on Community Preventative Services, 2007).

## Return on Investment

"A review of WSHP studies from the 1980s and early 1990s estimated ROI savings of $1.40 to $3.00 saved per dollar spent on programs" (Goetzel, Juday, & Ozminkowski, 1999).

## Conclusion

It is abundantly clear that much progress has been made in the development of WHP programs in the United States over the past four decades. Much of that development can be directly linked to and in many ways has been powerfully influenced by four key factors. First is the overall global awakening to the importance and role of individuals and societies in supporting and advancing the concept of health for all. In the United States this was particularly true with the publication by the U.S. government of a series of objective documents focusing on the development of behaviors that could directly impact lifestyle-linked chronic diseases. The second factor, which was closely linked to the first and which took root in many corporate settings, was the emergence of the field of health promotion. Perhaps more than anything else it was the innovative work of a select group of progressive corporations that laid the foundation for today's WHP programs.

A third key factor in the development and refinement of WHP programs in the United States was research that clearly indicated that with quality programming, health and economic objectives could be met and numerous positive benefits could be derived for individuals, corporations, and society at large. Today, given the outcomes of this third factor, there is now a fourth that can best be described as the "migration factor." Whereas in the past, many business components were thought to be separate from or completely unrelated to health promotion programs, progressive worksites of today are bringing together, or migrating, many different aspects of existing human capital management activities to build comprehensive WHP programs and are deriving very desirable outcomes.

## Summary

Over the past four decades, there has been continuous development of WHP programs in the United States. Beginning predominately as exercise programs for select senior corporate personnel, programs soon grew to include more employees and then, in some cases, even dependents and retirees. As programs increased in size, they were also expanded to offer activities beyond exercise, so as to address specific health risk factors through special interventions such as smoking cessation, weight management, and stress reduction. These developments were followed and evaluated in order to determine both program effectiveness and their costs and benefits with respect to return on investment.

Unlike those in most other countries, the development of WHP programs in the United States has always been linked to the delivery of healthcare services, as most workers receive such benefits through their employer. Thus, given the ever-increasing cost of health care, corporations have intensified their approaches to both programming strategies and evaluation methodologies. Outcomes associated with some of the best practice strategies have been reviewed by several leading health promotion researchers, resulting in the identification of key program components that best lead to desire results.

Several national organizations have developed recognition programs that are used to identify truly outstanding programs and reward such programs for exemplary practices. Reviewing such programs has proven to be very helpful for program planners. Moreover, given the current trends with respect to program development, it is clear that there will be a continued growth in both the number and the complexity of such programs in the coming years.

## Review Questions

1. What are the central healthcare-related issues facing the U.S. population?
2. What differentiates the U.S. healthcare funding system from that of most of the world? How is it funded? Regulated? Managed?
3. How does the U.S. culture of individualism and ambition affect population health and health-promotion efforts?
4. What are two of the primary factors driving U.S. workplace health-promotion programs? Explain each thoroughly.
5. What is the operational empowerment philosophy of many corporate health programs in the United States? What does this philosophy mean?
6. Several outcome indicators of U.S. workplace health-promotion programs are described in the systematic review provided. If outcome indicators are positive, why are U.S. workers still unhealthy?

## References

About HRSA. Health Resources and Services Administration (HRSA), an agency of the U.S. Department of Health and Human Services. (n.d.) Retrieved February 2010, from http://www.hrsa.gov/about/default.htm

Aldana, S. G. (2001). Financial impact of health promotion programs: A comprehensive review of the literature. *American Journal of Health Promotion, 15,* 296–320.

Anderson, G. (2004). *Chronic conditions: Making the case for ongoing care.* Baltimore, MD: John Hopkins University.

Bureau of Labor Statistics. U.S. Department of Labor. (2009) Physicians and surgeons. In *Occupational outlook handbook, (2010–11 ed.).* Retrieved February 2010, from http://www.bls.gov/oco/ocos074.htm

Centers for Disease Control and Prevention. (2006). Prevalence of doctor-diagnosed arthritis and arthritis-attributable activity limitation—United States, 2003–2005. *Morbidity and Mortality Weekly Report, 55*(40), 1089–1092. Retrieved from http://www.cdc.gov/mmwr/preview/mmwrhtml/mm5540a2.htm

Centers for Disease Control and Prevention. (2008a). *BRFSS prevalence and trends data.* Retrieved from http://apps.nccd.cdc.gov/brfss/page.asp?cat=AC&yr=2007&state=US#AC

Centers for Disease Control and Prevention. (2008b). Cigarette use among high school students—United States, 1991–2007. *Morbidity and Mortality Weekly Report, 57*(25), 686–688.

Centers for Disease Control and Prevention. (2008c). *National diabetes fact sheet, 2007.* Retrieved from http://www.cdc.gov/Diabetes/pubs/factsheet07.htm

Centers for Disease Control and Prevention. (2008d). Prevalence of self-reported physically active adults—United States, 2007. *Morbidity and Mortality Weekly Report, 57*(48), 1297–1300. Retrieved from http://www.cdc.gov/mmwr/preview/mmwrhtml/mm5748a1.htm

Centers for Disease Control and Prevention. (2008e). Youth risk behavior surveillance—United States, 2007. *Morbidity and Mortality Weekly Report, 57*(SS04), 1–131. Retrieved from http://www.cdc.gov/mmwr/preview/mmwrhtml/ss5704a1.htm

Centers for Disease Control and Prevention. (1990). Healthy People 2000: National health promotion and disease prevention objectives for the year 2000. Conference Report. *MMWR, 39,* 689, 695–697. Retrieved February 2010, from http://www.healthypeople.gov

Centers for Disease Control and Prevention. (2000). *Healthy People 2010.* Retrieved February 2010, from http://www.healthypeople.gov/

Centers for Disease Control and Prevention. (2010). *Healthy People 2020.* Retrieved Feburary 2010, from http://www.healthypeople.gov/HP2020/

Centers for Disease Control and Prevention. (n.d.). *Emergency department visits.* Retrieved from National Hospital Ambulatory Medical Care Survey: 2006 Emergency Department Summary, tables 1, 10, 12, 21, 25, http://www.cdc.gov/nchs/data/nhsr/nhsr007.pdf

CIA. (2010). *The world factbook.* Retrieved February 2010, from https://www.cia.gov/library/publications/the-world-factbook/

Cigna. (2008). *The 2008 health leadership series: Absenteeism and presenteeism.* Prepared by the Segmentation Company for Cigna. Retrieved February 2010 from newsroom.cigna.com/images/56/AP%20Findings-A.ppt

Cost of presenteeism surpasses absenteeism. (2007, January 26). *Newswire Today.* Retrieved from http://www.newswiretoday.com/news/13213

Crimmel, B. L. & Sommers, J. (2008, July). Employer-sponsored health insurance for large employers in the private sector, by industry classification, 2006. *Medical Expenditure Panel Survey, Statistical Brief No. 211.* Retrieved February 2010, from http://www.meps.ahrq.gov/mepsweb/data_files/publications/st211/stat211.pdf

Erfurt, J. C., & Foote, A. (1990). Maintenance of blood pressure treatment and control after discontinuation of work site follow-up. *Journal of Occupational Medicine, 32,* 513–520.

Goetzel, R. Z., Anderson, D. R., Whitmer, R. W., Ozminkowski, R. J., Dunn, R. L., & Wasserman, J. (1998). The relationship between modifiable health risks and health care expenditures: An analysis of the multi-employer HERO health risk and cost database. *Journal of Occupational and Environmental Medicine, 4,* 843–57.

Goetzel, R. Z., Juday, T. R., & Ozminkowski, R. J. (1999). What's the ROI? A systematic review of return on investment (ROI) studies of corporate health and productivity management inititatives. *AWHP's Worksite Health, 6,* 12–21.

Goetzel, R. Z., Shechter, D., Ozminkowski, R. J., Marmet, P. F., & Tabrizi, M. J. (2007). Promising practices in employer health and productivity management efforts: findings from a benchmarking study. *Journal of Occupational and Environmental Medicine, 49,* 111–30.

Goetzel, R. Z., & Ozminkowski, R. J. (2008). The health and cost benefits of work site health-promotion programs. *Annual Review of Public Health, 29,* 303–323.

Heaney, C., & Goetzel, R. Z. (1998). A review of health-related outcomes of multi-component worksite health promotion programs. *American Journal of Health Promotion,11,* 290–307.

Henry J. Kaiser Family Foundation. (2009). *Trends in health care costs and spending.* Retrieved February 2010, from http://www.kff.org/insurance/upload/7692_02.pdf

Henry J. Kaiser Family Foundation and the Health Research & Educational Trust. (2009). *Employer health benefits report.* Retrieved from http://www.kff.org/insurance/ehbs091509nr.cfm

Koop, C. Everett. (2010). *The health project. national health awards.* Retrieved February 2010, from http://www.sph.emory.edu/healthproject/koop/work.html

Kreuter, M. W., & Strecher, V. J. (1996). Do tailored behavior change messages enhance the effectiveness of health risk appraisal? Results from a randomized trial. *Health Education Research, 11,* 97–105.

Kung, H. C., Hoyert, D. L., Xu, J. Q., & Murphy, S. L. (2008). Deaths: Final data for 2005. *National Vital Statistics Reports 2008, 56*(10). Retrieved from http://www.cdc.gov/ nchs/data/nvsr/nvsr56/nvsr56_10.pdf

Lalonde, M. (1974). A new perspective on the health of Canadians. *Canadian Institutes of Health Research.* Retrieved February 2010, from http://www.cihr-irsc.gc.ca/e/29975.html

Lemco, J. (1994). *National health care: Lessons for the United States and Canada.* Ann Arbor, MI: University of Michigan Press.

Linnan, L., Bowling, M., Lindsay, G., Childress, J., Blakey, C., Pronk, S., et al. (2008). Results of the 2004 national worksite health promotion survey. *American Journal of Public Health, 98,* 1503–1509.

Miller, J. W., Naimi, T. S., Brewer, R. D., & Everett-Jones, S. (2007). Binge drinking and associated health risk behaviors among high school students. *Pediatrics, 119,* 76–85.

Naimi, T. S., Brewer, R. D., Miller, J. W., Okoro, C., & Mehrotra, C. (2007). What do binge drinkers drink? Implications for alcohol control policy. *American Journal of Preventive Medicine, 33,* 188–193.

National Center for Health Statistics. (2007). *Health, United States, 2007 with chartbook on trends in the health of Americans.* Retrieved from http://www.cdc.gov/nchs/data/hus/hus07.pdf

National Center for Health Statistics. (2008). Hospital ambulatory medical care surgery: 2006 emergency department summary. Retrieved February 2011, from http://ps.mcicvermont.com/appdocs/lps/National%20ED%20%20statistics%20%5B1%5D.pdf

O'Donnell, M. (2001). *Health promotion in the workplace* (3rd ed.). Albany, NY: Delmar Cengage Learning.

Ogden, C. L., Carroll, M. D., & Flegal, K. M. (2008). High body mass index for age among U.S. children and adolescents, 2003–2006. *Journal of the American Medical Association, 299,* 2401–2405.

Ogden, C. L., Carroll, M. D., McDowell, M. A., & Flegal, K. M. (2007). Obesity among adults in the United States—no change since 2003–2004. *NCHS data brief no 1.* Retrieved from http://www.cdc.gov/nchs/data/databriefs/db01.pdf

Ozminkowski, R. J., Goetzel, R. Z., Wang, F., Gibson, T. B., Shechter, D., Musich, S., et al. (2006). The savings gained from participation in health promotion programs for medicare beneficiaries. *Journal of Occupational and Environmental Medicine, 48,* 1125–32.

Occupational Safety and Health Administration. (1970). *Occupational safety and health act of 1970.* Retrieved February 2010, from http://www.osha.gov/pls/oshaweb/owadisp.show_document?p_id=2743&p_table=OSHACT

Peixotto, B. (n.d.). Health, safety, and wellness focus. In *Wisdom at work: Retaining experienced RNs and their knowledge case studies.* Retrieved February 2010, from http://www.rwjf.org/files/research/revlewincsllbeanoutdoor.pdf

Pelletier, K. R. (1999). A review and analysis of the clinical and cost-effectiveness studies of comprehensive health promotion and disease management programs at the worksite: 1995–1998 update (IV). *American Journal of Health Promotion, 13,* 333–45, iii.

Peterson, T. R., & Aldana, S. G. (1999). Improving exercise behavior: An application of the stages of change model in a worksite setting. *American Journal of Health Promotion, 13*, 229–232.

Potter, J. E. (2010, February 25). Five myths about the U.S. postal service. *The Washington Post.* Retrieved February 2010, from http://www.washingtonpost.com/wp-dyn/content/article/2010/02/25/AR2010022504888.html

Serxner, S., Anderson, D. R., & Gold, D. (2004). Building program participation: Strategies for recruitment and retention in worksite health promotion programs. *American Journal Health Promotion, 18*, iii, 1–6.

Society for Human Resource Management. (2009). *Cost of presenteeism surpasses absenteeism.* Retrieved February 2010, from http://www.shrm.org

Task Force on Community Preventative Services. (2007). *Proceedings of the task force meeting: Worksite reviews.* Atlanta, GA: Centers for Disease Control and Prevention.

U.S. Census Bureau. (2002). *Statistics about business size from the U.S. Census Bureau.* Retrieved from http://www.census.gov/epcd/www/smallbus.html

U.S. Department of Health and Human Services. (2007, November 27). *HHS launches childhood overweight and obesity prevention initiative.* Retrieved February 2010, from http://www.hhs.gov/news/press/2007pres/11/pr20071127a.html

U.S. Department of Health and Human Services. (n.d.). *Centers for Medicaid and Medicare service.* Retrieved February 2010, from www.cms.hhs.gov

U.S. Department of Health and Human Services. (1980). *Healthy people: Surgeon general's report.* Retrieved from http://www.surgeongeneral.gov/library/reports/

U.S. Department of Health and Human Services. (2010). *The surgeon general's vision for a healthy and fit nation 2010.* Retrieved February 2010, from http://www.surgeongeneral.gov/library/obesityvision/obesityvision2010.pdf

U.S. Department of Health and Human Services. (1980). *Promoting health/preventing disease: objectives for the nation.* Retrieved February 2010, from http://www.eric.ed.gov/ERICWebPortal/custom/portlets/recordDetails/detailmini.jsp?_nfpb=true&_&ERICExtSearch_SearchValue_0=ED209206&ERICExtSearch_SearchType_0=no&accno=ED209206

Weaver, R. (2006, December 27). *Cost of presenteeism surpasses absenteeism.* Retrieved February 2010, from http://ezinearticles.com/?Cost-of-Presenteeism-Surpasses-Absenteeism&id=397305

WELCOA. (n.d.). *Seven benchmarks.* Retrieved February 2010, from http://www.welcoa.org/

White House, Office of the First Lady. (2010). *First lady Michelle Obama launches let's move: America's move to raise a healthier generation of kids.* Retrieved February 2010, from http://www.whitehouse.gov/the-press-office/first-lady-michelle-obama-launches-lets-move-americas-move-raise-a-healthier-genera

White House, Office of the Press Secretary. (2010). *Presidential memorandum: Establishing a task force on childhood obesity.* Retrieved February 2010, from http://www.whitehouse.gov/the-press-office/presidential-memorandum-establishing-a-task-force-childhood-obesity

World Health Organization. (1978). Declaration of Alma Ata. *International Conference on Primary Health Care, Alma-Ata, USSR, 6-12 September 1978.* Retrieved February 2010, from http://www.who.int/hpr/NPH/docs/declaration_almaata.pdf

World Health Organization. (1986). The Ottawa charter. Retrieved February 2010, from http://www.who.int/healthpromotion/conferences/previous/ottawa/en/

World Health Organization. (2006). *Constitution of the World Health Organization.* Retrieved February 2010, from http://www.who.int/governance/eb/who_constitution_en.pdf

World's most admired companies. (2009). *Fortune.* Retrieved February 2010, from http://money.cnn.com/magazines/fortune/mostadmired/2009/full_list/

Wu, S. Y., & Green, A. (2000). *Projection of chronic illness prevalence and cost inflation.* Santa Monica, CA: RAND Corporation.

# Index

*Boxes, figures, and tables are indicated with b, f, and t following the page number.*

## A

## C

## D

## F



## G

## H

## I

## J



## K



## L

## M

## N

## O

## P

## T



## U